Garfield County Libraries
New Castle Branch Library
402 West Main • P.O. Box 320
New Castle, CO 81647
(970) 984-2346 Fax (970) 984-2081
www.garfieldlibraries.org

"I feel like a different person now and have so much energy. I am happy and grateful for life."

By the age of forty I was in a negative spiral downward, physically, emotionally, and mentally. For a type-A, successful attorney, this was difficult for me. I went through a number of tests, because my body hurt all over and felt like it was falling apart. My short-term memory was almost entirely gone.

I developed a stammer and couldn't find words anymore. My mind and body were failing so quickly that I believed I was developing both Alzheimer's and rheumatoid arthritis. However, after seeing several specialists, my tests came back negative. I was at a point where I could only accomplish one thing a day, because I ran out of gas so easily. I struggled with depression for many years and during this time I became even more short-tempered, irritable, and unenthusiastic about life. I tried several times unsuccessfully to get off the medications.

Finally, I was introduced to Dr. Hyman and decided to follow his advice. What I uncovered surprised me. My mitochondria weren't functioning properly, my body was unable to detoxify, so the toxins were building up and I had serious heavy metal poisoning with mercury levels in the upper sixties, and my lead and uranium levels were also very high (normal levels of mercury in the urinary chelating test are below four). After going through his detoxification program, changing my diet, making lifestyle changes to reduce stress and handle it better, and eliminating the heavy metals, my mental clarity came back, my aches and pains went away, and I ended up losing forty pounds.

I feel like a different person now and have so much energy. I am happy and grateful for life. My mind has changed and I can think clearly without being in a fog. Now the only medication I take is for my hypothyroidism. I enjoy my life, my husband, and my children so much more now. Thank you for saving my life.

Jackie Tepper
Stamford, CT

"She was normal again and wasn't hitting or raging on her sister."

When both of my daughters were young, they witnessed their father collapse on the kitchen floor and die. Emma, who was three at the time, reacted the most. Even after attending bereavement groups and seeing counselors, I started to see her acting in ways that were not normal.

She became extremely physical and full of rage. Digging her nails into me and hitting and kicking her sister constantly without remorse was an everyday experience. She had a difficult time socializing at school. Teachers wanted me to put her on medication, and doctors wanted to do brain scans. It wasn't until I was introduced to Dr. Hyman that it all made sense.

Dr. Hyman thought that the stress from witnessing her father's death knocked her immune system out of whack. After doing a series of tests we uncovered two very important keys to her emotional and psychological turmoil. The first was an overgrowth of bacteria and yeast in her gut. Dr. Hyman said it was the worst he had seen in a person who didn't have any real gut symptoms. The second was an intolerance to gluten and dairy.

After we treated the yeast overgrowth with antibiotics and got gluten and dairy out of her diet for two weeks, I couldn't believe the transformation in my daughter. She was normal again and wasn't hitting or raging on her sister. It wasn't easy to make the transition and change the way we eat, but the difference was undeniable. If I would slip and feed her macaroni and cheese or the little yellow Goldfish, she would be bouncing off the walls. Her teachers cannot believe the huge improvement, and she isn't seeing a therapist anymore.

Lisa R (mother)
Medford, NY

"I didn't fully understand how bad I felt, until I felt better."

For years my health was in decline. It got to the point where I felt like I had the flu all the time with a low-grade fever. I started gaining weight even though I wasn't eating a lot, I had zero energy, and my social life suffered because I didn't want to go anywhere or do anything after work except go home to lay on the couch. I took antidepressants and battled with chronic sinus infections.

After going to every doctor I could see including an endocrinologist, all they would do is throw antibiotics at me or suggest surgery. For years I thought it was just the stress of graduate school until my family jumped in and voiced their concern, and committed to helping me get to the bottom of whatever it was that was making me feel so awful.

Finally, I met Dr. Hyman and after listening to my story he did a series of tests to uncover that I had severe mercury poisoning with levels at two hundred sixty (normal levels of mercury in the urinary chelating test are below four) and a significant thyroid imbalance. Going through his plan changed my life.

The minute he told me about my mercury poisoning, I instantly had hope that I wasn't going to feel lousy for the rest of my life. After time and with patience, I feel like myself again and I am happy to be here. I spent years feeling miserable. Now, even the small things like my hair and skin feel like they used to. I didn't fully understand how bad I felt, until I felt better. I am a walking testimony of Dr. Hyman's work.

Kaki Martin
Cambridge, MA

"I felt foggy and thick—like I was thinking through a marshmallow."

All of my life I was very athletic, on the go, full of energy, and could sleep better than anyone I knew. Over the past twenty years I saw a steady decline, which I thought was due to aging until I started getting real scared.

The first major concern was on a family bike ride when I physically couldn't hold the brakes. My hands and feet were not doing the things that I was telling them to do. After that experience and waking up every night with severe cramping, I knew something was wrong. But even the best neurologists and endocrinologists were telling me I was fine.

I knew these symptoms weren't normal. I felt foggy and thick—like I was thinking through a marshmallow. What I learned (which no doctor could tell me) is that the various systems in my body couldn't eliminate the toxins I'd received from foods, the environment, and the amalgams in my fillings.

In addition to the toxins, my mercury levels were dangerously high, which compromised my immune system and compromised me neurologically. After going through Dr. Hyman's program, detoxifying, removing my fillings, and eliminating the mercury, I now have my life back (at least 90 percent given my age of forty-five). I sleep great again, have more focus, recently started a new business, competed in three triathlons last year, and, more important, I recognize me again.

Natalie Karp
Roslyn, NY

"We didn't know there was a fog until we started eliminating the heavy metals."

Up until two years of age, Jackson was developing at a normal level. He was up to twenty words, but suddenly started to regress. When we took him to see our pediatrician he was down to five words, three months later he couldn't say one.

After seeing a speech doctor and psychologists he was diagnosed with pervasive development disorder, or autism. We knew we had to do something because he wasn't getting any better. He was irritable and would throw tantrums all the time.

It wasn't until we discovered Dr. Hyman that we started to put the pieces of the puzzle together. After going through Dr. Hyman's program we found that our son had several food allergies, heavy metal poisoning, and severe gut inflammation and imbalances in his gut bacteria as well as yeast overgrowth.

After learning about this we changed his diet right away and within days of removing dairy we saw results. We saw more concentration. With the B_{12} supplements our son developed more verbal skills and was able to focus. What's amazing is that we didn't know there was a fog until we started eliminating the heavy metals (using chelation). After Jackson went through chelation he became much more alive, responsive, and verbal.

Marc R (father)
New York, NY

"His teachers told me he was like a completely different kid."

As a young child Clayton had trouble staying on task, was easily frustrated, and rarely slept through the night. Once school started and we had other children to compare him to, it became clear these issues were pronounced. We reluctantly had him repeat kindergarten, and sought the help of a local doctor who specialized in educational testing. When the results came back, we were left with a diagnosis of ADHD, but were given very few options other than medication to deal with it.

Over the course of the next year he continued to struggle and we eventually made the decision to start him on medication. It worked well, but like all medicine it came with a high price. Evenings were a challenge, as he suffered through rebound effects. His appetite was poor and he continued to have trouble sleeping. His concentration at school was improved, but he often had sinus infections, complained of stomach problems, and frequently broke out in hives for reasons we couldn't pin down.

We took Clayton to Dr. Hyman and for the first time had real, understandable answers for what had been happening to our son. Problems with gluten, yeast, and mercury toxicity were all correctly identified. Through changes in diet and nutritional support we were able to address not only the attention issues but all of his other physical symptoms as well. For the first time in his life, Clayton became focused, his health improved, and he slept through the night. A few months later I noticed a striking improvement in his handwriting, which before had been all but illegible. His teachers told me he was like a completely different kid.

Nearly two years later, our son has fully embraced this new model of taking care of himself. He packs his own lunch, manages social situations where foods he is sensitive to are present, and makes choices that keep him consistently healthy. I am extremely grateful to Dr. Hyman for his knowledge and compassionate support during our family's continued journey toward optimum health.

Audrey Lampert (mother)
North Granby, CT

Also by Mark Hyman

The Detox Box

Ultraprevention

UltraMetabolism

The UltraSimple Diet

The UltraMetabolism Cookbook

The

UltraMind

Solution

Fix Your Broken Brain by Healing Your Body First

The Simple Way to Defeat Depression, Overcome Anxiety, and Sharpen Your Mind

Mark Hyman, M.D.

FOREWORD BY MARTHA HERBERT, M.D., PH.D.
Assistant Professor of Neurology,
Harvard Medical School
Director, Transcend Research Program,
Massachusetts General Hospital

Scribner
New York   London   Toronto   Sydney

This publication contains the opinions and ideas of the author. It is intended to provide helpful and informative material on the subjects addressed in the publication. It is sold with the understanding that the author and publisher are not engaged in rendering medical, health, psychological, or any other kind of personal professional services in the book. If the reader requires personal medical, health, or other assistance or advice, a competent professional should be consulted.

The author and publisher specifically disclaim all responsibility for any liability, loss or risk, personal or otherwise, that is incurred as a consequence, directly or indirectly, of the use and application of the contents of this book.

SCRIBNER
A Division of Simon & Schuster, Inc.
1230 Avenue of the Americas
New York, NY 10020

First Scribner hardcover edition December 2008

SCRIBNER and design are registered trademarks of The Gale Group, Inc., used under license by Simon & Schuster, Inc., the publisher of this work.

For information about special discounts for bulk purchases, please contact Simon & Schuster Special Sales at 1-800-456-6798 or business@simonandschuster.com

Manufactured in the United States of America

5   7   9   10   8   6   4

Library of Congress Control Number: 2008032677

ISBN-13: 978-1-4165-4971-0
ISBN-10:   1-4165-4971-4

For my children, their children, their children's children,
and for all children—they depend on us to ask why and
act on the answers, however difficult.

CONTENTS

INTRODUCTION TO
THE ULTRAMIND SOLUTION

❖

BY MARTHA HERBERT, M.D., PH.D.
Assistant Professor of Neurology, Harvard Medical School,
and Director of Transcend Research Program,
Massachusetts General Hospital

In the twenty-first century the watchword of biology is "systems." As our technologies race ahead in sophistication, we are being flooded with evidence for the integration of functions in our brains and bodies. Things are very connected, and they are very interdependent. Gone is the single gene acting by itself; it has been replaced by networks. And gone is genetics acting by itself—this has been replaced by integration across levels. Genomics, proteomics, metabolomics, and many more "omics" are all intertwined. This is the new "systems biology."

What does this have to do with our health? In the twentieth century, medicine chopped the body up into specialties—neurology, cardiology, gastroenterology, and endocrinology. Specialists zoomed into their corner of the body; but who was minding the whole picture? Very few doctors have had that skill. Systems biology demands a fresh approach, and that's where Functional Medicine comes in. Rather than treating the body as a collection of separate organ systems, it looks at how our cells and systems flourish and how they get into trouble. Functional Medicine is the practical interface for systems biology in clinical care. It looks for system problems so it can catch things early and treat root causes rather than symptoms.

In the twenty-first century it is also becoming clear that the brain is deeply linked to the body, and that the brain and body profoundly shape each other. If the brain is in the body, and the body systems are in trouble, the brain will be in trouble too. Many of the systems commonly unwell in the body will also be unwell in the brain. Dr. Hyman uses Functional Medicine to show that if you treat these unwell systems, you help your body and that helps your brain too.

The chemical imbalances underlying "psychiatric illness" can now be seen as linked to more systemic chemical, metabolic problems, which can be treated at the bodily level. While just treating the brain chemistry can lead to drug dependence, treating systemic chemistry can fix the brain chemistry imbalance and lead to real sustainable healing.

With the onslaught of so much stress and so many chemical and other environmental challenges, it's no wonder that our body systems are challenged, and that our brain function is not what it should be. Dr. Hyman's seven keys to UltraWellness offer a clear approach to supporting and healing our core functional systems. While more research is important, we know enough to deal intelligently with these challenges right now, and Dr. Hyman shows not only why but how.

For the great enemy of truth is very often not the lie—deliberate, contrived, and dishonest—but the myth—persistent, persuasive, and unrealistic. Too often we hold fast to the clichés of our forbears. We subject all facts to a prefabricated set of interpretations. We enjoy the comfort of opinion without the discomfort of thought.

—JOHN F. KENNEDY

Be open minded, but not so open minded that your brains fall out.

—GROUCHO MARX

Why Diseases Don't Matter

In opening this book on the brain and mood, my guess is you are surprised by the absence of any chapters on familiar diseases like depression, anxiety, attention deficit/hyperactivity disorder (ADHD), autism, or Alzheimer's disease. Instead you find chapters on nutrition, hormones, inflammation, digestion, detoxification, energy, and calming the mind.

If diseases as we know them were a useful way to think about what is wrong with our brains, our moods, and our thinking, then I would have written a book about them. But they are not useful.

Instead this book is an exploration of what is really wrong with our brains. It is about the real causes and solutions for our mental suffering and the epidemics of depression, anxiety, dementia, autism, and attention deficit disorder we see in today's world. If you have been diagnosed with "mental disorders" or "brain diseases," I will tell you what you really need to know about the cause and cure for your suffering. Diseases as we currently define them will no longer be relevant, as we understand the basic common molecular mechanisms at the root of your symptoms.

I challenge you to put aside your beliefs about your suffering, and discover how medicine has evolved without anyone noticing. This book is about that change, and the possibility of renewal for you.

INTRODUCTION

How to Use This Book

Welcome to your brain.

You have just picked up the instruction book for the rest of your life.

Here is what you will find in these pages.

Part I: An Accidental Psychiatrist's Approach to the Epidemic of Broken Brains

In Part I you will learn about our epidemic of "broken brains"—both the scope and the cause of the problem facing us in the twenty-first century. And you will learn why the solutions to this problem are available today but nearly ignored.

You will also learn why fixing your body is the best way to fix your broken brain and why the foundations of modern psychiatry and neurology are based on myths.

Then you will learn why you are suffering from brain damage—all the myriad causes of injury to the soft, custardlike, three-pound wonder that is your brain.

Part II: The Seven Keys to UltraWellness

In Part II, you will learn how imbalances in the seven basic core systems of your body—nutrition, hormones, immune function, digestion, detoxification, energy metabolism, and mind-body—explain all the symptoms and diseases we think are "brain" problems. In truth, these are simply imbalances in the body that show up in the brain.

You will also find specific quizzes for each of the seven key systems to help you identify your unique imbalances.

Part III: The UltraMind Solution

Part III is a practical how-to, step-by-step program to fix your broken brain using the UltraMind Solution. You will learn how to:

✛ Eat right for your brain
✛ Tune up your brain chemistry with supplements
✛ Exercise, sleep, relax, and train your brain
✛ Live clean and green

Part IV: Balance the Seven Keys to UltraWellness and Optimize the Six-Week Plan

In Part IV, you will learn how to customize the UltraMind Solution to help correct the unique imbalances you discover through the quizzes in Part II.

You will also learn how to partner with your health-care practitioner when needed to correct the unique imbalances that prevent you from leading a whole, complete, joyful, and fulfilled life.

The UltraMind Companion Guide

Before you get started on the program, I wanted to let you know I have created a companion guide that is designed to make your path to an Ultra-Mind as simple as possible.

Go to www.ultramind.com/guide and download *The UltraMind Solution Companion Guide.* It is packed with tips and techniques that make what you are about to experience even easier.

PART I

The Accidental Psychiatrist's Approach to the Epidemic of Broken Brains

CHAPTER 1

BROKEN BRAINS

A Twenty-first Century Epidemic

Discovery consists of seeing what everybody has seen and thinking what nobody has thought.

—ALBERT VON SZENT-GYÖRGYI NAGYRAPOLT, 1937
Nobel Laureate in Physiology and Medicine,
the scientist who isolated vitamin C

Your brain is broken. You know it. You feel it. You hide it. You fear it. You have been touched by an epidemic. It deprives children of their future, the elderly of their past, and adults of their present.

No one is talking about this invisible epidemic. Yet it's the leading cause of disability, affects 1.1 billion people worldwide[1]—one in six children, one in two elderly—and will cripple one in four people during their lifetime.[2]

I am talking about the epidemic of broken brains.

We refer to our "broken brains" by many names—depression, anxiety, memory loss, brain fog, attention deficit disorder or ADD, autism, and dementia to name a few.

This epidemic of brain breakdown shows up in radically different ways from person to person so that they all seem like separate problems. But the truth is that they are all manifestations of a few common underlying root causes.

These seemingly different disorders are *all* really the same problem—imbalances in the seven keys to UltraWellness.

Conventional treatments don't help, make things worse, or provide only slight benefit.

That's because conventional treatments use the wrong model to heal these disorders.

There is another way to fix your broken brain, and it is not what you have heard or might think.

Just as brain problems all stem from the same root causes, they all have the same solution—*The UltraMind Solution.*

I know this as both doctor and patient. My own brain broke one beautiful late August day in 1996. I became disoriented and terrified and descended into a spiral of helplessness and hopelessness.

Let me tell you my story.

My Broken Brain

Learning, thinking, and speaking were always easy for me. My brain never failed me. In college, I learned thousands of Chinese characters. In medical school, the intricate patterns and names of our anatomy—the bones, muscles, organs, vessels, and nerves—mapped effortlessly into my mind, and the complex pathways of physiology and biochemistry were clear after one lecture and reading my notes.

I ran four miles every day to medical school. I took detailed notes in my classes, able to simultaneously listen to, remember, and write down nearly every word my professors spoke.

At the end of the day I ran back again to my apartment, did yoga for an hour, ate a freshly prepared whole-foods meal, and studied without distraction or loss of focus for three hours every night. Then I crawled into bed, fell peacefully asleep within five minutes, and slept deeply for seven hours.

The next day I got up and did it all over again.

That rhythmic life broke down, as it does for all physicians in training, when I entered the hospital and started pushing my body and mind beyond their limits with regular thirty-six-hour shifts on top of an occasional sixty-hour shift (Friday morning to Monday evening!).

When I went to practice as a small-town family doctor in Idaho, I worked a shortened schedule of only eighty hours a week, seeing thirty patients a day, delivering babies, and working in the emergency room.

From Idaho, I went to work in China for a year, breathing in the coal-soaked, mercury-laden air, before I landed back in Massachusetts, working a crazy schedule of shifts in an inner-city emergency room.

Then suddenly (or so it appeared at the time), my brain broke—along the with rest of my body.

Sitting with patients, I often couldn't remember what they had just said, or where I was in eliciting their story. I tried to take careful notes and keep track, but I couldn't focus on conversations, couldn't remember anyone's name. I started taking pictures and writing down personal details about my patients to serve as my peripheral memory so I wouldn't embarrass myself the next time I spoke to them.

During lectures I had to give as part of my job, I would get lost in the middle of a sentence and had to ask the audience what I had just said. When I read a book, I had to go over passages again and again just to glean any meaning. At night, I read my children bedtime stories but had to robotically mouth the words, because I couldn't simultaneously read aloud and understand what I read.

Sleep eluded me. Exhausted and bone weary, I would lie down in bed at night and remain sleepless for hours. After finally drifting off, I would wake the next morning feeling as if I had never slept.

Depression and anxiety, which I had never known before, became constant companions.

At times I felt I couldn't go on any longer. My capacity for pleasure and laughter faded into a distant memory.

The worse my body felt, the worse my brain functioned. If my stomach was bloated and swollen and I had diarrhea, I couldn't think or sleep. If my tongue was inflamed or my eyes swollen and red, I became depressed. If my muscles ached and twitched, I couldn't focus. If I felt bone-weary fatigue, I would forget what I was saying or why I had just walked into a room.

Some doctors said I was depressed and recommended antidepressants. Psychiatrists suggested antianxiety drugs. My family doctor prescribed sleeping medication. A neurologist told me I had ADD and I needed stimulants. Others said I had chronic fatigue and fibromyalgia. All I knew was that my brain was broken, my focus gone, my mood depressed, my memory fleeting, and my body wasn't working.

All at once, I couldn't pay attention, remember, or experience joy and happiness. It was as if I had suddenly "contracted" three terrible diseases—attention deficit disorder, depression, and dementia. How could my brain have failed me? The part of me that was strongest suddenly became my weakest link. What had happened?

What I experienced was extreme and I hid it from the rest of the world, except for a very few close friends. I faked it and pulled myself through each day.

But after that summer day in August when my brain broke, weary and fighting brain fog, I began searching for answers.

Piece by piece, cell by cell, body system by body system, I discovered the source of my broken brain. By combing through the literature, consulting with dozens of scientists and doctors, and experimenting with my body and mind, I slowly put myself back together.

It wasn't one thing that broke my brain. It was everything piled higher and higher until my brain and body couldn't take anymore. It seemed sudden but was the end of a long series of exposures to toxins, stress, and a strange infection.

The trail led back to mercury poisoning from living in Beijing, China, breathing in raw coal used to heat homes for 10 million people, eating endless childhood tunafish sandwiches, and having a mouthful of "silver" or mercury fillings. I was also missing a key gene needed to detoxify all this mercury, which compounded the problem. I found out about this later through careful testing.

Years of sleepless nights delivering babies and working in the emergency room *destroyed my body's rhythms, which I tried to bolster with quadruple espressos, giant-size chocolate chip cookies, and mountains of Chunky Monkey ice cream (I reasoned that was healthy because of the bananas and walnuts!).*

Then one late summer day in 1996 I ate or drank something up in a wilderness camp in Maine that infected my gut. That was the straw that broke the camel's back.

This book is the story of my healing. It is also the story of the discoveries I made that hold the answer to our current epidemic of broken brains. It offers a solution to your suffering just as it did to mine.

How many of you feel what I felt, at least to some degree?

- Maybe you fear losing your job because you're tired, unfocused, inattentive, and your memory is failing so you can't properly perform your tasks at work.
- Do you feel depressed, hopeless, disconnected, and disengaged from your life?
- Do you see your relationships breaking down because you are mentally and emotionally absent or numb?
- Perhaps you struggle to focus so you can help your children with their homework and guide them through life, but feel sure you aren't living up to your duties as a parent.
- Do you lie awake at night, tormented by the grief and pain of living half a life, and then worry about how you will find a way to wake up early in the morning just so you can get your kids to school?
- Do you forget to meet friends or go to appointments, and then can't figure out how in the world you forgot?

If so, you aren't alone. You have been affected by the broken brain epidemic, a terrifying and life-threatening chronic illness that has been largely unaddressed by the medical community, leaving millions of people to suffer alone, trapped in their deteriorating minds.

Our Looming Silent Epidemic of Broken Brains

Obesity is obvious. You can't hide it. But mental illness and memory loss are suffered silently, hidden from view. Yet they touch nearly everyone either directly or indirectly; personally or through family members and friends.

Our broken brains cause many problems—anxiety, depression, bipolar disease, personality disorders, eating disorders, addictions, obsessive-compulsive disorder, attention deficit disorder, autism, Asperger's, learning difficulties, and dyslexia.

Broken brains take many shapes, including psychotic disorders such as schizophrenia and mania, as well as all the neurodegenerative diseases of aging, especially Alzheimer's, dementia, and Parkinson's disease.

In addition, there are brain dysfunctions that fall on the lighter side of the broken brain continuum. While many psychiatrists and neurologists wouldn't qualify these problems as treatable diseases, they still cause unnecessary suffering for many. These include chronic stress, lack of focus, poor concentration, brain fog, anger, mood swings, sleep problems, or just feeling a bit anxious or depressed most of the time.

Broken brains show up in two major ways: psychiatric disorders—problems that most blame on emotional trauma—and neurological disorders—problems most consider to be caused by neurological impairment, not emotional malfunctioning.

Whether you suffer from a psychiatric disorder like depression or a neurological disorder like Alzheimer's, the simple fact is this . . .

Our brains don't work well.

We suffer from bouts of depression that darken our days and make our lives feel empty and meaningless. We have irrational fears that torment us day in and day out. We live under the constant pressure of stress that never seems to cease. We lose our grip on reality. We can't focus at work. We can't remember what we are taught in school. And our memories just get worse and worse every day.

Because they are so pervasive, broken brains are one of the primary issues keeping many in today's society from being optimally healthy and feeling vitally alive—an experience I call *UltraWellness*, which is something you are going to learn how to achieve in this book.

If you think this isn't a serious problem or it only affects a few people, think again.

- Psychiatric disorders affect 26 percent of our adult population or more than 60 million Americans.
- More than 20 percent of children have some type of psychiatric disorder.[3,4]
- More than 40 million people have anxiety.
- More than 20 million people have depression.
- One in ten Americans takes an antidepressant.
- The use of antidepressants has tripled in the last decade.
- In 2006, expenditures on antidepressants soared to over $1.9 billion.

- Psychiatric disorders like depression and anxiety are expensive.[5] They are among the top five most costly medical conditions, including heart disease, cancer, trauma, and lung disorders. The cost to our health-care system exceeds $200 billion a year, which is over 12 percent of total health-care spending.[6]
- Alzheimer's disease will affect 30 percent (and some experts say 50 percent) of people over eighty-five years old, which is the fastest-growing segment of the population. It will affect 16 million people by 2050.
- Attention deficit hyperactivity disorder is a label we now give 8.7 percent of children between the ages of eight and fifteen.[7]
- More than 8 million, or one in ten, children now take stimulant medications like methylphenidate (Ritalin).[8]
- Autism rates have increased from 3 in 10,000 children to 1 in 166 children—an elevenfold increase—over the last decade.[9]
- Learning disabilities affect between 5 and 10 percent of school-age children.[10]
- The indirect costs of all these broken brains to society are mammoth. They include loss of productivity at school, home, or in the workplace, accounting for a loss of over $80 billion a year.

There is something wrong with this picture. Nearly one in three of us suffers from a broken brain. Is this a normal part of the human condition? No. It isn't.

The problem is that we've been looking for answers to these problems in the wrong places—in the corners of our past, in the chemical "imbalances" in our brains, in the latest drug or therapeutic approach.

This is especially true of psychiatry and neurology, the two specialties that typically treat "brain disorders."

Neurologists and psychiatrists focus on treating your brain using medications or psychotherapy. In fact, most psychiatrists and neurologists focus solely on their favorite organ, the brain, and ignore the rest of the body.

But what if the cure for brain disorders is *outside* the brain? What if mood, memory, attention and behavior problems, and most other "brain diseases" have their root cause in the rest of the body—in treatable imbalances in the body's key systems? What if they are not localized in the brain? If this is true, it would mean our whole approach to dealing with brain disorders is completely backward.

Indeed, it is.

Why Traditional Neurology and Psychiatry Typically Don't Work

Psychiatry has its roots in the notion that previous life experiences or traumas control mood and behavior. This is the legacy of Sigmund Freud—that all mental illness is the result of childhood experiences.

Yet only about 10 percent of us are nutritionally, metabolically, and biochemically balanced enough to fully benefit from psychotherapy.

What's more, years of psychoanalysis or therapy will not reverse the depression that comes from profound omega-3 fatty acid deficiencies,[11] a lack of vitamin B_{12},[12] a low-functioning thyroid,[13] or chronic mercury toxicity.[14]

Certainly, if the body is back in balance, working with the emotional and spiritual dimensions of our suffering is critical and necessary. But it is a very hard road to follow without addressing how our genes, diet, and environment interact to change our brain chemistry and detract from the optimal function and balance of our body and mind.

If you have a significant biological imbalance, psychotherapy is a distraction and a waste of time.

And *many* of us suffer from biological imbalances . . .

Sensing this, modern psychiatry has moved into an elaborate attempt to control brain chemistry with drugs, as if all mental illness were a brain chemistry imbalance and all we have to do is match the right drug (or drugs) to the mental illness.

Is Depression a Prozac Deficiency?

Is this the answer to our epidemic of broken brains—more and better medication? Do we really need more antidepressants, stimulants, antipsychotics, and memory medications?

Are we defectively designed so that we cannot be happy, or concentrate or remember things, without pills? Is depression a Prozac deficiency? Is ADHD a Ritalin deficiency? Is Alzheimer's an Aricept deficiency?

I think not.

Yet the use of these drugs is skyrocketing. Psychiatric or psychotropic medications are the number-two selling class of prescription drugs,[15] after cholesterol medication. And the rate of increase in the use of psychiatric medications in the last decade is meteoric (such as a 1,000 percent increase in the use of stimulant medication in children).

If treatments like these were completely effective and free of side effects, I would welcome them to provide relief from suffering for millions. But they do not work well (or at all) for many.

Let's take the example of antidepressants.

Most patients who take antidepressants either don't respond or have only a partial response. In fact, success is considered a 50 percent improvement in half the symptoms. And this minimal result is achieved in less than half the patients taking these medications.

That's a pretty dismal record. It's made worse by the fact that 86 percent of those who do find some relief from their symptoms have one or more side effects, including sexual dysfunction, fatigue, insomnia, loss of mental abilities, nausea, and weight gain!

No wonder half of the people who try antidepressants quit after four months.[16]

A recent study in *The New England Journal of Medicine* discovered that drug companies selectively published studies on antidepressants. They published nearly all the studies that showed benefit and almost none of the studies that showed they don't work.[17]

This kind of underreporting warps our view, leading us to think that antidepressants (and other psychiatric medications) do work when they don't. This hiding of the real and complete data on antidepressants has fueled the tremendous growth we have seen in psychiatric medications.

The problem is actually worse than it sounds because the positive studies hardly show benefit in the first place. In double-blind studies of antidepressants (where people are given either the medication or a sugar pill) 40 percent of people taking a sugar pill got better, while only 60 percent taking the actual drug had improvement in their symptoms. Looking at it another way—80 percent of people get better with just a sugar pill.

I'll admit, the approach is half right. Chemical imbalances lead to problems. But the real question that manipulating brain chemicals with drugs begs is never asked . . .

Why are those chemicals out of balance in the first place and how do we get them back to their natural state of balance?

These drugs don't cure the problem. They cover over the symptoms.

To cure the epidemic of broken brains we have to ask a new set of questions:

✥ How do we find the cause of this epidemic?

✥ Are we defectively designed, or is it our toxic environment, our nutrient-depleted diet, and our unremitting stress affecting our sensitive brains? Is it the result of imbalances in our body?

✥ Are more drugs *really* the answer, or is there a way to address the underlying causes of this epidemic so that we can regain our mental (and physical) health and live whole, functional, fulfilling lives?

There is an answer to brain problems, but it's not more drugs or psychotherapy. Although these tools can be a helpful bridge during your recovery from a broken brain, they won't provide long-term solutions.

The secret that promises to help us fix our broken brains lies in an unlikely place, a place modern medicine has mostly ignored.

The answer lies in our body.

CHAPTER 2

THE ACCIDENTAL PSYCHIATRIST

Finding the Body-Mind Connection

Do you see what you believe or do you believe what you see?

—SIDNEY BAKER, M.D.

I wasn't sad, hopeless, forgetful, and unable to focus because I had depression, attention deficit disorder, or dementia. It was because I was toxic, inflamed, nutritionally depleted, my gut was a mess, my hormones were out of balance, my cells were unable to make energy, and I was stressed out from being a single parent.

It wasn't until I learned how to rebuild all these broken systems and heal my body that I got my brain back.

The solution I found is the same one I am going to teach you.

It is the UltraMind Solution.

To learn how to fix your brain you are going to have to accept a radically new way of thinking about health—one that most doctors today still struggle to understand. The crux of it is embodied in a simple truth:

Everything is connected.

Your entire body and all of the core systems in it interact as a single sophisticated symphony. You are one whole person, and all the pieces of your biology and your unique genetic code interact with your environment (including the foods you eat) to determine how sick or well you are in this moment.

This means your body-and-mind are connected as well.

The body-and-mind are a single, dynamic bidirectional system. What you do to one has enormous impact on the other. What you do to your body you do to your brain. Heal your body and you heal your brain.

Change your body and you will fix your broken brain.

Your thoughts, beliefs and attitudes, traumas, and life experiences directly influence your biology. We know that stress and other psychological factors can have a major impact on your health. Now we understand that 95 percent of all illnesses are either caused by or worsened by stress. What you think can influence how sick or well you are. The mind influences the body.

This is known as Mind-Body Medicine. It is an important contribution to the field of science and is researched by major institutions such as Harvard and Stanford.

Sadly, most physicians do not apply this knowledge in their practices. They accept it. But rather than using the power of the mind to heal, they disdainfully say that people with psychological influences on their health have "psychosomatic illness," or "somatize," meaning that their "physical" symptoms are all in their head.

Even worse, *somato-psychic* medicine (or how the body affects the mind) is hardly on the radar.

The body directly and powerfully influences the brain. Nutritional status, hormonal imbalances, food allergies, toxins, and digestive, immune, and metabolic imbalances, primarily influence mood, behavior, attention, and attitude.

You already know about this body-mind connection, even if you have never consciously considered it. Just take a moment to think about how your own body has affected your mind over your lifetime, and then extrapolate that to more serious conditions.

- Have you ever felt anxious, irritable, jittery, fearful, or even had a panic attack only to have a can of cola or muffin and feel better right away? Why were you anxious? Because your blood sugar was plummeting, and when that happens your body is programmed to respond as though it is a life-threatening emergency.
- Do you feel foggy and mentally sluggish after eating a large meal?
- Have you ever felt stressed and anxious and then taken a long walk or ridden your bike a few miles only to feel calm and relaxed afterward? Why did this happen? Because you burned off the stress chemicals, adrenaline and cortisol, which made you feel anxious.
- Have you ever felt angry and irritable because you have been deprived of sleep? Have you felt happier and that you had fewer problems after a great night's sleep?
- Have you ever had the flu and tried to focus and read a book or

concentrate on anything only to find it difficult, perhaps even impossible?

∴ Have you ever hallucinated or been delirious with a high fever?

These are basic examples of the body-mind connection that many of us have experienced. But there are so many other things that occur inside of you that affect your brain and mind of which you have no awareness.

Did you know that premenstrual mood swings are the result of fluctuating hormone levels, or that your winter blues are the result of vitamin D deficiency, or that your lifelong melancholy may be the result of mercury poisoning from hundreds of tuna fish sandwiches you've eaten over your lifetime, or that your obsessive-compulsive disorder could be the result of a bacterial infection?

These obvious and not so obvious interactions between your body and your mind are only the tip of the iceberg.

Consider for a moment that depression, anxiety, insomnia, attention deficit disorder, and obsessive-compulsive disorder—not to mention the hundreds of other mental disorders described by psychiatrists in the *Diagnostic and Statistical Manual of Mental Disorders* (*DSM-IV*)—may be primarily caused by imbalances in the body and have very little to do with the meaning, metaphors, and myths we associated with them. It is a perfect system for describing your symptoms, but useless for helping you find the cause.

Interestingly, there are a few conditions recognized and treated by conventional medicine that clearly show how problems in your body cause "diseases" in your brain, but the implications are ignored.

For example, when someone with late-stage liver disease develops something called "hepatic encephalopathy" or temporary insanity from liver failure, the treatment is not antipsychotics, but antibiotics to clear out the bacteria in the intestine, which produce brain-destroying toxins that can no longer be detoxified by the liver.

Imagine, treating insanity with antibiotics.

Similarly, we know that alcoholics become "crazy" with a condition known as Wernicke's encephalopathy from vitamin B_1 (or thiamine) deficiency, which can be cured by giving them a vitamin.

And we know that an antibiotic for a streptococcal infection can cure some children who suffer from obsessive-compulsive disorder. The condition is called PANDAS or Pediatric Autoimmune Neuropsychiatric Disorders Associated with Streptococcal Infections.

Yet physicians typically don't stop to consider whether or not other mental disorders may be related to imbalances in gut function, the immune system, problems with detoxification, or an imbalance in any of the body's other key systems.

I think this is because doctors tend to see what they believe and often don't believe what they see, even when it is right in front of them.

What happens in the body influences the brain, as we never imagined it could. The implications for treatment of mental and brain disorders are staggering. A whole new array of possible causes and treatments are open to us.

Changing your diet, nutrient levels, circadian rhythms or sleep patterns, the substances you use, the amount of exercise or playtime you have, getting rid of toxins in your system, balancing your hormones, correcting imbalances in your digestive tract, boosting your cells' ability to produce energy, and fixing food sensitivities or allergies can *all* radically transform your mood and brain function.

With that in mind, consider the following:

- ❖ Can lifelong depression be cured?
- ❖ Can children completely recover from autism?
- ❖ Can dementia be reversed?

Conventional medical wisdom says no. We don't see many cases in the medical literature where people recover from autism, reverse dementia, or are cured from lifelong depression.

But just because psychiatrists and neurologists aren't reporting dramatic recoveries like these employing the "normal" methods used to treat such disorders doesn't mean the disorders aren't treatable. In conventional approaches, partial relief of symptoms is sometimes possible. But cures or dramatic recoveries? You may hear doctors say, *Where is the evidence?*

The idea that psychiatric or neurological "diseases" like depression, anxiety, Alzheimer's, Parkinson's disease, and dementia can be effectively treated, not by administering psychoactive medication, but by altering dietary and lifestyle influences and repairing the body's systems, which affect the entire Body–Mind System in which the brain functions, is resisted by conventional psychiatry and neurology.

The forces that distort our view, and keep conventional doctors locked in their way of seeing and thinking, are complex. One factor is the enormous influence drug companies have by way of funding and setting the research agenda, developing treatments, withholding important data that contradicts their worldview, controlling medical education, "educating" doctors, and marketing to consumers.

Other factors are our medical institutions and our financial reimbursement systems, which are founded on outdated ideas of separate diseases and medical specialties. Abandoning those ideas would threaten their economic viability and perhaps even their existence.

And our medical training reinforces the illusion of separate body systems by training doctors in specialties and subspecialties—there are doctors for every inch of your body. But there are very few who understand how the whole body works as one complete ecosystem.

Even when we see research or miracles in practice (dismissed as spontaneous remissions) that contradict our worldview, it is very difficult to integrate. It is ignored or brushed aside in favor of our current paradigm. In fourteenth-century Europe it would have been very hard to convince anyone that the world is round. It looks flat so it must be flat. Similarly, doctors today can't see what is quickly becoming obvious.

I recently presented a lecture at Harvard outlining the case of a boy who recovered from autism using the approach in *The UltraMind Solution*. I documented in great detail his story, and showed how when his abnormal tests and biology returned to normal, his brain and behavior stabilized, and he lost his diagnosis of autism.

The pediatrician present explained away his recovery as an example of spontaneous remission. One of the other physicians at the lecture, who knew my work, said facetiously, "The only problem is that Dr. Hyman has twelve cases like this of 'spontaneous remission' in his practice."

Unfortunately, too many doctors have the same mind-set as that pediatrician: don't confuse me with the facts. My mind is made up.

Nevertheless, the recent discoveries about how behavior, mood, and mental functioning are linked to our biology are one of the greatest advances in twenty-first-century medicine. These discoveries are growing to meet other advances, which show how our thoughts, feelings, and life experiences literally shape our brain and influence our biology.

Such research holds the answer to the epidemic of mood, behavior, attention, and memory problems that are rampant in today's society.

What I am suggesting in this book is a revolutionary new method for treating broken brains—"mental disorders" and "brain diseases"—that is based on cutting-edge science and medicine; one that marks a radical departure from classical psychiatry and neurology and the methods these fields typically use to treat their patients.

The brain is not disconnected from the rest of the body as many practitioners of conventional medicine would have you believe, and the solution to the epidemic of broken brains is *not* found in more psychoactive medications or better therapy.

The brain is mostly downstream from the real causes, which are found in the biology of your whole body. Brain problems or "disorders" are almost always systemic disorders, and the cure will be found outside the brain—in your body.

My goal in writing *The UltraMind Solution* is to show you the new landscape of how brain function, mind, mood, and behavior are created by changes in your body and your biology. I want to show you how to use that information to cure or dramatically improve the rising tide of "broken brains," including conditions like depression, anxiety, bipolar disease, psychosis, attention deficit disorder, autism, dementia, Alzheimer's, Parkinson's disease, and more.

Even if you don't have one of these "diseases" and feel "fine," feeling fine is less than what you could feel. You should and can feel alert, focused, happy, energetic, unstressed, and mentally sharp. That is, if you know how to care for your brain.

That is what I will teach you in this book.

My goal for all of you is to live your life as you were meant to live it—a life full of energy, vitality, pleasure, and happiness. This is the state of Ultra-Wellness, and it is available to everyone if you know how to take advantage of it. The key to this is a balanced mind and body, which will allow you to experience the joys and the sorrows of life as you meet them, directly and fully.

Consider the experiences of just a few of my patients:

- A fifty-three-year-old man with lifelong bipolar disease and crippling depression on a multidrug cocktail who had relief from depression for the first time in thirty years after tuning up his brain function with folate and vitamins B_{12} and B_6.
- A three-year-old boy with violent behavior who calmed down after balancing his blood sugar and clearing out toxic bacteria from his intestinal tract.
- A twenty-three-year-old woman with lifelong anxiety and depression that lifted after she quit eating foods that she was allergic to.
- A seventy-year-old man who was losing a grip on his memory and had been diagnosed with early dementia, who after getting

all the mercury out of his body, came back to life and was able
to work and function.

❖ Or the little boy with autism, who began to talk and connect socially, after getting rid of gluten and casein (wheat and dairy) from
his diet and treating yeast in his gut.

How can you explain these "miraculous" cures? It's simple. Brain function is directly influenced by what you eat, and by nutritional deficiencies,
allergens, infections, toxins, and stress. These problems are taken care of by
rebalancing the seven keys to UltraWellness. This, in turn, leads to an Ultra-
Mind.

The solution to this epidemic is getting to the root of the problems by
examining how our ancient genes interact with our environment to create
systemic imbalances that affect our most prized and sensitive organ—the
brain.

The UltraMind Solution will show you how to correct the causes of the
imbalances in your brain. Those causes often result from imbalances in
other systems in your body. This book will teach you how to achieve optimum mental health and brain health without drugs or psychotherapy.

This approach is the future medicine, and will soon become the foundation for diagnosing and treating mental illness and brain diseases. It will be
the standard way we achieve optimal mental health and brain function.

The last twenty years of research in the field of the brain have concen-
trated on what makes it able to remember or forget, be happy or sad, feel
anxious or calm, and stay focused or be inattentive. Studies have uncovered
a few simple underlying factors that explain why things go wrong and how
to fix them.

But it can take more than twenty years for scientific findings like these to
be incorporated into most physicians' practices, and it may take even longer
since they threaten the very foundation of our scientific paradigm.

You don't have to wait another twenty years to take advantage of what
we know now.

What the years of investigation have revealed is that our troubles with
mood, behavior, attention, and memory don't come from bad parenting or
bad genes, but from imbalances in seven key underlying systems in the body.

And here's the really big news:

These "diseases" really do not exist.

"Mental disorders" and "brain disorders" are simply the names of common responses our bodies have to a variety of insults and deficiencies.
Fixing those underlying problems by rebalancing the seven keys may

allow the brain to heal, the body-mind and mind-body to come back into balance.

When even one of these seven core systems is out of balance, illness of all kinds can result, ranging from heart disease to diabetes to weight gain to the brain disorders you have come to this book looking to heal.

Helping people balance these seven key systems is the foundation of my medical practice. It is what I did to fix my broken brain and it is how I have helped thousands of patients from all walks of life achieve a state of health they never dreamed possible.

Every day I witness miracles.

Giving you a practical way to understand, identify, and fix imbalances in each of the seven key systems of your body (just as I do in my practice) so you can make a miraculous recovery of your own is the purpose of *The UltraMind Solution*.

This book makes available for the first time the results of new research and knowledge of the brain, mood, and body in a practical guide for everyone young and old, hyper or calm, forgetful or not. It is designed to give you the information and tools you need to treat the roots of your broken brains, and by doing so overcome their devastating effects and take a big step closer to UltraWellness.

How did I learn about this?

How I Became an Accidental Psychiatrist

I call myself the "accidental psychiatrist." I never set out to be a brain or mood expert. In fact, my focus was more on how the body works as a whole system. And people saw me not to treat depression or autism or Alzheimer's, but to deal with chronic complaints and illnesses of the body.

People make appointments to see me from far away, often after seeing many physicians, dissatisfied with more medications and more diagnoses. They come with a deep inner knowledge that something is out of balance—they just don't know how to find it by themselves. So many of my patients are willing to begin exploring the landscape of their bodies and minds in a new and deeper way.

Because of this I have had the unique opportunity to be a medical detective, hunting down clues and exploring the entire landscape of human biology and systems. I worked for almost ten years as the co-medical director of Canyon Ranch, and now for many years as the founder and medical director of the UltraWellness Center (www.ultrawellnesscenter.com).

Over the years as I worked to correct the fundamental imbalances that are the cause of all disease (the seven keys to UltraWellness, which you will learn about in a moment), I discovered that mood and brain disorders would often magically disappear as I treated a patient's physical problems.

Rather than dismiss this finding, I found it curious and began to investigate how treating digestive problems could cure depression, or how detoxifying a patient from mercury could bring back their memory. I investigated each of my patients carefully by listening to their stories of transformation and by examining the existing rich medical literature on this subject, which is mostly ignored.

Many years ago I treated a woman with a bacterial infection in her gut from a bug called Clostridia (which produces a molecule called DHPPA, which has neurochemical effects) with an antibiotic. Not only did her digestive symptoms clear up, but also her lifelong depression, which was resistant to treatment with medications like Prozac, lifted almost overnight.

Experiences like these as well as my own struggle with a chronic illness allowed the mysterious world of how the body influences the brain to open up to me.

Hence I became an "accidental psychiatrist."

Since then I have found remarkable patterns and connections that link the body to the mind. The wonder of the body continues to delight and amaze me, as I understand more clearly how the entire body and the mind is one interacting, interlocking, networked system.

Nowhere is this truer than in how the brain is connected to the rest of the body.

Through the prism of one boy's story told below, you will learn how powerful this approach can be for fixing your broken brain. This one story, and this boy's two homework assignments done two months apart, will clarify the bidirectional communication between the brain and the body more than any complicated explanation of biochemical pathways.

While this is a story about one boy, the story of his imbalanced system and how it affected his brain is repeated millions of times over in America. Each story has its personal flavor, and each person may have different imbalances in physiology. But the overarching principle that ties together all brain disorders is simple.

Brain disorders resulting in altered mood, memory, behavior, and attention are a result of imbalances in the seven key systems of your body that determine whether you are well or ill, whether you are living a life of UltraWellness or a diminished life of poor mental and physical health.

Here is Clayton's story . . .

Clayton: A Case Study in the Body-Mind Effect

An exasperated professional woman finally found her way to my office with her twelve-year-old son, Clayton. Clayton, labeled with a multitude of both psychological and physical diagnoses by a number of highly specialized physicians, seemed to be a walking embodiment of "bad luck—poor kid."

In the realm of psychiatry Clayton was "diagnosed" with attention deficit hyperactivity disorder (ADHD), a behavioral disorder. He could not focus in school, "zoned out," and was disruptive. Like many other children labeled with ADHD or on the autism spectrum, Clayton's writing was nearly illegible.[1] On the other hand he excelled in math.

Physically, Clayton was diagnosed with asthma, suffered from "environmental" allergies, sinus congestion, postnasal drip, sore throats, eczema, nausea, stomach pains, diarrhea, headaches, anal itching, canker sores, muscle aches, muscle cramps, hypersensitivity to noises and smells, sneezing, hives, itchy skin with bumps, and frequent infections. He slept poorly and had trouble breathing when he did sleep. He also suffered from anxiety, fearfulness, and carbohydrate cravings.

All of his symptoms were being treated with seven different medications prescribed by five different doctors. These included Ritalin for ADHD, allergy medicine, and inhalers for his asthma and hives, acid-blocking medication for his stomach problems, and painkillers for his headaches.

This is quite a drug cocktail for a twelve-year-old. Yet he still didn't experience much relief from his physical, mental, or behavioral symptoms. But this is how we approach things in medicine—divide it all up into parts, farm them out, and pile on the pills. What a life for both Clayton and his family!

Most psychiatrists not only lack the training to address any physical issues but also feel these are irrelevant to the mental "diagnosis" at hand. I, however, believe these physical ailments are the most important findings and these clues will provide the causes and appropriate treatment to repair disordered brain function.

Today the list of medications and the untested cocktails and combinations have grown to frightening proportions. Children who present with mental, behavioral, or emotional problems like the ones Clayton had now get antipsychotic medications, like Risperdal; antiseizure medications, like Trileptal; and antidepressants, like Prozac—all on top of stimulant medications, like Ritalin, Concerta, and Adderall.

I recently visited a local school nurse. After seeing a large box on the floor filled with empty pill bottles, the nurse told me that 63 percent of the children were on some type of medication.

My challenge is to organize symptoms according to how they are influenced by the seven keys of UltraWellness, not by chopping them up into separate diagnoses. That is how I lead my patients to an UltraMind.

Clayton's UltraMind Solution

As we dug below the surface we found and treated the causes of Clayton's symptoms—imbalances in the seven keys to UltraWellness that form the basis of the UltraMind Solution. Here is what we found and what we did. Clayton's story represents, to one degree or another, all of our stories. It illustrates both the despair and the delivery from our epidemic of broken brains.

Let's look at some of the essential keys affected in Clayton's case.

Nutritional Deficiencies

Like most kids, and especially those on the spectrum of ADHD and autism, Clayton lived on and craved junk food. His typical diet included trans fat, food additives,[2] and an overload of carbohydrates and refined sugar. This has been associated with ADHD.[3] Blood tests confirmed significant deficiencies in many important fats, vitamins, antioxidants, and minerals. Clayton had no omega-3 fats and very low levels of tryptophan, vitamins B_6, A, and D, antioxidants (vitamin E and beta carotene), zinc, and magnesium.

Omega-3 fats, eicosapentanoic acid (EPA) and docosahexanenoic acid (DHA), are essential for brain function. In fact, 60 percent of the brain consists of DHA. A lack of these fats is strongly associated with ADHD,[4] as well as eczema and immune deficiency.

Tryptophan is an amino acid (building block of protein) needed to make serotonin, the chemical in the brain for a relaxed and happy mood, and melatonin, the chemical for sleep. *Vitamin B_6* is crucial to converting tryptophan into serotonin. Clayton's unstable mood, sleep disturbance, and ADHD were clues to a B_6 deficiency. Some of his prescription medications were actually further depleting his B_6 supply.[5]

A clear indication of low *vitamin A* and *omega-3 fat deficiency* were "bumps" on the back of his arms called hyperkeratosis pilaris.[6] His low level of *vitamin D* led to lowered immunity.[7] Deficiencies of other vitamins such as *vitamin E* and *beta carotene* indicated he ate a diet high in junk food and low in vegetables and whole grains.

Low levels of *zinc* are associated with lowered immunity, poor heavy metal detoxification, and ADHD. This was consistent with Clayton's frequent infections, eczema, and allergies[8] as well as the hyperactivity symptoms. Low-*magnesium* levels lead to headaches; anxiety; insomnia, muscle spasms, cramps, and aches; and hypersensitivity to noises.[9]

Nutrients have a multifactorial effect and work in synergy. It is important to attempt to correct all the deficiencies; as you can see, they all interact and overlap.

Immune and Inflammatory Imbalances

Clayton had asthma, allergies, hives, sinusitis, itchy skin, canker sores, a history of intolerance to baby formula, diaper rash, and frequent ear infections. These are all clear evidence of *immune* and *inflammatory imbalances.*

These should not be thought of as separate conditions but rather *one* immune system highly annoyed by one or more triggers such as food or environmental allergens, molds, toxins, chronic low-grade infections, or perhaps a combination of these factors.

Special testing for delayed, low-grade food allergies (IgG food sensitivity) showed Clayton's immune system (and likely his brain[10;11]) was reacting to eighteen foods, including dairy, peanuts, yeast, citrus, and especially gluten, all of which created more inflammation.[12]

Gluten can trigger a low-grade, chronic immune response that inflames the brain and many other systems. Canker sores were just another clue pointing to celiac disease or gluten intolerance.[13] Indeed, his IgG antigliadin antibodies were elevated (indicating an autoimmune reaction to gluten found in wheat, rye, barley, spelt, oats, and tritacle). In a later chapter, you will learn more about why gluten was a major clue in Clayton's healing process.

Digestive Imbalances

Nausea, diarrhea, stomachaches, anal itching, and sensitive stomach were clear symptoms of Clayton's *digestive imbalances.* The use of frequent antibiotics for the many infections led to a yeast overgrowth and abnormal gut flora. This resulted in a *leaky gut* (also called intestinal permeability). This condition gives way to the above-mentioned food allergies, systemic allergies, and inflammation.[14] So we can see why his immune system was so angry.

Detoxification Imbalance

Metal toxicity indicates poor detoxification. Tests showed that Clayton had high levels of **mercury** and **lead**. His exposure was probably similar to other children of his age; however, he nutritionally and/or genetically could not eliminate the metals from his body and stored them in his tissues.

Mercury has been associated with myriad gastrointestinal as well as autoimmune and cognitive problems.[15] Children born between 1989 and 2001 were all exposed to mercury in the form of thimerosal in the multitude of vaccines they were given at a very early age (this mercury preservative was removed from the vaccines in 2001). As you will learn, other sources of mercury include coal-burning industrial plants, many large predatory ocean fish, river fish, and even "silver" dental fillings.

Lead toxicity has been associated with cognitive and behavioral problems in children.[16] In a recent groundbreaking study, lead toxicity and environmental toxins were clearly linked to ADHD.[17] By living in a polluted world, playing with toys made in China and coated with lead paint, and crawling around on the floor where shoes drag in the lead pollution from the outside, Clayton was exposed to the dangers of the industrial revolution.

He may also have suffered from other environmental toxins like mold toxins from the black mold in his house and food additives we could not measure.

Clearly, Clayton's problem was not a Ritalin deficiency or bad parenting! The cause of all these problems lay in the dietary and environmental pollutants that throw the seven underlying systems in our body out of balance.

The Simplicity of Treatment

It is not any *one* thing that caused Clayton's ADHD, abnormal handwriting, hives, asthma, or stomachaches. It was the total load of all the stresses on his system interacting with his unique genetic susceptibilities, which thus led to his abnormal brain function and health problems.

Clayton's treatment was disarmingly simple.

By deliberately and carefully working to find the cause or *source of the irritation to his system* (nutritional deficiencies, toxic foods, food allergies, gluten, environmental toxins, food additives, yeast overgrowth) and identifying *the missing ingredients* needed to restore normal physiological function (a multivitamin, omega-3 fats, vitamin B_6, zinc, magnesium, vitamin D, healthy gut bacteria, and 5-hydroxytryptophan for sleep and anxiety), Clayton's health and brain function could finally start to normalize.

I recommended a whole-foods diet free of additives, sugar, trans fats, processed foods, and his particular allergic foods—gluten, dairy, citrus, peanuts, and yeast. This is the diet on which the UltraMind Solution is founded.

Then we got rid of the low-grade yeast problem he developed after years of taking antibiotics (it showed up as anal itching) with an antifungal medication.

Lead and mercury toxicity was addressed using DMSA, dimercaptosuccinic acid, an FDA-approved medication to remove lead from children. This part of the treatment was postponed until his gastrointestinal health was restored. This was important so Clayton could properly eliminate the metals as they were chelated (pulled out) of his tissues.

My approach is simple: the first step is to *take out the bad stuff;* remove what's irritating you. You need to find all the tacks under your feet to be pain free; removing only one tack will not make you 50 percent better. The second step is to *add the good stuff;* add the specific vitamins, nutrients, and other "ingredients" you need to thrive. These differ from person to person.

The Result of Clayton's Treatment

Clayton and his mother were diligent and determined to make changes. At his two-month follow-up visit, Clayton had discontinued all medications, including Ritalin, antihistamines (Zyrtec and Tagamet), bronchodilators, steroid inhaler, Tylenol (acetaminophen), and Advil (ibuprofen).

His mood and behavior returned to that of a typical twelve-year-old. His attention improved, his disruptiveness at home and in school disappeared, and his irritability and anxiety vanished completely.

Clayton found himself free from all his chronic symptoms for the first time in his life. His hives, asthma, chronic runny nose, anal itching, stomachaches, nausea, diarrhea, headaches, muscle cramps, and sensitivity to loud noises all completely resolved. He was also able to finally fall asleep and stay asleep throughout the night. Clayton also began to succeed in school both socially and academically as he never had before.

Clayton did not have a neurological or psychiatric "disease." He had a "broken brain" caused by nutritional imbalances; toxicity; and altered immune, neurotransmitter, and digestive function. Treating those root causes and correcting the imbalances led to the resolution of all his symptoms.

Some of these findings and resolutions are subjective; therefore, for those skeptics, one irrefutable objective finding underscores the effectiveness of this approach and "proves" the powerful effect the body has on the mind and brain.

Clayton's dysgraphia, or abnormal handwriting, completely resolved within two months of treatment (see Figures 1 and 2 below and on page 31). Here is his homework before the UltraMind Solution and two months later.

Before Treatment

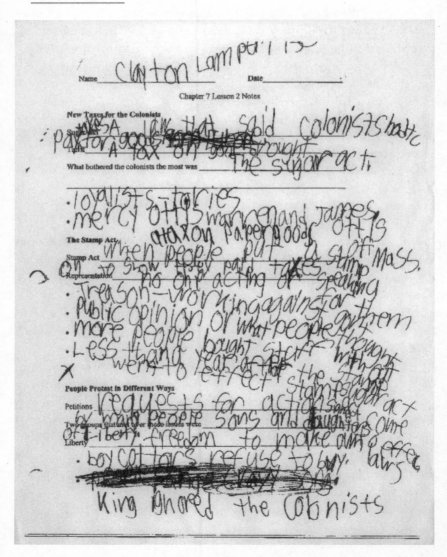

Figure 1: Clayton's handwriting before treatment

After Treatment

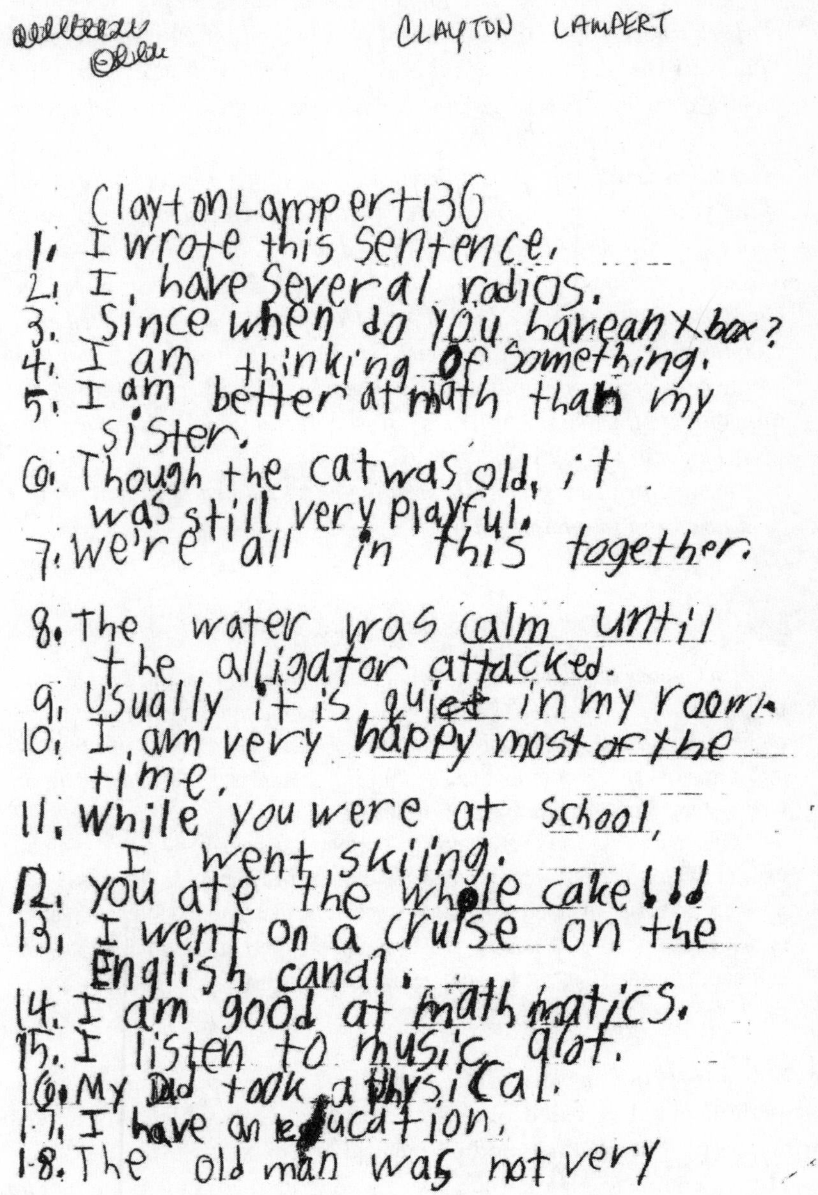

CLAYTON LAMPERT

Clayton Lampert136
1. I wrote this sentence.
2. I have several radios.
3. Since when do you have an Xbox?
4. I am thinking of something.
5. I am better at math than my sister.
6. Though the cat was old, it was still very playful.
7. We're all in this together.

8. The water was calm until the alligator attacked.
9. Usually it is quiet in my room.
10. I am very happy most of the time.
11. While you were at school, I went skiing.
12. You ate the whole cake!!!
13. I went on a cruise on the English canal.
14. I am good at mathmatics.
15. I listen to music alot.
16. My Dad took a physical.
17. I have an education.
18. The old man was not very

Figure 2: Clayton's handwriting after treatment

Clayton's mother also sent me an e-mail reporting on her meeting with his school. The change was remarkable.

> We had a 504 meeting at Clayton's school this morning (where the teachers, school counselor, parents, and principal all get together to review "the plan" for kids with special educational needs—in Clayton's case prompted by the ADHD diagnosis). This was the first time in his entire schooling history that everything seems to be going well. The input from his teachers was that he is "a different kid" than they saw in the first half of the year and that they're amazed by the difference. The school nurse hasn't seen him since March (and he used to be in her office several times a week). The school psychologist said his social skills are very good, age appropriate, and that she sees no problems at all. She also noted that Clayton seems very proud of himself and his new health and that he's taking good ownership of all the changes in his diet. He even seems to be shrugging it off when the other kids at school tell him he's an "alien" because he doesn't drink soda.
>
> This was just such a fantastic meeting and I wanted to pass along the good news and say thank you!

HOW DO YOU KNOW WHAT WORKED?

Many of my colleagues argue that it is impossible to know what the most important factors were in Clayton's treatment or in similar treatments I offer to other patients. These people are stuck in the one-disease, one-drug model of thinking. It is an example of reductionistic thinking that misses the whole point of how systems work—of how the body works.

As evident in Clayton's case, many symptoms are caused by a multitude of irritants and a variety of irritants cause a multitude of symptoms. Success is not possible unless all the factors are addressed. If we just stopped food allergens, or just gave zinc, or just treated yeast, or just stopped food additives, or just stopped trans fats, Clayton would not have gotten better.

This story is not an isolated anecdote, but a story repeated over and over in medical practices based on Functional Medicine, which is where the principles of UltraWellness and UltraMind originate.

This case (and so many others like it) suggests that priority be given to research that teases out the subtleties of how to apply this approach to our epidemic of brain and psychiatric disorders. Instead we continue to research more "traditional" models for treating these problems.

I am no longer the "accidental" psychiatrist. I know as I treat the body the brain will heal. And that's no accident.

And I want to tell you what I have learned and show you how to take advantage of this science now. I want to give you the tools you need to apply this Functional Medicine approach to your own life so you don't have to wait twenty years for medical practices and the scientific community to catch up with what we already know today.

The question that remains is how to treat these underlying causes, so you can rebalance your health and empower your brain.

What was I able to help Clayton achieve by identifying and treating the underlying factors that were driving his illness, and how did I do it? How can you use this same approach to help you overcome the "broken brain" that is so debilitating you?

A New Road Map for Treating Disease: The Seven Keys to UltraWellness

A new road map has emerged for how the human body works and how to treat illnesses—whether they are mental or physical. This road map is not based on the traditional ways of naming and diagnosing disease (or the ICD-9 disease classification system that you will learn more about in chapter 3) but on the underlying, core, interlocking, physiological systems that, in fact, underlie all disease.[18]

No one element can explain Clayton's constellation of symptoms, but his particular puzzle tells a unique story when taken as a whole. And while there may be similar patterns in other children with ADHD, his pattern is unique to him. Another child with ADHD might have different imbalances and require different diagnostic tests and therapies.

My medical school training gave me the ability to diagnose thousands of different separate diseases. Diseases that I suggest don't really exist in the way we think they do. We give names to disease like depression or ADHD, but that just helps us group people together who have the same symptoms for the purposes of giving them all the same drug therapy. But what if I were to tell you that new scientific discoveries tell us that there is no such thing as depression?

What we see as the symptoms of depression are reflections of a few common interconnected imbalances in the body that have nothing to do with the medical specialties as we know them. Depression is not a psychiatric illness, but a systemic disease. To treat it we need to address the whole system—the ecosystem of your body.

That means we need to understand how the *whole* body operates as a system, not just how different pieces of the body operate independently from one another. We need to treat people, not body parts; we want to treat the causes of disease, not symptoms.

I was trained according to the dogma of separate medical specialties—for heart problems you see the cardiologist, for stomach problems you see the gastroenterologist, for joint pain you see the rheumatologist, for skin problems, the dermatologist. You just don't ask the skin doctor about your joint pain. If you do ask, he or she will cut you off and tell you to see the joint doctor.

The road map I was given in medical school to navigate through the territory of illness was the *wrong* map. It taught us to diagnose disease and then assign standardized treatments no matter who was suffering. This is the wrong approach. It's a map that sends us in the wrong direction.

Not only are your joint pains, skin rash, irritable bowel, and depression all connected, but the *only* way to find your way out of this mess of chronic disease (which affects 162 million people) is by using a new map—one that allows us to see how everything is connected.

This is what the rich new method called Functional Medicine offers. Functional Medicine (www.functionalmedicine.org) applies the science of systems biology in a practical setting. It *is* the revolutionary new system I have been talking about. It's a fundamental change in our thinking, a whole different paradigm, like the world-is-round-not-flat shift. It changes our approach to the very way we think about illness and the human body.

With it, we can truly treat and cure disease.

Unlike conventional medicine, Functional Medicine personalizes treatment based on a patient's unique needs. We are all different. We have a different genetic makeup. As a result our bodies react to our environment in different ways. Understanding this allows us to develop unique methods to treat *people*, not diseases.

At the heart of this paradigm shift are the seven keys of UltraWellness, the same keys that make up the UltraMind Solution.

All medicine can be simplied into a few basic principles and concepts or natural laws that explain all disease and suffering. These concepts are the seven keys or core systems of the body.

In Part II I will explore how each of these keys affects your mood, behavior, attention, memory, and overall brain function, and supply quizzes that will help you identify which of these keys is out of balance for you so you can optimize and heal your brain.

This will give you a personalized road map for your journey back to health and wellness. It will help you heal from your broken brain and from a host of other symptoms you may be suffering with.

I would like to give you an introduction to the keys now, as they are critical for understanding how the whole program works. As you read this, keep in mind that these keys are not really separate but interconnect and interact in a dynamic, fluid web.

THE SEVEN KEYS: STAYING IN BALANCE

KEY #1: OPTIMIZE NUTRITION

We are made of the stuff we eat. Our biology, biochemistry, and physiology need certain raw materials to run optimally—the right balance and quality of protein, fats, carbohydrates, the right vitamins and minerals in the correct dose for each of us and all the colorful pigments in plant foods, called phytonutrients, that support our well-being and function. Nearly all of us are nutritionally imbalanced in one way or another.

KEY #2: BALANCE YOUR HORMONES

Our hormones, including insulin, thyroid, sex hormones, stress hormones, and many more, are a symphony of molecules. They have to work in harmony for you to be healthy.

KEY #3: COOL OFF INFLAMMATION

We must protect and defend ourselves from foreign invaders or abnormal cells inside our own body. When this is over- or underactive, illness occurs. Inflammation of the brain is a central theme for almost all psychiatric and neurologic conditions, as well as most chronic disease. If you have a broken brain it is almost certainly inflamed.

(continued)

KEY #4: FIX YOUR DIGESTION

Digesting, absorbing, and assimilating all the food and nutrients we eat is critical for health. Our digestive systems must also protect us from internal toxins, bugs, and potential allergens, as well as eliminate wastes. Breakdown anywhere in this process creates illness.

KEY #5: ENHANCE DETOXIFICATION

Our bodies must eliminate all of our metabolic wastes and toxins, which we take in from the environment through our food, air, water, and medications. The toxic burden in the twenty-first century is overwhelming and often our bodies can't keep up. This leads to illness.

KEY #6: BOOST ENERGY METABOLISM

Life is energy. Once no more energy is produced in your cells, you die. The process of extracting energy from the food you eat and the oxygen you breathe is the most essential process of life. Keeping that metabolic engine running smoothly and protecting it from harm are essential for health. Loss of energy is found in almost all brain disorders.

KEY #7: CALM YOUR MIND

A life of meaning and purpose, a life in balance with connection, community, love, support, and a sense of empowerment, are essential for health. The overwhelming stresses of the twenty-first century, including social isolation, overwork, and disempowerment, create enormous strain on our nervous system, leading to burnout and breakdown.

By treating imbalances in these seven keys we now have a way to cure, stop, slow, and reverse this looming epidemic of "brain" disorders (as well as virtually all the diseases we see in the twenty-first century).

But what creates these imbalances?

Are these seven key systems out of balance because of poor diet, allergens, infections, stress, and toxins?

Or are they out of balance because they are missing the essential raw materials for life and health—whole, real food rich in phytonutrients and fiber, vitamins and minerals, oxygen, clean water and air, light, sleep, exercise, deep relaxation, love, connection and community, meaning, and purpose?

More to the point, I want to know how these factors influence a person's unique genome and their gene expression, creating their unique set of problems. You see, your genes are not fixed but capable of dynamically responding to information or instructions that come from your diet, lifestyle, and environment. The "information" you send your genes determines whether you stay well or get sick, and just how well you function day to day.

This is the study of *nutrigenomics* (the science of how food affects your genes), and it is the other critical piece of this new road map for healing disease outlined in *The UltraMind Solution*.

A New Approach to Understanding Food: Nutrigenomics

The most powerful tool you have to change your brain and your health is your fork.

Why?

Food is not just calories or energy. Food contains information that talks to your genes, turning them on or off and affecting their function moment to moment.

Food is the fastest-acting and most powerful medicine you can take to change your life.

This discovery is called *"nutrigenomics."*

Think of your genes as the software that runs everything in your body. Just like your computer software, it only does what you instruct it to do with the stroke of your keyboard.

The foods you eat are the keystrokes that send messages to your genes telling them what to do—creating health or disease.

Imagine what messages you are sending with a double cheeseburger, large fries, and a forty-eight-ounce cola. Consider what messages you might send instead with deep red wild salmon, braised greens, and brown rice.

The science of nutrigenomics allows us to personalize medicine—not everyone with the same problems needs the same prescription. Your individual genetic makeup determines what you need to be optimally healthy.

You have only about thirty thousand genes. But you have more than 3 million little variations in those genes called SNPs (single nucleotide polymorphisms). Those variations make up who you are. And they make your individual needs slightly different from my individual needs. We all have different needs for food, vitamins, rest, exercise, stress tolerance, or ability to handle toxins.

This book is a map to help you personalize your road to UltraWellness based on your strengths and vulnerabilities—your individual needs.

By analyzing where you are out of balance in the seven keys to Ultra-Wellness and then applying the science of nutrigenomics to help reestablish balance, we can create treatments matched to each person's individual needs.

That is what you will learn how to do in this book.

Using this method, I now approach each encounter with a patient from a general framework that is completely different from the one I learned in medical school. I create a treatment plan that is not reproducible for a group of people with the same symptoms, but is, of necessity, created anew for each patient.

What I do is actually quite simple.

The first step is to *take out the bad stuff* (the things that create imbalance, such as a nutrient-poor, processed diet; toxins; allergens; infections; and stress); remove what's bugging you. If you have ten tacks in your foot, you can't take out one, pop an aspirin, and hope to feel better. You need to find and take out all the tacks; taking out just one of them won't make you better.

The second step is to *add the good stuff* (high-quality whole foods, nutrients, water, oxygen, light, movement, sleep, relaxation, community, connection, love, meaning, and purpose), and the body's natural intelligence and healing system will take care of the rest. This is the foundation of *The UltraMind Solution*.

That's all there is to it. Using this simple, yet comprehensive, method allows me to treat virtually *all* diseases, whether they are "in the brain" or "in the body." And it works for one simple reason: the body and the brain are one system.

Unfortunately, common myths founded in classical psychiatry and neurology and promoted for decades by society have blinded us to the simple but profound truth Functional Medicine has unveiled.

And we must understand these myths before we can be free of them.

CHAPTER 3

THE MYTHS OF PSYCHIATRY AND NEUROLOGY

. . . scientists cannot see the way they see with their way of seeing.[1]

—R. D. LAING

We are so used to looking at things in a certain way that we cannot see a different way of looking at the brain, behavior, and mood. As we begin to discover the nature of how the brain works and how its function is intimately connected to the rest of the core systems in the body, the medical myths that we have labored under, and that have blocked us from truly seeing the origins of problems with our mood, memory, attention, and brain health, are falling away.

Let's review these myths and put them to rest.

The Myth of Diagnosis: If You Know the Name of Your Disease, You Know What's Wrong with You

This myth is pervasive throughout medicine not just in psychiatry and neurology, and it is *the* single biggest obstacle to changing the way we do things and finding the answers to our health problems.

The problem is simply this—we are in the naming and blaming game in medicine. It is what we were trained to do. Find the name of the "disease," then match the drug to the disease. You have "depression," so you need an "antidepressant." You are "anxious," so you need an "antianxiety" medication. You have bipolar disease or mood swings, so you need a "mood stabilizer."

Unfortunately, this approach or method of thinking is outdated, increasingly useless, and often dangerous. In some ways it's even tyrannical. Once you have a label, you are put in the group of people who have the same label, and it is assumed you carry the attributes of this group.

For example, a group of psychologists, psychiatrists, and lawyers headed by Dr. David Rosenhan, a Stanford University professor of law and psychology, pretended to be hearing voices and got themselves admitted to psychiatric hospitals across the country.[2]

Once they were admitted to the hospitals, they resumed acting normally. The hospital staff and physicians then viewed all their "normal behavior," such as note taking, as "abnormal." It was only the regular "crazy" patients who could tell them apart!

The same thing happens to you once we assign *you* a label like depression, schizophrenia, ADHD, or dementia. We throw you in the same group with everyone else who has that diagnosis and assume you all have the same problem, even if evidence is found to the contrary.

But these labels or diagnoses are just *names* we associate with a collection of symptoms. This name has *nothing* to do with *why* you have those symptoms—with the root causes of the "disease."

Here's another example. When you go see a psychiatrist or psychologist, you are given the label "depression" if you meet the criteria agreed upon by the psychiatric community and outlined in the classic manual of the American Psychiatric Association, the *Diagnostic and Statistical Manual of Mental Disorders IV (DSM-IV)*.

Here is the list of features for depression from the *DSM-IV*:

❖ Depressed mood most of the day, nearly every day, as indicated by either subjective report (e.g., feels sad or empty) or observation made by others (e.g., appears tearful). (In children and adolescents, this may be characterized as an irritable mood.)

❖ Markedly diminished interest or pleasure in all, or almost all, activities most of the day, nearly every day.

❖ Significant weight loss when not dieting or weight gain (e.g., a change of more than five pounds of body weight in a month), or decrease or increase in appetite nearly every day.

❖ Insomnia or hypersomnia (sleeping too much) nearly every day.

❖ Psychomotor agitation or retardation nearly every day.

❖ Fatigue or loss of energy nearly every day.

❖ Feelings of worthlessness or excessive or inappropriate guilt nearly every day.

❖ Diminished ability to think or concentrate, or indecisiveness, nearly every day.

❖ Recurrent thoughts of death (not just fear of dying), recurrent suicidal ideation without a specific plan, or a suicide attempt, or a specific plan for committing suicide.

There are even subtypes of depression such as mild, moderate, and severe, with and without psychotic features, chronic, catatonic, melancholic, atypical, and more outlined in a similar manner.

And there are literally thousands of different distinctions like these made for the major "mental diseases" cataloged in the *DSM-IV*. They include disorders of childhood, delirium, dementia, or cognitive disorders, substance abuse disorders, schizophrenia and other psychotic disorders, mood disorders, anxiety disorders, personality disorders, eating disorders, and sleep disorders.

But this description of depression (and of all the other mental disorders in the *DSM-IV*) is *only* of the symptoms we observe. These descriptions tell us nothing at all about *why* those symptoms occur, or how people with *exactly* the same symptoms may have them for many different underlying reasons and need different and individualized treatment as a result.

At a recent dinner for Research! America (an advocacy group for research and dissemination of research) in Washington, D.C., I sat with the surgeon general and the director of the National Institutes of Mental Health, Thomas Insel, M.D. The discussion around the dinner table focused on the limitations of our current approach of breaking down the body into its component parts to understand how things work.

I asked Dr. Insel what he thought of the *DSM-IV.* He said that it has 100 percent accuracy, but 0 percent validity—that it provides a perfect way to describe symptoms, but has nothing to tell us about the underlying biology for what causes them.

He proposed a new model of psychiatry, called "Clinical Neuroscience," which would encompass the entire spectrum of things that affect the mind and the brain. We discussed the need for the medical establishment to move beyond its current limited model of diagnosis (both in psychiatry and the rest of medicine). It no longer reflects the science or our understanding of how the body works.

The future of medicine is personalized treatment, not "one size fits all." The outdated method of naming the disease and then assigning a drug to fix it clearly isn't working.

Unfortunately, few in the medical industry today seem to understand this. The truth is that medical practice is virtually predicated on the myth of diagnosis.

I want to help you understand how serious this problem is, because it is the basis of everything I am explaining in this book. It is not trivial because it changes *everything* about how we think about disease and what to do about it.

There is a two-volume book medical professionals use called the *ICD-9* (*The International Classification of Diseases*). It is the bible of medical diagnosis. It is the system used by medical insurance companies and Medicare to decide who gets paid. Doctors have to "name" the disease they are treating based on the *ICD-9* to collect their money from these agencies!

The book contains the name of every single disease known. There are more than 12,000 diseases listed. The *ICD-9* gives the impression that all these diseases are separate and distinct.

There is only one problem. They are not.

A very few fundamental problems exist that explain nearly every disease. It doesn't matter what specialty your disease falls under. As Pierre Laplace, the eighteenth-century mathematician and astronomer, said in his *Mecanique Celeste,* a very few fundamental laws can explain an extraordinary number of very complex phenomena.[3]

These underlying problems are the link between *all* of the diseases in the *ICD-9*. In almost every one of the diseases listed in that "bible," the same few things go wrong. And those same few problems are all interconnected. One affects the other in a giant web of biology. Pull on one part of the web, and the whole web moves.

This web is built of the seven keys of UltraWellness. These keys are the underlying causes of *all* illness. And they are the keys that lead to an UltraMind.

These are the common pathways for all disease. Wherever you look, whatever problem you have, once you learn how to analyze these seven keys, you will find they are the root of all your health problems.

That's all we need.

Once we learn how to navigate health and disease using these concepts, we can throw the two-volume *ICD-9* manual in the garbage, because it is the wrong road map for the territory of illness.

This new road map turns the myth of diagnosis on its head, and in doing so reveals one of the most radical concepts that emerges from this new medical approach: the *name* of the disease bears little relationship to the *cause* of the disease.

One Disease, Many Causes—One Cause, Many Diseases

One disease can have many, many different causes, *all* of which manifest the same symptoms. Take depression, for example. It may be caused by many different factors, yet the symptoms we see are the same across the board. The

DSM-IV accurately describes these symptoms (100 percent accuracy), but it says nothing at all about the causes (0 percent validity).

Imagine a room full of people with depression. They all meet the *DSM-IV* criteria for depression, and they would all be prescribed antidepressants for their "disease."

However, neither this diagnosis nor the treatment provided takes into account their genetic individuality. It doesn't tease out the reasons each of them became depressed in the first place.

These problems arise because the real causes of depression are not addressed with antidepressants.

It may be there are many "depressions," not just one generic "depression." These "depressions" may be the result of a multitude of causes: folate, B_6, or B_{12} deficiency; low thyroid function; "brain allergies"* to foods; an autoimmune† response to gluten that inflames the brain; mercury poisoning; abnormal proteins called gluteo- or caseomorphins from poorly digested food that alter brain chemistry; brain inflammation from a hidden infection; blood-sugar imbalances; low testosterone or other sex hormones; a deficiency of omega-3 fats; or adrenal-gland dysfunction from excessive stress among many other possible causes.

These are some of the real causes of "depression" as well as many other mental illness and neurological conditions. Without addressing core, underlying issues like these, we can never have optimal brain function or mood.

There is really no such thing as the "disease" called depression, just many different systemic imbalances that cause the symptoms we collectively refer to as "depression." One disease, many causes . . .

On the other side of the spectrum, there can be one factor in a person's diet, lifestyle, environment, or genetic makeup that can cause dozens of different and seemingly unrelated "diseases."

Gluten, the protein found in the most common grain eaten in America—wheat—as well as barley, rye, oats, spelt, triticale, and kamut, is an excellent example. Gluten is one common factor that can create so many illnesses and diseases it would be hard to count them all.

The reasons are many. They include our lack of genetic adaptation to grasses, and particularly gluten in our diet. Wheat was introduced into

---

* Brain allergies are reactions to food that can take many forms, including mood disorders, attention deficit disorder, autism, insomnia, and just plain brain fog.
† Autoimmunity is an abnormal immune response to the body's own tissues. It usually occurs because of "molecular mimickry," which is where the body confuses some of its own tissue with a foreign invader. In this case, antibodies against gluten also attack your own tissue.

Europe during the Middle Ages, and 30 percent of those of European descent carry the gene for celiac disease (HLA DQ2 or HLA DQ8),[4] which increases susceptibility to health problems from eating gluten. Keep in mind that American strains of wheat have a much higher gluten content (which is needed to make light fluffy Wonder Bread).

A recent review paper in *The New England Journal of Medicine* listed fifty-five "diseases" that can be caused by eating gluten.[5] These include many neurological and psychiatric diseases such as anxiety, depression, schizophrenia, dementia, migraines, epilepsy, and neuropathy (nerve damage).[6] Gluten has also been linked to autism.[7]

Besides making the brain inflamed, gluten can be broken down in the gut into odd little proteins that are almost like psychedelic drugs (opium-like peptides called gluteomorphins). These change brain function and behavior.

Gluten also contains significant amounts of *glutamate,* a molecule that accelerates, activates, excites, and damages brain cells through a special brain receptor or docking station called the NMDA (N-methyl-D-aspartate) receptor. Overactivation of this receptor by glutamate is implicated in many psychiatric disorders.[8] Glutamate is called an excitotoxin (a substance which overexcites and kills or damages brain cells).

Gluten can cause brain dysfunction by three different mechanisms—inflammation, odd morphine or psychedelic proteins, and as an excitotoxin.[9]

So gluten, we see, can be the single cause behind many different "diseases." These diseases are not treatable with better medication, but simply by 100 percent elimination of gluten from the diet. One cause, many diseases . . .

One disease caused by multiple factors, one factor that causes multiple diseases? How could this happen? It completely upsets our current thinking. And it should!

But the reason this is true is simpler than you might think.

We are all unique, biochemically and genetically, and have different responses to the same insults. In one person gluten may cause arthritis, in another it can cause depression. Depression may be caused by gluten in one person; in another it may be caused by B_{12} deficiency.

The beauty of Functional Medicine, the seven keys to UltraWellness, and the science of nutrigenomics is that they take these factors into account to help create health for each individual.

Medicine has been looking for answers in the wrong place. Finally, science has provided a gateway to a different way of thinking about mental illness and brain disorders. We need to get out of the name-it, blame-it, and tame-it game—the myth of diagnosis—and start thinking about how the body works, how to personalize our approach, and how not to suppress symptoms but to restore normal function.

The UltraMind Solution leverages all of these new methods of understanding health and illness to help you sort through the real causes of your broken brain and get to the root of the problem, not just stay stuck with the name of your disease and the limited options available for treating it in this outdated paradigm.

The Myth of Medication: Drugs Are the Answer to Mental Illness

I want to let you in on a little secret . . .

Depression is *not* a Prozac deficiency.

The real problem with conventional medical training is that doctors are not trained to be healers, but to be pharmacologists (except for surgeons). This problem is a direct consequence of the myth of diagnosis. We are trained to name the disease, and then assign a medication to treat it.

But if the causes of a disease can be radically different in a given group of people, why should we believe that a "one-size-fits-all" prescription of medications would work to treat those underlying causes of the disease?

Medications can be lifesaving, and are incredibly useful if given in the right dose, for the right person, at the right time, for the right reason. But the problem in medical practice today is that our *only* tools are medications. The old adage, "If all you have is a hammer, everything looks like a nail," applies to medicine today.

The best or right treatment for any particular condition may be ignored, because all we have studied and used are medications.

If you are sleep-deprived you can increase alertness and energy with a stimulant medication, but the "right" treatment is sleep. If you are depressed because your intestine is inflamed and you are not absorbing vitamin B_{12}, Prozac may help you feel a little better, but the treatment is fixing your gut and replacing B_{12}.

This all seems obvious enough, and in fact is common sense, but it is *so* far away from how doctors are trained and how we currently practice medicine.

Our goal in medicine should be to find the right "medicine" for each person, without prejudice, whether it is a drug, a nutrient, diet change, detoxification, a hormone, exercise, or exorcism! We must embrace whatever works, and inquire into its effectiveness with all our scientific, economic, and political resources.

Let's take a look at the main categories of medicine for the brain: antidepressants (such as Prozac), stimulants (such as Ritalin), and tranquilizers (such as Valium and major tranquilizers such as Risperdal). Do they work? Are they safe? What problems are associated with them? Is there a better alternative to medications like these, one that addresses the underlying causes of mental illness and brain dysfunction?

These mood-altering drugs are the fastest-growing segment of the pharmaceutical market, and as a group constitute the second-biggest class of medication in total sales and prescriptions. In children alone over the three-year period from 1997 to 2000, the use of antipsychotic medication increased by 138 percent, atypical antidepressants by 42 percent, and SSRIs (selective serotonin reuptake inhibitors—they are the most commonly prescribed antidepressants) by 18 percent.[10] The global use of ADHD medication rose 300 percent from 1993 to 2000.[11]

What's worse is that the use of untested and potentially unsafe combinations of psychotropic drug cocktails has increased 500 percent in children. The authors of the study that pointed this out warned that our prescribing practices are not in sync with our current knowledge.[12] In other words, our current research *does not* support these drug-cocktail combinations.

Concerns about overuse extend to adults as well as children. In fact, Eli Lilly, the maker of the antipsychotic drug called Zyprexa, has already paid $1.2 billion to settle thirty thousand lawsuits from people who claim that Zyprexa caused them to develop diabetes or other diseases, and is also alleged to have promoted Zyprexa for unapproved off-label use, which it denies. Drug companies cannot actively promote drugs for off-label uses, but doctors can prescribe them for such uses. (For example, Zyprexa is approved for schizophrenia but doctors also prescribe it for anxiety.)

Do we really need medications to keep us from being sad, hyper, anxious, or psychotic?

Today modern psychopharmacologists dispense drugs like candy despite their limited effectiveness. Often these drugs are administered in untested cocktails and combinations, which may occasionally be helpful, but come with more side effects.

Consider the rather astonishing example of antipsychotics or major tranquilizers (including Risperdal, Zyprexa, Seroquel, and Geodon). This class of medications is one of the biggest-growing sectors in drug sales.

Antipsychotic usage has shown a 10 to 20 percent rate of increase per year over the last few years and today sales of these drugs total about $12 billion a year.

Traditionally such medications were reserved for psychosis, defined as an inability to distinguish what's real from what's imagined. Hearing voices and thinking that aliens are visiting your bedroom at night are examples of psychosis.

But now, with little hesitation or scientific evidence, antipsychotics are given to children with behavioral problems, autism, and ADHD, and to adults with depression, anxiety, obsessive-compulsive disorder, bipolar disease, dementia, and Parkinson's disease.

These drugs can lead to serious side effects. Besides acting like a chemical straitjacket and making people dull, slow, and stupid, they increase the risk of obesity, diabetes, stroke, blood clots, and more serious conditions known as neuroleptic malignant syndrome (where your body literally burns up with fever and your muscles are destroyed) and tardive dyskinesia (uncontrolled repetitive, involuntary, and purposeless movements such as lip smacking, rapid eye blinking, grimacing, and spasms in the legs).

Have we suddenly all gone crazy?

What most consumers don't understand is that drug testing is often very limited before drug approval. New drugs are tested on a few hundred to a few thousand people often for a very limited time (usually a few weeks to a few months). Then they are released on the market, supported by more than $30 billion in pharmaceutical advertising dollars (or about $25,000 a year for each one of the 737,000 physicians in America).

Once approved, these drugs can be prescribed for *any* use.

We in the medical industry call these "off-label uses."

For example, the drug may be approved *only* for use in schizophrenia (as in the examples of antipsychotics above). But doctors can prescribe it for anyone they like—from someone who is overly anxious to someone with obsessive-compulsive disorder to a child whose behavior is out of control.

Once the drug is approved, there is no official tracking of its risks or benefits to the millions who are prescribed the drug. It's left up to patients or doctors to self-report problems.

This leaves the public very vulnerable. Doctors are using the only tools they know how to use, but that's the way they get into trouble.

Unfortunately, it appears that drug companies often see any backlash or lawsuits as simply part of their "research and development" expenses of their drugs.

Bloomberg News reported in December 2006:

Nationwide, several lawsuits accuse drug companies of engaging in deceptive marketing by overstating the effectiveness and understating the risks of newer anti-psychotics. The suits also claim companies promoted the drugs for unapproved uses. Mississippi, Louisiana, Alaska and West Virginia sued Eli Lilly & Co. this year on behalf of their Medicaid health programs for the poor. They said the company fraudulently touted the antipsychotic Zyprexa for unapproved uses. Indianapolis-based Lilly settled about eight thousand personal-injury complaints for $700 million in 2005 and faces four thousand more claims.

We are a drug-addicted society, and we are overprescribed medication when there are better solutions. According to *The Journal of the American Medical Association,* in an average week 81 percent of Americans use at least one medication, 50 percent take at least one prescription drug, and 7 percent take five or more drugs. Of those over sixty-five years old, 12 percent take at least ten medications and 23 percent take at least five medications.[13]

This bias toward medication sadly distracts us from finding the real or best answers to our ailments.

Unfortunately, the billions of dollars that pour into the pharmaceutical industry every year are not spent researching or promoting changes in diet, nutrient therapies, detoxification, addressing food allergies, and other potentially beneficial treatments. Instead, our economy thrives on products and services that make us sick or benefit from our illness (drugs, processed foods, fast foods, and companies that thrive by adding to our environmental toxic load).

Who knows where we would be if such research were being done.

The next frontier in medicine, psychiatry, and neurology is realizing that depression is not a Prozac deficiency, ADHD is not a Ritalin deficiency, and schizophrenia is not a Zyprexa deficiency.

We have the tools and knowledge now to make an enormous difference in this epidemic of mental and brain disorders by looking deeper and thinking differently.

Getting off medications can be difficult, comes with certain risks, and must be done under a physician's supervision. I don't recommend anyone stop using their medications suddenly, but I do suggest that by following the plan to optimize your brain function and address the underlying causes of mood disorders and brain dysfunction in *The Ultra-*

Mind Solution, many people can get off their medications with their physician's help and feel better and healthier than ever.

Fix your body and you will fix your brain.

The Myth of Psychotherapy: You Can Talk or Meditate Away Your Mood and Brain Problems

---

We must all learn to deal with the infestation of ANTS in our brains if we want to be happy. The ANTS are "automatic negative thoughts," or our beliefs, attitudes, and ways of thinking and being that move us away from well-being. Counseling, therapy, coaching, cognitive behavioral therapy, and even psychoanalysis can be essential components of an overall plan for mental health.

But if you are mercury poisoned, or deficient in folic acid, or have low-thyroid function, or drink twelve cups of coffee a day, or eat half a pound of sugar a day (the amount consumed by the average American), or have an inflamed brain from eating gluten, it is very difficult to talk or meditate your way out of your suffering.

I believe you must address the biological causes of the problems *first* before psychotherapy can be effective. Fix your biology. Then get psychotherapy and do your soul work.

Addressing the underlying imbalances in your body that cause brain dysfunction will allow you to venture more deeply and successfully into the exploration of your mind and your soul.

We all want to fully wake up, be happy, and completely feel the joys and pleasures of love, work, and play that give life its meaning and purpose.

But we can achieve that only by working on both our biology and our biography!

We can use the best of psychoemotional and behavioral therapies, but we *must* optimize brain function through improving nutrition; stabilizing immune function, hormone, and neurotransmitter balance; enhancing detoxification; normalizing digestive function; and boosting the energy in our cells.

The Brain-Body Separation Myth: Your Brain Is Protected from Your Body

---

The idea that the brain and the body are separated is a solid, well-established belief. All doctors are trained in the absolute nature of the blood–brain barrier—a wall of tightly packed cells lining the smallest blood vessels of the brain, called capillaries, and a back-up defensive team of astrocytes (star-shaped cells of the glia) that holds this tightly packed wall together.

This barrier is designed to keep out toxic influences and infections, but let metabolically necessary ingredients like sugars, fatty acids, and amino acids through.

Because we know this barrier exists, we believe that what happens in the brain stays in the brain and what happens in the body stays in the body. Like an iron curtain, that barrier is never breached.

There is only one problem with this theory.

The blood–brain barrier is really just a partial barrier.

We now know the brain can become leaky and the barrier permeable under many conditions—poor nutrition, stress, infection, digestive imbalances, toxic injury, and allergy. The brain, in fact, reads what is happening in the rest of the body even under normal conditions of life.

What you do to your body you do to your brain.

Let's take a brief look at childhood autism and Alzheimer's to illustrate the frailty of the myth that the brain is walled off from the body.

Autism: A Body Disorder That Affects the Brain

Dr. Martha Herbert is an assistant professor of neurology at Harvard Medical School and the director of TRANSCEND (Treatment, Research, and Neuroscience Evaluation of Neurodevelopmental Disorders). Her work in autism is paradigm-shifting scientific research and thinking.

Rather than ignoring the almost universal *physical* complaints found in autistic children, most of which have been described in the scientific literature since the 1940s, she explains how they could be at the root of the brain and behavioral symptoms found in autistic children.

In her groundbreaking article in *Clinical Neuropsychiatry* entitled "Autism: A brain disorder, or a disorder that affects the brain?"[14] she explains how the incoherent brain connections found in children with autism, which show up as the inability to talk, connect with other people, or produce odd repetitive behaviors, have their root *not* in the brain but in problems with the digestive system and the immune system.

These breakdowns in the body, which lead to behavioral problems, occur because of genetic susceptibilities, which are amplified by environmental stresses and toxins.

Why, she asks, do 95 to 100 percent of autistic children have gastrointestinal dysfunction, or 70 percent of them have immune system abnormalities? After examining all the accumulated research on autism, including her own work on brain imaging and the structure and function of the brain in autistic children, she concludes that autism is *not* a brain disorder, but a *systemic* disorder that affects the brain.

In fact, she challenges the idea that there is only one kind of autism. She says there may be many "autisms," because each child has unique genetic and environmental factors that can lead to the same symptoms and behaviors. (This goes back to the myth of the diagnosis—having the name of the problem doesn't tell you about the cause or causes.)

Dr. Herbert noticed that brains of autistic children are bigger, swollen perhaps. These swollen brains are filled with activated immune cells and inflammatory molecules.[15] Where is this inflammation coming from?

It starts outside the brain.

She describes autism as a "metabolic encephalopathy." In nonmedical language that means that all the information and noise from outside the brain—from the gut, from the immune system, and from toxins—are causing the brain to malfunction.

This is a 180-degree turn from conventional thinking. If an altered response to a microbe or bug in the body by the immune system can affect brain function, or if a molecule made in the gut can change behavior or perception, then of course the brain is in communication with the rest of the body.

With autism we see clearly the effects of systemic imbalances in the body on the brain and mind. And what holds true of autism holds true of brain disorders like depression, Alzheimer's, and a host of others as well.

A Sweet Brain: Slow as Molasses

Also out of Harvard is the work of pioneering neurologist Dennis Selkoe,[16] who has linked sugar and its ability to create insulin resistance, metabolic syndrome (or prediabetes), and diabetes to Alzheimer's disease.

In fact, some researchers are calling Alzheimer's "type 3" diabetes. People with type 2 diabetes have four times the risk of getting Alzheimer's compared to those without diabetes.

We will explore this connection between diabetes and Alzheimer's a little later in Part II when I discuss hormonal imbalances, but the take-home message here is that our diet, the sugar and processed food we eat, has a clear effect on our brain.

If your brain was walled off from the rest of your body, then how could this happen? The answer is that your brain is not walled off, and is in fact intimately connected to everything else going on in your body.

We know that even people with prediabetes have a higher risk of cognitive decline, poor memory, and loss of brain function.[17] So when you have that soda, some imaginary barrier does not protect your brain.

How could we really believe that our brains could tolerate half a pound of sugar a day on average and be healthy?

There are *many* other examples of how great an influence the body (and what you put in your body) can have on your brain, some more of which you will learn about over the course of this book. But here is the bottom line . . .

All broken brains have their root in the body. They are not localized to that three pounds of custardlike gray stuff between your ears!

The body and brain interact as one system. Don't be deceived. The barrier between them is no iron curtain. It is more like cheesecloth.

The Brain Cell Myth:
Once You Lose Brain Cells, They Are Gone Forever

We all learned that once you lose brain cells, that's it, they're gone forever. We thought too many nights partying in college, or long-term stress or trauma, which injure the brain, were irreparable. And *clearly* brain damage and loss of brain activity from stroke or even cerebral palsy cannot be recovered.

Or so we thought . . .

Some of the most exciting research on the brain in the last decade has clearly shown that the brain can heal, renew, repair, and regenerate itself. You *can* make new brain cells (neurogenesis), you can wake up and activate damaged brain cells, and you can improve connections between brain cells (neuroplasticity), all of which lead to improved cognitive function and remarkable recoveries.

This discovery has now been replicated over and over. It is a whole new field of scientific inquiry called "neurogenesis," or the creation of new brain cells.[18]

We have long known of the brain's ability to stretch. It is what we call plasticity. You can train areas of your brain to take over lost function and make enormous accommodations even under very extreme circumstances.

I know a little girl who was born with half a brain, and though she has some small motor problems and a few little quirks, if you met her you would never know she only had one half of her brain.

But brain regeneration and renewal go far beyond that. The implications for reversing dementia and affecting mood disorders are staggering.

If it's true that you can grow new brain cells, the question really becomes: how do we accelerate and facilitate the process of neurogenesis? How do we help our brains heal and grow?

The key areas that regenerate are the hippocampus, a walnut-sized area of the brain that controls much of our mood and memory, and the olfactory (smell) center of the brain. We now know that hormones, growth factors (fertilizer for brain cells), new learning, neurotransmitters (brain messenger chemicals), and physical exercise can promote new brain cell formation.

We also know that stress, drugs, toxins, and anything that causes inflammation can damage the hippocampus, kill brain cells, and reduce neurogenesis.

The key to optimal brain health is doing more of the things that help generate new brain cells and less of the things that kill brain cells.

For example, we know that the stress hormone cortisol injures the hippocampus, damages brain cells, and leads to memory loss and dementia. Conversely, we know that reducing cortisol levels with relaxation increases the size of the hippocampus through neurogenesis.

So the next time you get stressed out, think about how you are killing your brain cells and take a deep breath instead.

Remember, there is hope to rebuild your brain and reverse conditions we thought permanent, such as autism and dementia, as well as depression and other mood disorders. You just need to know how to do it.

The first step is understanding that the myths outlined in this chapter are just that—myths. If you are suffering from a "mental illness" like depression, anxiety, or bipolar disorder, a "brain disorder" like Alzheimer's disease, or simply suffer from a bad mood, there are underlying root causes that are putting your system out of balance and creating these conditions.

Just because you got labeled or diagnosed with a disease does not mean you know what's wrong with you. You probably don't need more and better medications to overcome your "illness." Psychotherapy may help, but on its own it's unlikely to be as effective.

Fix your body and you will fix your broken brain and boost your brain power. The body-and-brain are *not* walled off from each other. What you put in your body affects your brain. In fact, it may mean the difference between growing new brain cells and living with the same old diminished brain you are living with right now.

The second step is taking the "tacks" out of your brain—eliminating environmental and dietary factors that have been proven to cause your "broken brain."

These are the *real* causes of your mood, memory, and cognition problems, and it is only by eliminating or reducing them that you will rebalance your body and restore your brain function.

CHAPTER 4

WHY YOU ARE SUFFERING FROM BRAIN DAMAGE

Learning How to Protect Your Brain

A new scientific truth does not triumph by convincing its opponents and making them see the light, but rather because its opponents eventually die, and a new generation grows up that is familiar with it.

—MAX PLANCK

Our brains are the most sensitive organs in our bodies, and they respond immediately and almost instantly to insults.

So stop insulting your brain.

Most of us have no clue that sitting around on our couch watching TV hurts our brain. So does losing a few hours of sleep at night, drinking a can of cola, having that Starbucks grande latte, getting the flu vaccine, having those two glasses of chardonnay, taking a few Rolaids for heartburn, eating strawberries grown on a conventional farm, having a fight with our spouse, and talking on our cell phones for a few hours a day.

Save your brain. Learn what harms and what enhances it. Understand why you are brain damaged and how to prevent—even reverse—it. The data is in. We know what the harmful influences are on brain function. We know how these influences alter our mood; promote depression, anxiety, ADHD, autism, dementia, Parkinson's; and more.

I will review all of these insults in detail in Part II. There I will show you how different environmental influences, dietary factors, and other toxins can influence and create imbalances in each of the seven key systems in your body, and, as a result, affect your brain and your overall health.

For now, I want to summarize the big picture so you can begin to understand the environmental and dietary influences that affect your brain, how your brain is getting damaged, and how you can protect and care for it in the future.

Toxic Foods

There are two toxic foods that everyone should eliminate from their diet today, *immediately*. In fact, go right now to your cupboard and throw out everything with these two ingredients because they damage your brain (and the rest of your body as well). But be prepared. There may be nothing left in your cupboard.

High-Fructose Corn Syrup
(and Any Form of Sugar or Refined Carbohydrate)

High-fructose corn syrup (HFCS) is an insidious chemical that has crept into our food supply in recent years. Though it was completely unknown until 1980, we now make 17.5 billion pounds of it and consume sixty-six pounds per person every year.

This is a potent form of sugar that is sweeter than regular sugar, increases appetite,[1] promotes obesity more than regular sugar,[2] and is more addictive than cocaine.[3] It also leads to diabetes and an inflamed brain.

It is now the main form of sweetener in all processed and junk foods from cola to energy snack bars, from yogurt to turkey slices, from bread to salad dressing, and even ketchup.

In case an inflamed brain and an addicition stronger than cocaine doesn't convince you, here are a few other reasons HFCS (and other forms of sugar) is harmful to the brain:

- ❖ Sugar uses up your body's store of vitamins and minerals without providing any in return.
- ❖ High sugar consumption is tied to so many mental disorders it's hard to list them all. They include lower IQ, anxiety, aggressive behavior, hyperactivity, depression, eating disorders, fatigue, learning difficulties, and premenstrual syndrome.[4]
- ❖ Sugar causes crusting in your brain. Think about that sugary crust on crème brûlée or a crusty bread or crispy chicken skin. Sugar in these foods (and in your body) reacts with proteins and forms little crusts or plaques called AGEs (advanced glycation end products). These crusty sugar-protein combos gum up your brain, leading to dementia, and damage most cells and tissues along the way.

So get off the sugar and save your brain.

Trans or Hydrogenated Fats[5]

Trans fats come from processed foods, baked goods, most fried foods, margarine, and virtually any product that comes from a factory. They damage cells, increase inflammation, and interrupt normal brain function in everyone from children with ADHD to adults with depression or dementia.[6]

By eliminating these two foreign, man-made, mood- and mind-altering toxic substances from your diet, you radically transform your health overnight. In fact, if you put down this book right now and do nothing else, you will have made a major impact on your health.

Protect Your Head

Brain trauma, even a slight concussion, can have long-term consequences for your brain. Not only can it affect your ability to learn, focus, and concentrate, but it can increase your risk of dementia and Parkinson's disease.

If you have a gene called apo E4, found in about 25 percent of the population, you are 2.5 to 5 times more likely to get Alzheimer's. And if you have a history of head trauma and have that gene, your risk of getting the disease increases tenfold.

So protect your brain. Protect your kids' brains. Avoid contact sports like football and heading the ball in soccer. Wear helmets for any high-risk sport such as biking, roller blading, skateboarding, snowboarding, or even skiing.

Your Brain Loves Sleep

We live in a sleep-deprived world. A hundred years ago we slept eight to nine hours a night, now we average six or seven hours a night. According to a report done by the National Institute of Medicine on sleep, 50 to 70 million Americans are regularly deprived of sleep or suffer from sleep problems. This may be good for Starbucks' bottom line, but not for your brain.

Sleep is when your body repairs and heals. Extreme sleep deprivation leads to psychosis, as demonstrated in military recruits. Moderate- and long-term sleep deprivation leads to depression, attention deficit disorder, problems with learning and memory, not to mention 100,000 car accidents a year—especially by teenagers.

Lack of sleep has even been linked to Alzheimer's disease.

If that doesn't get you to sleep more, then you should know that sleep deprivation makes you gain weight by increasing the hormone grehlin, which increases hunger, and lowering your appetite-suppressing hormones (known as PYY). You eat more to compensate for lack of sleep and you crave more sugars and refined carbohydrates as a result.

Sleep deprivation also increases stress hormones such as cortisol, which kills brain cells in the memory and mood center called the hippocampus.

Sleep is not a nuisance or a luxury. It is part of regular maintenance and repair. Getting enough sleep can mean the difference between a tired, foggy, unfocused, forgetful brain and one that is attentive, sharp, and fully tuned into the world around you.

Sedentary Lifestyle

If you are a couch potato or one of those people who, when they feel like exercising, lie down until the feeling goes away, then consider this: when you don't exercise you have lower levels of IGF-1,[7] an indicator of growth hormone (the repair and youth hormone) and lower levels of BDNF (brain-derived neurotropic factor), which is like super fertilizer for your brain. These chemicals are the brain's way to make new brain cells (neurogenesis) and improve connections between existing brain cells (neuroplasticity).

Running, lifting, or just dancing around releases more IGF-1, which goes into your brain and stimulates more BDNF.[8] The memory and mood center in the brain, the hippocampus, is the most sensitive to this fertilizer for the brain. That means when you exercise, you can improve the area of your brain that is most sensitive to changes in memory and mood, and when you don't, you won't.

Our bodies (and brains) were designed to thrive with exercise, not without it. Exercise has been found to improve cognitive performance, enhance memory, reverse depression, slow or stop mental decline associated with aging, and prevent dementia.

In a study by the University of Illinois of third and fifth graders, the fittest kids were also the ones with the fittest brains.

Exercise also builds new neural connections, rewiring your brain for better mood and cognitive function, making your brain run faster, smoother, and more efficiently.[9]

When you exercise you also increase levels of dopamine, which helps you focus, and serotonin, which calms you down. Exercise can give you the same neurotransmitter and mental benefits as Ritalin and Zyprexa without the risk or side effects. In fact, exercise beats or equals Prozac or psychotherapy as an antidepressant in head–to–head studies.[10]

So get moving!

Don't Stress Your Brain Out

Why don't zebras get ulcers? According to Dr. Robert Sapolsky from Stanford, they spend their days grazing in the savanna until a lion comes along, run like crazy until one gets caught, and then they all go back to grazing while the lion has his dinner.

Relax, sudden stress, relax. That's why they don't get ulcers.

They don't live in a state of chronic stress. We do. We stew in our own stress juices—namely cortisol, which kills brain cells, shrinks the brain, and leads to dementia. It also causes crippling depression and other mood disorders.[11]

Any chronic psychological or emotional stress damages your brain: a divorce, a fight with your spouse, worrying about finances, or your job. Most of us don't even know we are stressed—it's like not realizing someone is standing on your foot until the person gets off.

The good news is that relaxing is good for your brain and can increase BDNF. People who meditate regularly actually have increased brain size and cortical thickness,[12] along with better mood and cognitive function.

But drinking a beer, watching TV, or practicing retail therapy in the mall won't do the trick. You have to learn tools to actively relax such as meditation, yoga, deep breathing, hypnosis, laughter therapy, biofeedback, making love, exercise, and sleep.

All these can reduce stress hormones and burn off excess brain-damaging cortisol. Practice at least one of these activities daily. I will teach you how to do that in Part III of this book.

Toxic Drugs

The four top things purchased in American supermarkets are all mood-altering drugs. They are:

- ✧ Sugar—(see this chapter for effects)
- ✧ Caffeine—which increases anxiety and depression[13]
- ✧ Alcohol—large amounts (four glasses a day or more) can double your risk of dementia.[14; 15] Small amounts such as a few glasses a week (but *not* daily) may reduce the risk of dementia by

35 percent.[16] Alcohol also depletes mood-boosting B vitamins, is a brain toxin, and slows down brain metabolism.[17]

❖ Nicotine—constricts blood flow to the brain; cigarette smoke contains four thousand toxins[18] and leads to depression.[19]

All these drugs damage your brain. Addiction to any of them *seriously* damages it. The more often you partake of these mood-altering substances, and the longer you use them, the more damage you do. Occasional, moderate use is harmless. Regular use is a guarantee of premature brain aging and mood disorders.

Other Drugs of Abuse

Newer brain-imaging studies such as SPECT scans, which look at brain function and blood flow, clearly show the harmful effect of substance abuse.[20] Dr. Daniel Amen, who has pioneered this work, is responsible for the famous images of "your brain" and "your brain on drugs." All substances like cocaine, methamphetamines (speed), heroin, inhalants, marijuana, LSD, ecstasy, and more have adverse effects on short- and long-term brain function.

This is a SPECT scan of a normal brain.

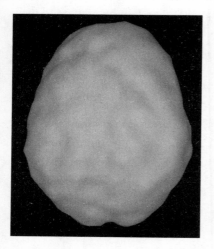

Figure 3: SPECT scan of a normal brain

This is a SPECT of a brain on methamphetamines (the same class of drugs as Ritalin).

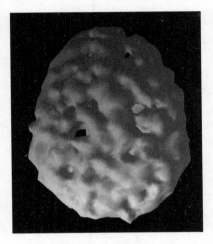

Figure 4: SPECT scan of a brain on methamphetamines

Any questions?

Medications

Eighty-one percent of Americans take at least one medication per week. Are you one of those people who pop an acid-blocking pill for indigestion, a cholesterol-lowering medication, acetaminophen for your joint pain, ibuprofen for your headaches, or a birth-control pill? Or are you getting the flu vaccine every year?

We are a pill-popping society and we believe drugs are safe and have been adequately tested for long-term effects.

Remember that most drugs go on the market after being tested for a few months on only a few hundred to a few thousand people. Long-term effects don't become apparent, except of course in the long term, after millions have been exposed.

We know that drugs have many *effects*. The ones we like, we call "drug action." The ones we don't, we call "side effects." In fact they are all "effects" of the drugs. And many of these effects damage your brain.

I have some big concerns regarding some of the most common medications. What concerns me as much as what we know now is what we don't know.

The past decade has seen a litany of products that have fallen from grace—Vioxx, Avandia, Rezulin, Seldane, Baycol, CETP inhibitors, Premarin, and more. Which drugs that millions consume today will be the fallen heroes of tomorrow?

I am certainly not against medications or their intelligent use. But they should be used carefully, with full awareness of *all* their effects whether that's "drug action" or "side effects."

Most medication is prescribed for conditions that are better treated by diet, nutritional therapies, and lifestyle changes.

Here are the top drugs on my radar that have potentially harmful effects on the brain, and deplete critical nutrients that are required for optimal brain function and health. For a complete list, I highly recommend the *Drug-Induced Nutrient Depletion Handbook*. Most doctors are worried about supplements interfering with medication. This rarely occurs. But few doctors worry about severe nutrient depletion, which can lead to long-term harm from well-known "side effects" of common medications.

> *A word of warning:* Do not stop any medication prescribed by your doctor. You should talk to him or her and learn how to treat your condition with lifestyle first. If you have to use medication, learn how to use the lowest dose and compensate for the "side effects" with the right nutrients. If you can go off medication and choose to, you should do so gradually under a doctor's supervision.

CoQ10-Lowering Medication

Coenzyme Q10 is lowered by common drugs including the cholesterol-lowering statins (Lipitor, Zocor, Pravacohl), beta-blockers (Toprol, Inderal), and antidiabetic drugs (the oral hypoglycemic drugs like Glucotrol and Micronase).

Coenzyme Q10 is made by the same enzyme in your body (HMG-CoA reductase) as cholesterol. So if you take a statin, you shut down your production of coenzyme Q10, which is necessary to make energy for your cells.[21] If you are taking these medications, seek alternatives. If you must take them, be sure to add 100 to 200 mg of coenzyme Q10 to your supplement regimen to replenish your depleted levels.

B Vitamin–Lowering Medication

The most worrisome class of medication for the brain in the long term, I believe, is the acid-blocking drugs.[22] These include Prilosec, Prevacid, Nexium, Aciphex, and Protonix.

Effects of Acid-Blocking Medication

* Prevents adequate protein digestion, which diminishes our ability to provide the amino-acid building blocks of neurotransmitters to help our mood, memory, and attention.
* Prevents mineral absorption, leading to decreased magnesium levels in the body. Magnesium deficiency is a major contributor to anxiety and mood disorders.
* Increases the risk of intestinal infections[23] and causes osteoporosis.[24]
* And most important, prevents absorption of B_{12},[25] leading to fatigue, memory loss, dementia, and depression.[26]

Other drugs that deplete B vitamins include aspirin, estrogens (including birth-control pills and steroids), diuretics or water pills, anticonvulsant drugs (seizure medication, also often used for mood disorders, such as Tegretol and Depakote), anti-inflammatory drugs like ibuprofen, and drugs for Parkinson's disease such as Sinemet.

Glutathione-Lowering Medication

There is one drug that stands above all others in quickly depleting glutathione—acetaminophen (Tylenol or Panadol). It is found in countless over-the-counter medications. People take it all the time without thinking about it. But the truth is that this drug is more toxic than most prescription drugs.

Glutathione is your body's last stand against toxins, inflammation, and free radicals. You will learn why these problems wreak havoc in your body in Part II, and how glutathione protects you against them.

For now, suffice it to say that glutathione is one of the single most important chemicals in the human body, and a deficiency in it can cause severe mental and physical health issues.

In addition to the environmental and dietary influences that deplete glutathione, half of us (and most of the people with broken brains) are missing a key gene, GSTM1, which helps the body rebuild its stores of glutathione. This only compounds the problem.

You can boost your own glutathione levels by eating foods from the broccoli and garlic families and taking a supplement called NAC (n-acetylcysteine), which helps rebuild your depleted glutathione.[27] It works to treat acetaminophen overdose in the emergency room, and prevent liver failure and death, and it will work to protect you.

And remember: acetaminophen can be dangerous, especially if consumed with alcohol. Take it only occasionally and only if you really need it.

Metal-Containing Medications

Aside from the inadvertent contamination of many calcium supplements with lead,[28] many medications have or have had metals put in on purpose! These metals can be literally poisonous to your body and brain.

For example, aluminum has been linked to a higher risk of Alzheimer's. It is found in antacids such as Gaviscon, Maalox, and Mylanta, which people swig like orange juice. It is also found in our water, cookware, foil wrap, and most underarm deodorants.

Up until recently, mercury, in the form of thimerosal, was the most common disinfectant placed in vaccines (and is still in most flu vaccines) and contact-lens fluid.

Other studies "prove" that mercury exposure from vaccines is harmless.[29] Or is it?

A recent CDC study in the *New England Journal of Medicine* appears to have been designed to show no harm. Notably:

1. They excluded all kids with autism from the study! These are the kids with the genetic susceptibilities to problems. These are the kids who *can't* detoxify. This is like doing a study to see if peanuts cause allergies, but excluding *all* kids with an allergy to peanuts from the study. It's just plain bad science.
2. They did *not* measure mercury levels in the bodies of the children—just their exposure. So if kids were good detoxifiers, of course they wouldn't have effects from the mercury. They should have measured the total body load of mercury in the children studied and *then* noted how that correlates to any neurologic or other effects. They also should have measured the genes involved

in detoxification of mercury, such as apo E4 and GSTM1. Again, this is just plain bad science.

3. The study itself and its accompanying editorial disclose, as potential conflicts of interest, that a number of the authors are either former employees or serve on an advisory board of, or were receiving grant support, lecture fees, or consulting fees from, the very manufacturers who put mercury in vaccines in the first place. That's like putting tobacco companies in charge of studies on the risks of smoking.

4. They didn't explain how it could be safe that between 1991 and 1999, little babies could have inadvertently received up to 125 times the EPA safe level of mercury as determined by the oral methyl mercury standard on any given day that multiple vaccines were given. This not only exceeded the EPA standard but also the FDA, Agency for Toxic Substances and Disease Registry, and World Health Organization safety standards.

This kind of unscientific "research" is the problem that keeps the medical industry (not to mention our economy) connected to practices that clearly don't promote health and well-being.

If thimerosal is as safe as studies like this attempt to suggest, why was it removed from use after fifty years from most childhood and adult vaccines in 2001 (except, of course, the ones we export to the third world)? You can find out which vaccines contain mercury by going to www.fda.gov/cber/vaccine/thimerosal.htm.

Mercury isn't safe. It's the second-most toxic subtance known to human biology on the planet. The only chemical worse is plutonium.

Yet mercury is everywhere in our society. Here are a few examples:

- ⁘ A mercury-containing powder called calomel was given to babies for teething pains in the 1940s and caused pink disease (a syndrome that included cognitive and psychiatric disorders that mimicked autism). Incidentally, calomel has been used since the early days of American history as a remedy for many diseases. It is what led to President Andrew Jackson's insanity.[30]

- ⁘ Most of us used a topical disinfectant called Mercurochrome (which was silently banned by the FDA in 1998 because it was no longer considered safe due to its mercury content) for all our wounds when we were young.

- ⁘ Mercury fillings or "silver" amalgams are still used in dentistry (except in most European countries, where they are banned, and

in Canada, where use is highly discouraged). Though highly controversial, the American Dental Association continues to support
their safety and use.

If mercury in fillings is stable and does not influence human health, why
do autopsy studies show the level of mercury in tissues (especially the brain)
directly correlates to the number of fillings in the mouth?[31] And why are
dental fillings considered toxic waste (whose disposal the EPA regulates)
when removed from your body (www.epa.gov/mercury/healthcare.htm)?
Why are they banned or restricted in Canada, Germany, and Sweden? And
why do studies show that the mercury migrates right through the teeth into
the bloodstream?[32]

Let me reiterate this: *mercury is the second-most toxic substance known to
human biology after plutonium.*

Do not underestimate what ingesting this poison, from medications, dental "silver" fillings, large marine fish like tuna or shark, or even environmental exposure can do to your body. Twenty-five percent of New Yorkers have
toxic blood levels of mercury from eating too much sushi and 15 percent of
American women of childbearing age have toxic levels of mercury in their
blood.[33] That means that 15 percent of the 4 million children born in the
U.S.A. each year or 600,000 children are exposed to toxic levels of mercury
in the womb.[34]

This is a serious health concern. Mercury will wreak havoc on your
body and your brain.

Toxic Chemicals

We are exposed to astounding amounts of brain pollution. More than
80,000 chemicals have been introduced into our society since 1900, yet
only 550 have been tested for safety (www.epa.gov/iriswebp/iris/stand
-al.htm). According to the U.S. Environmental Protection Agency (EPA),
about 2.5 billion pounds of toxic chemicals are released yearly by large industrial facilities.

Most toxicity studies (and remember there are only studies on 550
chemicals or 0.6 percent of the total amount of toxins floating around in
our environment) look at only one compound at a time.[35] But we are exposed to hundreds of different toxins, most of which can affect brain function. There are few studies done on the combined effects of this toxic
exposure on the brain.

In fact, a recent government survey ("National Report on Human Exposure to Environmental Chemicals," issued in July 2005, www.cdc/gov/exposurereport/) found an average of 148 chemicals in our bodies, and those were only the ones they tested.

We are exposed to hazardous wastes, emissions from local waste incinerators, solvents, heavy metals, ground-water pollutants including industrial heavy metal waste products such as arsenic, common materials such as phthalates (plasticizers found in all plastic bottles), and polybrominated diphenyl ethers (flame retardants).

A recent study of umbilical cord blood found 287 toxic chemicals, 217 of which are toxic to the brain and nervous system. And this is what infants are exposed to even before they take their first breath.[36]

And then there are the toxins found in our foods and homes (like certain cleaning agents or pest controls), all of which add to the total toxic load on our bodies.

We live in a sea of toxins. See chapter 10 for more details. For now, let's look at some of the more common toxic agents you are likely exposed to.

Additives and Toxins in Our Food

More than 3,500 different chemicals can be added to our food and more than 3,000 are in our homes.[37] Every one of them is legal, and you will be exposed to some or all of them, depending on how you live.

The average American consumes literally pounds of hormones, antibiotics, food chemicals, additives, artificial sweeteners, and MSG each year. Each one of these toxic chemicals has been shown to harm the brain.

The average person consumes a gallon of neurotoxic pesticides and herbicides each year by eating conventionally grown fruits and vegetables.[38] (And that's with people eating much less than the eight to ten servings they should be eating!) Remember, pesticides work *because* they are neurotoxic to pests—they attack their nervous system.

When children are exposed to toxic chemicals and pesticides, the stakes are higher. They are exposed to a higher relative dose of these toxins due to their low body weight, and their developing brains are more sensitive to insult.

One study showed children who regularly ate nonorganic foods purchased in an average grocery store had high levels of pesticides in their urine, while those who strictly ate organic food had almost none.[39] Other studies link early pesticide exposure to autism[40] and other neurobehavioral problems in children.[41]

A recent study in *Lancet*[42] clearly showed that food additives make children hyperactive. They took about three hundred normal children and split them into two groups. Each group was given an identical-looking colored drink. One was naturally colored and the other contained sodium benzoate and many other colors and additives.

The children who drank the tainted drink were all much more hyperactive. There is no benefit or role for these compounds in our diet, and much evidence of harm. They benefit the food industry by improving shelf life, taste, and "attractiveness." But they should not be in our food supply, period. Come eat the neon blue food!

These compounds (and the total load of all the other toxins we are exposed to) create changes in mood, aggressive behavior, depression, problems with attention and focus, sleep problems, reduced intellectual performance, and memory loss.

It isn't just consuming one red candy, blue cupcake, or the few drops of pesticide sprayed on our pint of strawberries once in a while. It is the consistent, repetitive, cumulative presence of these chemicals in our lives.

The evidence of harm is in. Do we need more to act?

The basis for a decision should not even be the evidence of harm (though we have more than enough); it should be the clear evidence of the absence of harm and complete safety. This is called the *precautionary principle,* otherwise known as better safe than sorry.

But we are living human guinea pigs, and our children are the most sensitive.

Why else would we be seeing epidemics of autism, mood disorders, and ADHD in children over the last thirty years?

Household and Environmental Toxins

In our everyday life we are exposed to and absorb many toxic chemicals into our bodies, especially VOCs, or volatile organic compounds.[43] These toxins seep out of our furniture made with formaldehyde and our sofas made with fire retardants and are in many regular household cleaning products. It is in the stuff we use to wash our dishes with, clean our tables with, wash our toilet bowls with, and clean our clothes in.

One of the "green" or environmental movement's biggest assets is that it is actually cheaper to create environments and buildings that support health, rather than those that make us sick. Eliminating these toxic chemicals from our homes and workplaces is not only environmentally more sustainable, it is economically more sustainable.

In fact, Kaiser Permanente, a large health maintenance organization in California, has gone green, declaring that all its buildings and building materials from now on will be environmentally sustainable. They project spending $24 billion by 2014 on new and existing buildings to create these environmentally sustainable and health-promoting facilities. And, they say, it will be cheaper than regular construction.

According to Mike Hrast, construction supervisor at the Modesto, California, Kaiser facility (still under construction at this writing), the company will save a minimum of $238,000 by implementing green standards just at this one facility.

Eventually we will get to a place in our society where environmental safety and sustainability will be "built into" our homes and workplaces. In the meantime, do an inventory of all the chemicals you are exposed to at work and at home and make a clean sweep.

Toxic chemicals have a clear impact on behavior and brain function, both short and long term.[44] Reduce or avoid your exposure to them. I recommend a book called *Green Housekeeping* by Ellen Sandbeck as a resource to cleaning up your home environment.

Toxic Molds

Mold exposure is also a threat to our brains. I have seen many patients whose brains malfunction from mold toxins (known as mycotoxins), common in homes and office buildings. Remember, that was part of Clayton's story in chapter 2 (page 28). His home was infected with toxic mold.

The suffering and symptoms caused by these molds are well described as "sick building syndrome."[45] These mold toxins cause nerve damage and provoke the body to produce autoimmunity or autoantibodies against its own nerves and brain tissue.

In a study in the *Archives of Environmental Health*,[46] scientists studied one hundred patients who had been exposed to toxic molds in their homes. The most common molds were Alternaria, Cladosporium, Aspergillus, Penicillium, Stachybotrys (also known as the toxic black mold), Curvularia, Basidiomycetes, Myxomycetes, Epicoccus, Fusarium, Bipolaris, and Rhizopus.

Sounds like an invasion!

These scientists found that more than 80 percent of the people living with these molds had immune system abnormalities, and 64 percent had respiratory system problems like sinus problems and wheezing.

More alarming was that 70 percent had severe symptoms of brain damage, including an inability to walk in a straight line with their eyes closed, difficulty standing on their toes, and short-term memory loss.

More alarming still was the finding, in 100 percent of patients, of autonomic nervous system abnormalities (this is the automatic nervous system that controls all your basic life functions like heart rate and breathing).

If that weren't enough, brain scans were abnormal in 86 percent of those studied and objective neuropsychological testing of brain function was abnormal in 100 percent of them. This included findings of short-term memory loss and impairment of executive function/judgment, concentration, and hand-eye coordination.[47]

So if you think you may be exposed to mold, be extremely aggressive in addressing it.

Toxic Metals

Unfortunately, we live not only in a sea of toxic chemicals but also of toxic metals, including mercury, lead, arsenic, cadmium, and aluminum.

Two of the most brain-damaging compounds known are both heavy metals—mercury and lead. The research on these is abundant and frightening. Dr. David Bellinger, a professor of neurology at Harvard Medical School, reviewed this research in his paper "Children's Cognitive Health: The Influence of Environmental Chemical Exposures."[48]

Lead was the first toxic heavy metal to be identified, and some action has been taken regarding lead exposure in our society. Before lead paint and leaded gasoline were banned, exposure levels were much higher. However, they are still a major problem.

Toxic metals, like lead and mercury, are highly persistent in the environment and can be carried far distances in the atmosphere, getting deposited far from their place of origin.

For example, coal-burning, lead- and mercury-belching smokestacks in China send their toxic load to the most remote and wild areas of America. Lead and mercury from facilities like these also end up on our driveways and streets and on our carpets and floors where children play. (That's not to mention all the lead-painted toys from China.)

Dr. Herbert Needleman examined the effects of lead on 2,146 children in first and second grade in Alabama.[49] He looked at lead levels in teeth, not in blood, to assess long-term exposure.

Not only did the children with the highest levels of lead have the lowest IQs, but they were also more distractible, dependent, disorganized, hyper-

active, and impulsive, and had difficulty following simple directions. There
were no children in the high-lead group that had IQs over 125, while 5
percent in the low-lead group did.

Dr. Needleman did a follow-up study[50] on these children that found the
lead-exposed children experienced serious consequences when they got
older. They faced a higher rate of high school dropout, a greater likelihood
of reading disability, lower class standing in high school, increased absen-
teeism, lower vocabulary and grammatical-reasoning scores, poorer hand-
eye coordination, longer reaction times, and slower finger tapping.

They were also more likely to have episodes of juvenile delinquency.

In the 1950s the American government set safe levels of lead at 60 micrograms per deciliter of blood as the upper limit of "normal." Considering
severe brain damage occurs at 100 micrograms per deciliter, and death at
150 micrograms per deciliter, this decision is perplexing.

The "safe" level was decreased to 40 in 1971, 30 in 1975, 25 in 1985, and
10 in 1991.

But recent studies show that the greatest drop-off in IQ scores happens
between a level of 1 and 10 micrograms per deciliter.[51] This is particularly
scary since more than 10 percent of poor and inner-city children have lead
exposure levels over 10 micrograms per deciliter!

Of course, children aren't the only population at risk. Lead exposure in
adults has been linked to severe depression and schizophrenia. One factory
that produced tetraethyl lead was known as the "House of Butterflies," because so many workers had hallucinations.

Lead exposure has also been linked to depression, irritability, interper-
sonal conflict, fatigue, anger, tension, and even decreased sex drive.

And it has been linked to degenerative changes in the brain on MRI. In
fact, evidence shows that much of what we think of as "normal" age-related
decline in mental and cognitive function is actually due to chronic lead toxicity and the resultant loss of brain function.[52]

Understand that since lead was removed from gasoline, and house paint,
blood levels of the average person have dropped tenfold in the last few decades.

However, lead is still dramatically higher in people today than it was in
those who lived before the industrial age. We continue to be exposed to it
in our soil and water, as well as from our own bones, where it is stored.

And it is lethal.

Blood lead levels were measured in a nationally representative sample
of 13,946 adult participants of the Third National Health and Nutrition

Examination Survey (NHANES III), recruited in 1988 to 1994 and followed for up to twelve years to track what diseases people developed and why they died.[53]

The NHANES III study found that any level over 2 micrograms per deciliter (not 10 or 40) in the blood caused dramatic increases in heart attacks, strokes, and death.

In fact, after controlling for all other risk factors including cholesterol, high blood pressure, smoking, and inflammation, the study found that the risk of death from all causes increased by 25 percent, deaths from heart disease increased by 55 percent, risk of heart attacks increased by 151 percent, and risk of stroke increased by 89 percent.

What was even more remarkable is that it is estimated that nearly 40 percent of all Americans have toxic levels of lead high enough to cause these problems.

The good news is that using chelation therapy (an underused medical treatment to help the body bind and excrete metals) has been effective in reversing many of these problems.[54]

So we know lead is an extremely toxic substance. What about mercury?

Well, I've already told you it's the second most toxic substance after plutonium. But in case that isn't enough . . .

Mercury, I believe (because of the hundreds of patients I have seen with mercury toxicity), is one of the most serious threats to our brain, and is responsible for or contributes to much of the modern epidemic of autism, ADHD, depression, dementia, and other versions of broken brains. Finding it and getting rid of it in my patients is one of the most effective ways I have to improve mood, attention, and memory.

Mercury is emitted from coal-burning industrial facilities at the rate of 2,900 tons (or over 6 million pounds) per year. As you consider that, keep in mind mercury is toxic at greater than 1 part per million, and that the EPA has declared the "safe" level of mercury exposure to be less than 0.1 micrograms/kilogram body weight/day.

That means we are in big trouble based on our exposure.

After testing mercury levels in thousands of patients, I believe that a large majority of us have some level of mercury toxicity.

Mercury has been implicated in severe neurologic injury. This was well demonstrated in the Minamata Bay exposures (from toxic dumping into the ocean) and the Iraq grain contamination disaster (mercury was applied to prevent spoilage of grain used for planting, but the grain was eaten by accident).

But mercury is also toxic at very low doses. We have already looked at mercury in dental amalgams and vaccines, but environmental exposures are also significant risks.

The largest is from consumption of large fish contaminated with mercury such as tuna, swordfish, shark, tilefish, and sea bass, as well as nearly all river fish.

Remember you are whatever you ate. Big fish eat smaller fish and so on. Toxins bioconcentrate up the food chain. The bigger the fish, the higher dose of mercury you are likely to get. So eat only fish that are small enough to fit in your frying pan. Sardines are my favorite.

Studies of fish-consuming populations directly correlate levels of mercury in the umbilical cord blood with lower IQ, attention deficits, and impairment in language and memory. So if you don't think the amount of mercury you are exposed to in the fish you eat is a problem, think again.

What's most frightening are autopsy studies on mercury-exposed people. Adult brains show damage in only a few areas—the ones responsible for dementia and depression. But if exposure to mercury occurred in the womb or early in life, it was deposited in the entire brain and completely disrupted normal brain development.[55]

Clearly exposure to toxic metals is damaging to the brain. We need to be very smart about reducing emissions and exposures, as well as treating heavy metal toxicity.

We will review the role of all toxins in our health in more detail in Part II, where I explain how problems with detoxification and toxic exposures are linked to most of the worst neurological disorders (like Parkinson's and Alzheimer's), mood or psychological disorders (including depression anxiety, insomnia, and more), as well as autism and ADHD.

Toxic Waves

Even though most of us are not willing (or able) to give up our computers, cell phones, wireless networks, microwave ovens, televisions, and other electronics, we have to ask if these electromagnetic devices are harming us. Even if you could give them up, you would have to think about the effects all the radiofrequency waves buzzing about from WiFi, cell towers, power lines, and electrical wires have on you.

We are electromagnetic beings. Just think about an EKG or EEG—these simply record the electrical activities of your heart and brain. We are very sensitive to electromagnetic fields of any kind, and excessive exposure to certain types of toxic waves may be extremely harmful to our health.

Before I briefly review the risks of electromagnetic fields (EMFs) on human health, I want to state that *the absence of evidence is not evidence of absence*. This is an area of enormous controversy and equally large knowledge gaps. But to think that because we haven't adequately studied the effects of "electropollution" it is not a problem may be a grave error. The data we do have is enough to make me very concerned.[56]

The few things we do know make me want to limit my exposure. This is an area where caution should be our guide.

For example, we know that EMFs alter cellular metabolism and generate free radicals that can be toxic to your brain and promote memory loss and dementia. Research shows higher rates of Alzheimer's in people exposed to EMFs.[57] Other studies link it to mood disorders and depression.[58]

EMFs also may be linked to an increase in cancers, especially brain cancer. Could having a radio-frequency-emitting device (otherwise known as a cell phone) held up to your brain for hours a day have an impact? Do you want to wait twenty years to find out?

We know that cell phone use does account for thousands of deaths every year from car accidents (because people don't pay attention to driving when they are on the phone).

There are 1.6 billion cell-phone users worldwide, with the number growing every day. And over half of the children in developing countries use them. What impact does this have on a developing brain?

While I do use a cell phone, I try to limit its use and use a safe headset such as one that has an air tube to diffuse the EMF (not a wireless one).

Cell phones are only the most obvious form of EMFs we are exposed to. As I mentioned at the start of this section, we are also exposed to toxic waves in many other forms. There are things you can do to reduce your exposure to these toxic waves and protect yourself, and you may not even have to give up all your electronics to do it. I will review how you can protect yourself and your family in Part III.

What you learned in this chapter is depressing, I know. But I don't believe in the proverb "What you don't know won't hurt you," at least when it comes to brain damage.

Clearly there are many environmental influences that can have a major impact on your brain health. These toxins affect us all from our food, our water, and our air, medications, chemicals, metals, molds, and electromagnetic radiation.

Everyday choices we make to protect ourselves will have an impact globally. The European Union, through new legislation (called REACH) designed to limit toxins in commercially produced goods, caused China to change its manufacturing practices. The European Union also demanded that Silicon Valley produce cells phones without toxic metals and they did.

Buying organic food, refusing vaccines with mercury, and buying deodorant without aluminum will create a ripple effect throughout our economy and environment.

You can make changes in your life and in your world with the choices you make.

What's more, you can make changes in your personal health. You can heal yourself from brain damage by improving your diet, limiting your exposure to toxins, and changing the way you live. You can *reverse* the effects of depression, anxiety, bipolar disorder, autism, Alzheimer's, ADHD, and more—if you know how to.

The UltraMind Solution is designed to give you a specific method to achieve that goal and by doing so take one more step toward that state of vital health I call UltraWellness.

You now understand the theoretical underpinnings of this approach. It's time to learn how to apply it in practice to fix your broken brain. Whether you are suffering from depression, lack of attention, autism, Alzheimer's, Parkinson's, or if you just deal with bad moods and brain fog, the UltraMind Solution will help you overcome these problems so you can achieve Ultra-Wellness.

PART II

The Seven Keys
to UltraWellness

CHAPTER 5

YOUR MOOD AND BRAIN POWER ARE NOT ALL IN YOUR HEAD

The Seven Keys to UltraWellness

In Part II, I will explain how seven key biological systems influence every feeling, thought, emotion, behavior, and memory we have (not to mention our physical health and weight). It is through understanding how these systems play a role in your health and your brain (the same thing) that you can take control of your brain health and recover from the debilitating effects of memory disorders, attention deficits, and mood disturbances. If you focus on your health first, your brain may take care of itself.

These factors must be addressed first because medication and psychotherapy are then rarely needed, and if used, will be dramatically more effective. These seven keys are the new way to repair, renew, and revitalize your brain and help return your life to balance and vibrant health.

I introduced you to the seven keys to UltraWellness, which form the basis of The UltraMind Solution in Part I. To refresh your memory, they are:

1. Optimize Nutrition
2. Balance Your Hormones
3. Cool Off Inflammation
4. Fix Your Digestion
5. Enhance Detoxification
6. Boost Energy Metabolism
7. Calm Your Mind

In the following seven chapters I will show you how each of these seven keys fits into the larger story of mental and physical health.

Each chapter contains quizzes to help you identify where you are out of balance. Are you deficient in omega-3 fats? Are you magnesium-deficient? Are you mercury toxic? Is your thyroid not functioning well? Is gluten inflaming your brain? Is sugar destroying your mood and brain? The quizzes will help you answer these questions.

In Part III, I give you my six-week plan on how to care for your brain for life. I will explain the basic "ingredients" you need to make a happy, attentive, sharp, clear, and engaged brain. This is the basic care plan for your brain.

In Part IV, I will show you how to customize the basic care plan for your brain based on your quizzes. Those quizzes give you the information you need to understand which of your systems are out of balance. You will learn how to bring each of your core systems back into a thriving and robust balance.

Do you need more omega-3 fats, or vitamin B_{12}, or thyroid hormone? Do you need to cool off an inflamed brain, or detoxify a toxic brain? I will help you find answers.

But regardless of the name of your disease, a mood disorder, a problem with attention or memory, a neurological disease, or even psychosis, what you learn in *The UltraMind Solution* will help you live the best, healthiest life you can.

Have Another (Drug) Cocktail?

I want to tell you a story about the typical patient I see with a whole list of problems—all apparently unrelated and all treated by different doctors. While this man's symptoms were partly controlled, he was anything but healthy. He was on a cocktail of four psychoactive drugs just to manage his life at forty-two years old!

Do people really need psychological "cocktails" of drugs just to help them deal with depression, anxiety, insomnia, and ADHD? Joe's story points to an answer.

*J*oe *was a forty-two-year-old man who thought he was healthy—despite being on four different drugs for mood and psychiatric problems. This list of medications was a bit scary for a guy in his early forties. He took one for depression (Lexapro), one for attention deficit disorder because he couldn't concentrate (Concerta), one for anxiety (Xanax), and one for sleep (Ambien). One new drug was piled on another over just a few years!*

He also took medications for asthma and frequent rounds of antibiotics over the years. He had psoriasis, reflux, irritable bowel syndrome, and chronic postnasal drip. His sex drive was low, and his anal area was always itchy. He got frequent sores and bumps on his tongue after eating certain foods. He also had sugar cravings and would frequently get weak and have episodes of very low blood sugar (hypoglycemia). He was about twenty-five pounds overweight—right around his middle—and his triglycerides were over five hundred (normal is less than one hundred). He had a fatty liver and prediabetes or metabolic syndrome.

Joe's diet was less than ideal. He ate a bagel or a processed protein bar in the morning with coffee. Lunch was usually a turkey wrap with lots of cheese, a few diet Cokes, and chips. Dinner was a little better, but he craved bread, pasta, and potatoes and had sweets after dinner because he craved them. He usually had two glasses of wine a day, three cups of coffee, and too many diet Cokes to count. He slept about five to six hours a night.

Looking at the seven keys to UltraWellness, we found many imbalances. His gut was inflamed, and he had a parasite and yeast overgrowth from years of antibiotic use. This led to food sensitivities to wheat and rye (the main gluten-containing grains). He had multiple nutritional deficiencies, including B_{12}, folate, vitamin D, chromium, and omega-3 fats—all very important for mood and a healthy metabolism.

So instead of treating any one disease or problem, I helped him by treating the imbalances in his life.

I helped him improve his diet, stop the refined carbohydrates and sugars, and eat more fiber and omega-3 fats. I also had him get off gluten and dairy—foods that were triggering inflammation in his gut. He cut way back on coffee and stopped drinking wine. And he started exercising and sleeping a bit more.

I gave him a multivitamin (with plenty of chromium), fish oil, and probiotics (healthy gut bacteria). I also treated him with high doses of folate and B_{12} to accommodate his genetic need for more. In addition to this, I gave him high doses of vitamin D to bring his levels back to normal and improve his mood and immune system. I treated his parasite and the yeast overgrowth with short-term medication.

After three months, I saw him again. This time he had lost twenty-five pounds, his triglycerides dropped from 597 to 80, and his cholesterol went from 275 to 198. His folate and B_{12} status was back to normal. His fasting blood sugar dropped from 101 to 84, which is normal, and his insulin levels dropped back to normal. His fatty liver was healed. And how did he feel?

Well, he had no more need for reflux medication or inhalers for asthma. Those symptoms were gone. Without my instruction (and despite my advice to the contrary), he stopped all four of his psychiatric medications because he was sleeping fine, was no longer anxious or depressed, and had no more problems with concentration or attention.

The science of Functional Medicine is ready for the doctor's office. It is possible for people to get to the root of their problems.

Asthma and reflux are not irreversible problems, but may be the result of food sensitivities to substances like gluten or dairy, or imbalances in the gut from parasites and yeast, or the product of a poor diet.

Similarly, depression (and other psychological issues like the ones Joe suffered) may be related to key nutritional factors, including sugar in the diet, and nutritional deficiencies such as folic acid, vitamin B_{12}, vitamin D, and omega-3 fats, as well as food sensitivities or gut problems—not a Lexapro deficiency.

With Joe, I once again found myself an accidental psychiatrist, witnessing remarkable transformations in patients by simply taking away the things that make them ill and giving them things that put them back in balance.

It is really that simple. The body's intelligence for healing does the rest. This is the essence of the UltraMind Solution.

CHAPTER 6

KEY #1: OPTIMIZE NUTRITION

The Key to Mental Health and Brain Health

The staple foods may not contain the same nutritive substances as in former times . . . Chemical fertilizers, by increasing the abundance of the crops without replacing all the exhausted elements of the soil, have indirectly contributed to change the nutritive value of cereal grains and of vegetables . . . They have, thus, contributed to the weakening of our body and our soul.

—ALEXIS CARREL, *Man the Unknown*

Optimal nutrition is the most important factor in keeping your brain healthy. Feeding your brain is not something most of us know how to do. What you put in your mouth provides all the raw materials to build the structure of your brain cells and keep all the communications systems running coherently so you can think, emote, learn, and remember. You have to start with the right food, and enough of the right nutrients for the brain to function well.

The problem is that most of us (including doctors) know very little about nutrition and even less about how and why vitamins and minerals are so essential for brain function and health. To restore optimal brain function and health, you need to know the *why*, not just the *what*, of what you are doing.

I know that the nutritional science I present in this chapter may feel a little dense, but you can understand it. Once you do, it will completely alter your perception of the role of food and nutrients in your physical and mental health forever.

This background knowledge will help you take full advantage of *The UltraMind Solution*. If you know what is happening in the body, why it goes wrong, and how to fix it, you are much more likely to incorporate changes in your diet, behavior, and habits in the long run. And it just may motivate you to take your vitamins and essential omega-3 fats every day.

This chapter will focus on the most important aspects of nutrition in the context of your brain function.

Bad Brain Food Versus Good Brain Food

In chapter 4, I explained the harmful effects of trans fats, high-fructose corn syrup and sugar, artificial sweeteners and food additives, as well as the dangers of hormones, antibiotics, pesticides, and heavy metals, in our food. I also reviewed the risks of caffeine and alcohol.

Common sense and scientific research both lead us to the conclusion that if we want healthy bodies and healthy brains we must put in the right raw materials: real, whole, local, fresh, unadulterated, unprocessed, and chemical-, hormone-, and antibiotic-free food.

There is *no* role for foreign molecules that interfere with our biology at every level. Enough said.

Let's look at what we *should* be eating—the stuff of life.

In the remainder of this chapter I am going to focus on the ingredients most relevant to the epidemic of broken brains, of mood, behavior, attention, and memory disorders. We will focus on the role of the following in brain health:

1. The essential fats
2. The key essential amino acids, which come from protein
3. Carbohydrates
4. Vitamins and minerals
   ∴ Special brain vitamins, including folate, B_6, B_{12}, and vitamin D
   ∴ Special minerals, including magnesium, zinc, and selenium.

In Part IV, we will review many other special nutrients essential for healthy brain function that work specifically in different key systems, such as acetyl-L-carnitine, n-acetylcysteine, or coenzyme Q10. These become more essential under certain conditions of life, such as stress or toxicity or age.

Let's start with fats.

Fats and Your Brain

❖

Does your oil need to be changed? Take the following quiz to find out.

In the box on the right place a check for each positive answer. Then find out how severe your problem is by using the scoring key below.

FATTY ACIDS QUIZ*

I have soft, cracked, or brittle nails. ☐
I have dry, itchy, scaling, or flaking skin. ☐
I have hard ear wax. ☐
I have chicken skin (tiny bumps on the backs of arms or on the trunk). ☐
I have dandruff. ☐
I feel aching or stiffness in my joints. ☐
I am thirsty most of the time. ☐
I am constipated (have less than two bowel movements a day). ☐
I have light-colored, hard, or foul-smelling stools. ☐
I have depression, ADHD, and/or memory loss. ☐
I have high blood pressure. ☐
I have fibrocystic breasts. ☐
I have premenstrual syndrome. ☐
I have high LDL cholesterol, low HDL levels, and high triglycerides. ☐

(continued)

I am of North Atlantic genetic background: Irish, Scottish, Welsh, Scandinavian, or coastal Native American.   ☐

---

* For your convenience, this quiz has been reprinted in *The UltraMind Solution Companion Guide*. Simply go to www.ultramind.com/guide, download the guide, and print out the quiz.

Scoring Key—Fatty Acids

Score one point for each box you checked.

Score	Severity	Care Plan	Action to Take
0–4	You may have a mild fatty-acid deficiency.	*The UltraMind Solution*	Complete the six-week program in Part III.
5–7	You may have a moderate fatty-acid deficiency.	Self-Care	Complete the six-week program in Part III and optimize your fatty acids using the self-care options in chapter 22.
8 and above	You may have a severe fatty-acid deficiency.	Medical Care	Do both of the steps above and see a physician for additional assistance. I have outlined some of the options you should discuss with your doctor in chapter 22.

Do you gather wild plants to eat or hunt for your meat? If not, you are likely one of the 99 percent of people in the twenty-first century who are deficient in the most important ingredient in our bodies for normal cell and brain function—omega-3 fatty acids.

The Greenland Inuit (a native tribe in Greenland) consumed between 15 and 19 gm of omega-3 fats a day from eating whale, walrus, seal, and arctic char. That may be how much we are designed to operate on. Most of us consume far less than 1 gm a day.

Omega-3 fats come from wild things—which means they are hard to find in today's society. In the modern world our only real source of omega-3 fats is fish, and most of the fish we eat are contaminated with toxins and mercury, which may lead to a host of problems you will learn more about in chapter 10.

Aside from controlling your gene function, regulating your immune system, and improving your metabolism, these fats are vital components of the cell membrane that covers every one of the 100 trillion cells in your body. Without omega-3 fats, the proper messages can't be communicated from one cell to another.

The two most important omega-3 fats to know about are eicosapentanoic acid (EPA) and docosahexaenoic acid (DHA). They are both necessary omega-3 fats. Since your brain is mostly fat, and 60 percent of your brain is specifically made of DHA, it is easy to see why they are so important. If you don't have enough, the brain doesn't work.

However, in the last 150 years we have seen an unprecedented change in our fat intake. Refined, omega-6, inflammatory oils, including corn, soy, and safflower oils, replaced omega-3 fats from fish, wild game, and wild plants.

The ratio of omega-6 to omega-3 fats has increased from 1:1 to 10:1 or 20:1 in our diets, and the effects have been disastrous. All of the major diseases of aging as well as the epidemic of "brain disorders" are directly associated with this change in our diet.

Today the only real sources of omega-3 fats are breast milk, wild fish and game, seaweed, algae, and eggs hatched from chickens fed only on flaxseeds and fish meal.

Our brains don't work without omega-3 fats. Period. That is why low levels of omega-3 fats have been linked to everything from depression and anxiety, to bipolar disease and criminal behavior, to schizophrenia, to attention deficit disorder and autism and learning disabilities, as well as dementia and many other neurological diseases.[1]

The omega-3 fatty acids from wild fish and certain nuts and seeds like flaxseeds play critical roles in our cognitive development and learning, visual development, immune and inflammatory function, fetal brain development, brain health, Alzheimer's disease, and mental illness, not to mention heart disease and cancer.

At a recent nutrition conference I listened to Joseph Hibbeln, M.D. (who is the scientist in the section dedicated to nutritional neurosciences at the National Institutes of Health), where he presented some startling data about the effect of fish oil or omega-3 fats on our mental health.

He told us that the flood of soy oils and seed oils like corn in our diet, which contain high amounts of linoleic acid (an unhealthy omega-6 fatty acid), promote inflammation and disease.

In our culture, this inflammatory fatty acid primarily comes from soy oil. Eighty percent of the fats consumed in the United States are linoleic acid, which comes from soy oil and other similar fats. Twenty percent are in the form of EPA, which comes from fish oil. (I believe we consume even less EPA.)

In Japan, 80 percent of the fat eaten is EPA, and only 20 percent is arachidonic acid (another unhealthy omega-6 fatty acid). That may be why the Japanese have less depression, dementia, and heart disease.

Consuming these harmful seed and soy oils instead of omega-3 fats changes our tissue composition in dramatic ways and damages our health.

Dr. Hibbeln explained that there has been a *thousandfold increase* in the consumption of soy oil over the last century. In fact, 20 percent of all calories consumed in America are from soybean oil and therefore 9 to 10 percent of all our calories are from linoleic acid instead of the omega-3 fats, which we should be eating.

It is interesting that 4 to 5 million years of human evolution occurred in a seafood-rich nutritional environment in which *seafood* was the main source of fats. There were no seed oils, which we now use to cook French fries, doughnuts, and packaged foods. We have to ask ourselves what happens to our mind and body when our nutritional environment radically changes this way.

This level of the soy oils in our diet is unsafe. Recent research has found that homicide mortality in the United Kingdom increased dramatically with the increase in consumption of linoleic acid from soy oil.[2] The same thing happened in the United States as well as in Australia, Canada, and Argentina. Conversely, the homicide mortality rates are inversely related to seafood consumption, meaning that the more seafood people eat in a society such as Japan, the less homicide they have.

Even more dramatic was a study published in the *British Journal of Psychiatry* in 2002 that looked at the reduction in felony-level violent offenses among prisoners with supplementation of omega-3 fats.[3] A placebo-controlled trial gave one group the recommended daily amounts of vitamins, minerals, and omega-3 fats and the other group retained their regular prison diet and lifestyle. By just providing vitamin and fish-oil supplements, there was a 35 percent reduction in felony-related violent crime in prison.

It has also been shown that a lack of fish consumption is universally related to depression. A one-year study found EPA was helpful in treating resistant depression.

Omega-3 fats are also helpful in treating postpartum depression. DHA from fish oils is a critical part of a mother's breast milk that helps neurological development in the fetus. Women who have higher levels of omega-3 fats in their tissues have lower rates of postpartum depression.[4]

Similarly, kids who have dyslexia, dyspraxia (difficulty writing), other learning disabilities, and attention deficit disorder are mostly omega-3 fat–deficient. Dopamine activity, which is critical for brain function in these children, is improved with essential fatty acid consumption. There have been controlled studies showing that giving fish oil to children with these kinds of problems improves reading and spelling in treatment groups and improves conduct in school because the nervous system is very dependent on these fats to function.[5]

Omega-3 fats are well known for their benefits in heart health, obesity, and diabetes. They help prevent heart attacks, arrhythmias, and strokes; reduce inflammation; and prevent blood clots. But their effects on the brain are just as critical.

Omega-3 fats may sound like a miracle cure, and they can be in some cases. I have seen patients completely recover from autism with cod liver oil (which contains omega-3 fats, and vitamins A and D).[6]

*O*ne of my patients, a twenty-year-old woman who hated seafood and avoided it her whole life, suffered from depression, learning disabilities, obesity, muscle pain, and chronic fatigue. Her blood tests showed severe omega-3 fat deficiency and an overload of inflammatory omega-6 fats. By giving her an oil change with high doses of fish oil (EPA and DHA), she recovered from her depression and cognitive struggles, her pain disappeared, and she lost sixty pounds.

But why the dramatic change with one simple supplement?

Don't make the mistake to think all the conditions listed above (or those discussed elsewhere in the book) can magically be cured with a little fish oil. Some may, but most conditions result from imbalance and deficiencies in many of the body's core systems. Nutrient deficiency is only one area where problems are created, and omega-3 fats are only one of those nutrients.

If you are omega-3 fat–deficient, B_{12} deficient, have mercury poisoning, low thyroid function, and eat foods you are allergic to, just fixing the omega-3 fat deficiencies won't cure the whole problem. You have to fix everything.

However, nutrient deficiency is a major contributor to *all* of the other health issues you may be experiencing, so figuring out what nutrients you are deficient in and reestablishing nutritional balance is an important step on your path to UltraWellness.

I am going to use the example of omega-3 fats to show you the myriad ways in which nutrients work in the body to normalize function and why their deficiency can cause so many diseases.

What Omega-3 Fats (and Other Fats) Do, and Why Deficiencies Wreak Havoc on Your Biology

Here are four key roles omega-3 fats play in your body and reasons why they are linked to so many different mood, memory, and attention problems (as well as most chronic diseases).[7] These fats are literally the stuff we are made of.

1. They build all cell membranes (along with a few other key fats called phospholipids—PC and PS).
2. They reduce inflammation, which has been linked to almost all brain problems such as autism, ADHD, Alzheimer's, and depression.
3. They balance blood sugar, which, as you will see in chapter 7, is essential for keeping your brain healthy.
4. They increase the activity of a key molecule in your brain called BDNF (brain-derived neurotropic factor), which acts like fertilizer for your brain, stimulating new cell growth and increased cell connections.

Let's take a closer look at our cell membranes, which form the covering of all your cells.

Healthy Cell Membranes: Happy Mood, Clear Focus, Sharp Memory

Omega-3 fats form the basic structure of *all* our cell membranes. And all life processes start and end at the surface of our cells. These surfaces are where all of the biological "communication" in your body takes place. Every instruction you need to survive is communicated from one cell to the next through your cell membranes. Think of the cell membranes as the ears of your cells. Without healthy cell membranes you will be deaf to the call of messages coming in.

You are only as healthy as your cell membranes. Changes in your cell membranes affect the health of your entire body. The healthier your cell membranes are, the healthier you will be. Let's focus for a minute on why this is true in the brain.

Your brain weighs only about three pounds, or 2 percent of your body weight, but it uses about 20 percent of the oxygen you breathe and about 20 percent of the calories you consume. Your brain contains 100 billion brain cells, with trillions of supportive cells to protect and defend them called glial cells (the immune cells of the brain).

Each brain cell is connected to every other brain cell by about 40,000 connections (called synapses). So let's see, 40,000 x 100,000,000,000. That is how many connections there are in your brain and they are all sending messages constantly!

Each of those connections meet at the cell membrane.

If those membranes are not healthy, the effectiveness and speed of communication slows down. That leads to poorer mental function, memory problems, and mood disorders. There are many things that affect the wiring and connections in the brain—in fact, all the keys explained in *The Ultra-Mind Solution* do. But the membranes of your brain cells are at the heart (or brain) of the matter.

Cell membranes are made of the following things:

1. *Fatty acids* (from wild fish and fish oil): the omega-3 fats (DHA and EPA) if you are eating well or taking fish oil, or shortening and lard, if you are not. (I discussed this above.)
2. *Phospholipids* (choline from egg yolks, soybeans, peanuts, lentils, sesame seeds, flaxseeds): fats that contain phosphorous, phosphatidylcholine (PC) and phosphatidylserine (PS) are the two most important.
3. *Cholesterol* (from eggs, shrimp, poultry): glue between molecules (see, you *need* cholesterol).
4. *Protein* (from legumes, whole grains, nuts, seeds, eggs, poultry, meat, and dairy): receptors, transporters, gates, signal transducers, etc. This is where all the communication signals from other parts of the body and the environment get processed. (I will be talking more about protein after we discuss phospholipids.)

Besides the omega-3 fats, which make up much of your cell membrane, there is another class of compounds called phospholipids, which are equally crucial for building membranes.

These fatty substances are critical for optimal brain function and the research has borne out the benefits of these nature-made molecules. If your cell membranes are your brain's ears, then PS and PC are your brain's "eardrums." They are the listening interface of every cell and receive the communications all of your other cells are sending. If your cells are not made of the right materials, you will be "deaf" and become not only dumb but also depressed and demented!

Your cell membranes are made up of the fats you consume. If those membranes are made of trans fats and beef fat, they become stiff and hard like lard or Crisco. As a result, communication gets stopped up. It's hard for things to get in or out—for information to pass smoothly from one cell membrane to the next—when your cell membranes harden this way.

If they are made from omega-3 fats and phospholipids your cell membranes become fluid and flexible, allowing easy communication from cell to cell. Think about the cold-water fish swimming in arctic waters. Their bodies have high levels of fat to preserve heat, but must be fluid so they can swim and move in icy waters. Your cell membranes need to be fluid and smooth like those fish.

The most abundant fats in your cell membranes are phospholipids. PS, in particular, is found in all cell membranes. In fact, it is in all cells in all life-forms. It is one of the building blocks of nature, and the human brain has extremely high amounts of it.

Using PS supplements has been proven effective in improving memory and cognitive function,[8] boosting mood and stress reduction,[9] improving attention, and reducing aggression in children with ADHD. And it has no side effects!

Unless you eat a lot of organ meats (like liver, kidney, and brains, often prized in traditional cultures), which is not a good idea because they store toxins, you may need to supplement with PS. I will discuss this in more detail in Part IV, where I give you my plan to optimize your brain with nutrients.[10]

The other main phospholipid is PC. The effects of PC are widespread throughout our bodies and brains. It is the most abundant molecule in your cell membranes. It helps make new brain cells, and helps maintain attention, concentration, memory, and mood, as well as boost detoxification. And it reduces the stress hormone, cortisol, which is harmful to the brain, as you will learn in chapter 12.

How does PC do all this?

It contains a vitamin called "choline," which is essential for producing acetylcholine. Acetylcholine is one of the major neurotransmitters responsible for memory, motor function, and the function of your autonomic nervous system, which regulates your unconscious bodily functions like breathing, heart rate, digestion, and all your organ functions.

PC is one of the raw materials that make up your body. Without it, you can't have healthy membranes, control your organ function, remember things, repair your brain, effectively eliminate toxins, or control inflammation. This chemical sets the stage for addressing any problem with mood, memory, attention, and behavior.

The best sources of choline are lecithin (essentially a dietary source of PC that comes from egg yolks and soybeans; it can be taken as a supplement), eggs, sardines, soybeans, nuts, and peanuts.

The *protein receptors* for all your brain neurotransmitters sit inside the fatty cell membrane. When the membrane is rigid, the receptors can't work and your brain doesn't function well. A fluid membrane improves the structure and function of protein receptors for neurotransmitters like serotonin (depression), dopamine (attention), acetylcholine (memory). Fluid membranes also improve the function of enzymes and ion channels in the membrane, leading to better cell communication and signals.

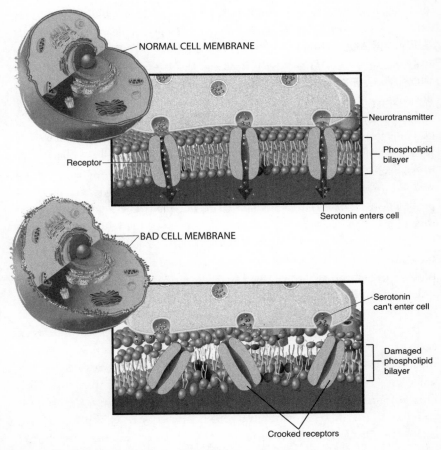

Figure 5: A normal cell membrane and a damaged cell membrane

Just eating a can of sardines (which are full of healthy omega-3 fats and phospholipids) will help your brain grow, improve connections, make mood chemicals work better, help cells communicate better, reduce inflammation, and improve the function of every cell in your body by giving them the fats they need to build smooth, fluid membranes that communicate information easily. And all that with a few bites of lunch!

To find out if omega-3 fat deficiency is a problem for you, you can go to http://efaeducation.nih.gov, enter your diet, and see the omega-3 content of your body. Or you can simply complete the quiz I gave you above to get a sense for whether or not you have nutritional deficiencies in this area.

Building healthy cell membranes is essential to fixing your broken brain. Jane's story is a great example.

Jane was a forty-two-year-old Ivy League college professor who found herself unable to think, focus, or remember scientific papers that had been a critical part of her world. Brain fog and a dark cloud of depression so limited her ability to function, that she went on disability leave.

By taking a careful history and doing some blood testing, I found that she was living in a house full of toxic molds. These molds produce highly toxic molecules as part of their defense mechanisms. They damage cells and cell membranes leading to all the symptoms Jane experienced.

We matched the molds found in her house to the mold antibodies and toxins in her blood. Based on that, she was able to get her insurance company to pay for the demolition and the rebuilding of her house.

Once we had her out of the toxic environment, we rebuilt her brain through a program of detoxification and an oil change with PC and omega-3 fats. She has now fully recovered and the brain fog and cloud of depression are gone.

So now you know what your cell membranes are made of and why it's important to keep them healthy. But how do messages flow from one cell to the next? That is where proteins and neurotransmitters come into the story.

Protein and Amino Acids: The Building Blocks of Neurotransmitters, the Language of Mood and Memory

Your brain is built from fat. The cell membranes are made of omega-3 fats, cholesterol, and the phospholipids PC and PS. You have learned why these are so important, but they are only half the story. Those trillions of cell membranes are the ears that "listen" for messages that tell your brain to be happy or sad, to focus or be inattentive, to forget or remember, to be sluggish or full of energy, to feel pain or pleasure, to relax or be stressed.

The other half of the story is protein, specifically the amino-acid building blocks of protein that get transformed in your body into the messengers, or *neurotransmitters,* which do the "talking" in your brain and throughout your body. Protein is also used to build the little *receptors,* or docking stations, for these neurotransmitters that are embedded in your cell membranes. So if your cells are going to "hear" anything at all, they need protein to help them do it.

All protein is built from special building blocks called *amino acids.* The *only* function of your DNA is to take these amino acids and string them together in chains to make protein. That's all it does!

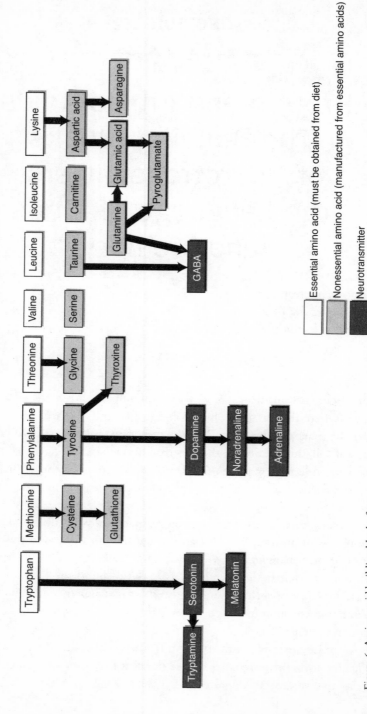

Figure 6: Amino-acid building blocks for neurotransmitters

All of the thousands of molecules in your body are built from only eight essential amino acids that we must get from our diet. These essential amino acids are the raw materials we use to make all our brain messenger chemicals or neurotransmitters and the receptors or docking stations on our cells that they land on to transmit their messages.

The only source of these amino acids is the protein you eat in your diet. Ideally the majority of this comes from fish, chicken, beans, nuts, and seeds. If you don't eat adequate protein at every meal, your brain can't work. You will be sluggish, foggy, anxious, unfocused, tired, and depressed.

The good news is that taking individual amino acids is extraordinarily effective and safe. So even if you aren't getting enough of the specific amino acids you need for optimal brain function, you can acquire them through supplements. And, if you have a genetic predisposition that requires you to take more of these amino acids than a normal diet would allow, you can *still* get them.

We will deal with how to properly supplement your diet with amino acids in Part IV of this book. Now, let's focus on the neurotransmitters your amino acids create, what they do, and their *critical* role in brain function, and talk about how nutritional deficiency leads to a dramatic breakdown in your neurotransmitters.

What Do Neurotransmitters Do?

Let's take a closer look at the neurotransmitters and their receptors, because at the end of the day without the proper balance of these molecules you cannot be happy, mentally alert, remember things, concentrate, or effectively do anything your brain is designed to do.

Neurotransmitters are the messenger molecules produced by nerve cells to communicate and control almost every function of your body. This is the way your brain "talks." Each nerve cell releases different neurotransmitters, which then have to find a spot, or "receptor," on another cell, bind to it, and communicate instructions for that cell. Once it is released, it can be recycled or broken down and destroyed.

Most of psychiatry and its tools—the drugs or psychopharmacology on which psychiatry is largely based—focus on mimicking or increasing the effects of these neurotransmitters in some way that works against the body's natural processes.

For example, antidepressants typically increase the availability of *serotonin* (the happy mood molecule) or *norepinephrine* (a stimulating and energy-giving neurotransmitter); stimulants increase *dopamine* effects (the pleasure

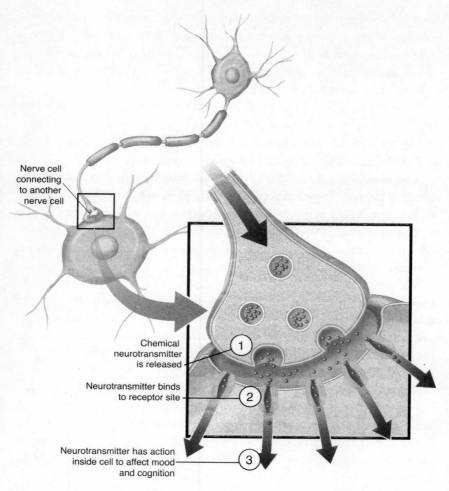

Nerve cell
connecting
to another
nerve cell

Chemical
neurotransmitter
is released

(1)

Neurotransmitter binds
to receptor site

(2)

Neurotransmitter has action
inside cell to affect mood
and cognition

(3)

Figure 7: A neurotransmitter "communicating" with another cell

and reward neurotransmitter that is responsible for attention and focus); Alzheimer's drugs increase *acetylcholine* (which is responsible for memory and focus); and anxiety drugs increase *GABA* (which puts the brakes on your excitatory neurotransmitters).

By increasing the availability of these neurotransmitters through medications, psychiatrists attempt to counteract the problems that low levels of these chemicals create in the body and mind.

Low levels of serotonin and norepinephrine show up as depression, low dopamine as attention and behavior disorders, low acetylcholine as Alzheimer's, and low GABA as anxiety. These are literally the chemical messengers of mood, learning, attention, memory, and overall brain function—they determine how you feel, how fast you learn, and how much you remember.

Artificially boosting these molecules in the brain with medication does not fix the cause of your broken brain. But here is the real problem with this kind of drug therapy: we are asking the *wrong* question!

Instead of asking which neurotransmitter we need more of or less of and then designing a drug to increase chemicals or block them as a means to generate this effect, we *should* be asking *why* these neurotransmitter levels are too low or too high in the first place.

Take serotonin, for example. This is the neurotransmitter that is responsible for a happy mood. The more serotonin in your bloodstream, the happier you will be. Imagine something wonderful happens to you one day—a job promotion, for example. Your brain sends out serotonin as a response to this event. It binds with receptors on your cells, delivering this message of happiness, and you feel amazing.

It has been shown that people who are depressed tend to make less serotonin than the "normal" population. As a result they experience less happiness and become depressed.

A billion-dollar drug sector has arisen in response to this need for more serotonin in depressed patients. Their answer is to create a drug that blocks serotonin from being reabsorbed back into the end of your nerve cells after it has sent its happy messages (which is what normally happens with the chemical). This leaves more serotonin around to create the same happy messages over and over again.

These drugs are called selective serotonin reuptake inhibitors (SSRIs). The chief among them is Prozac, and they are one of the top-selling classes of drugs in the world today.

But this whole industry is working at the wrong end of the problem.

We never ask why your serotonin levels are low in the first place or why your serotonin delivery system isn't working as it was designed to—sending the right messages but not being "heard" by your cells.

Do we have some basic defect that destines 25 percent of us to have a major depression at some point in our lives or millions more to have a "minor" depression?

The answers are available. (You *can* replenish serotonin from the ground up and help your receptors "listen" better, as you will learn in a moment.) But hardly anyone, except the tireless scientists who ask these questions, knows about it. Unfortunately, these scientists don't have billions of dollars to create television ads promoting their work like the makers of Zoloft or Prozac do!

This program is designed to support and enhance the creation and operation of your neurotransmitters and the receptors on which they dock and communicate their important information. If you are on psychiatric medications right now, the UltraMind Solution promises to enhance their effectiveness, and may allow you to come off them. If you aren't, it may offer you a solution to the mood, attention, and behavior problems you face without the need for medication.

To understand how this works, I want to introduce you to four of the most important neurotransmitters and explain how nutrition has an impact on their creation and performance.

Four Key Neurotransmitters: Dopamine, Acetylcholine, Serotonin, and GABA

These four key neurotransmitters can be subdivided into two major categories. Think of them as on and off switches for your brain. Those that excite and activate you, and those that make you calm and happy. Think of them as the gas and the brake pedals for your nervous system—the yin and yang of your nervous system.

Those that make you feel energized, excited, and stimulated, and help you focus, learn, and remember, are called *excitatory neurotransmitters*. The neurotransmitters in this category that I will discuss are dopamine (and its close cousins, epinephrine and norepinephrine) and acetylcholine.

Those that make you happy, relaxed, and peaceful are called *inhibitory neurotransmitters*. I will discuss GABA and serotonin here.

There are many other players, but the basic theme is that your nervous system has a gas pedal and a brake. The key is to keep all the brain molecules in balance. If they are in balance you are happy, focused, attentive, relaxed, and able to remember and learn effectively.

That is what the six-week plan in *The UltraMind Solution* is designed to do. Balance all the seven keys and your brain (and body) will be in balance.

Learning how these four neurotransmitters work and how to balance them is a key part of optimal brain function. So let's look at these major players:

- Dopamine and the Catecholamines (epinephrine and norepinephrine): Getting Focused
- Serotonin: Staying Happy
- GABA: Getting Relaxed
- Acetylcholine: Learning and Remembering

Dopamine and the Catecholamines: Getting Focused

Do you have low dopamine levels? Take this quiz to find out.

In the box on the right, place a check for each positive answer. Then find out how severe your problem is by using the scoring key below.

DOPAMINE QUIZ*

I feel down or depressed a lot and don't have the energy or desire to do anything. ☐
I am a low-energy kind of person mentally or physically. ☐
I struggle to get motivated to exercise. ☐
I have trouble concentrating or focusing on things. ☐
I tend to sleep a lot or have trouble waking up. ☐
I need substances such as caffeine, chocolate, "diet pills," or even cocaine to "wake" me up. ☐

---

* For your convenience, this quiz has been reprinted in *The UltraMind Solution Companion Guide*. Simply go to www.ultramind.com/guide, download the guide, and print out the quiz.

Scoring Key—Dopamine

Score one point for each box you checked.

Score	Severity	Care Plan	Action to Take
0–2	You may have a slightly low level of dopamine.	*The UltraMind Solution*	Complete the six-week program in Part III.
3–4	You may have a moderately low level of dopamine.	Self-Care	Complete the six-week program in Part III and optimize your dopamine levels using the self-care options in chapter 22.
5 and above	You may have a severely low level of dopamine.	Medical Care	Do both of the steps above and see a physician for additional assistance. I have outlined some of the options you should discuss with your doctor in chapter 22.

Dopamine is the pleasure and reward neurotransmitter. It is responsible for attention and focusing. It motivates you and stimulates you to engage in life. Its close cousins are the stimulating and energy-giving neurotransmitters epinephrine and norepinephrine.

All three are built from the amino acid *tyrosine,* which in turn comes from the essential dietary amino acid *phenylalanine.* Supplementing your diet with both of these amino acids can help mood, energy, and attention. You get these amino acids by eating high-quality protein such as beans, nuts, seeds, and lean poultry, fish, and eggs.

Dopamine levels are low in addicts, in people with low-energy types of depression as opposed to an agitated or anxious type of depression, and in people with ADHD. Stimulant drugs like Ritalin are designed to mimic dopamine effects. That is why they are prescribed to people with ADHD. Cocaine, speed, and a cup of coffee also mimic dopamine's effects. But taking any of these drugs over time (Ritalin included) depletes your body's ability to make your own dopamine, norepinephrine, and epinephrine.

This neurotransmitter is also low in Parkinson's disease. The flat, slow, and sluggish appearance of people with Parkinson's disease is because they can't produce enough dopamine.

If you have a dopamine receptor that isn't very good at "listening" to the signals, then any little stress or toxic influence like mercury can trigger a problem because toxins can interfere with the receptors' ability to listen to messages. Genetic variations in dopamine receptors have been found in people with autism and ADHD.[11; 12] So even if you have enough dopamine, the receptors may not work as well, leading to ADHD, autism, and mood disorders.

The good news is that we *can* improve the function of these receptors with proper nutrition (remember how fats influence neurotransmitter and receptor production) and vitamin supplementation (especially folate, B_6, and B_{12}, which you will learn more about a little later in this chapter). Both improve your cells' ability to "listen" as well as produce more neurotransmitters.[13]

That's why studies show that supplementing with the amino acid tyrosine, as well as essential fats (omega-3 fats, PC, and PS) and special nutrients (folate, B_{12}, and B_6), can improve depression, ADHD, and Parkinson's.[14] These nutrients give your body what it needs to function as it was designed, and to repair the damage that leads to conditions like these in the first place.

In fact, nutrients often work better than conventional medication and without side effects, because they are part of your brain's natural raw materials and design.

Tyrosine is a wonderful, safe, cheap way to boost dopamine levels. Even the military has researched it and uses it to boost physical and mental performance during stressful conditions.[15] (In fact, I am using it to help me stay focused and write this book!) And the amino acid phenylalanine can be very helpful in boosting the other energy-giving, motivating, and focusing neurotransmitter norepinephrine. You will learn more tips on how to do this in chapter 22.

Serotonin: Staying Happy

Do you have low serotonin levels? Take the following quiz to find out.

In the box on the right, place a check for each positive answer. Then find out how severe your problem is by using the scoring key below.

SEROTONIN QUIZ*

My head is full of ANTS (automatic negative thoughts). ☐
I am a glass half-empty person. ☐
I have low self-esteem and self-confidence. ☐
I tend to have obsessive thoughts and behaviors (such as being a
perfectionist or neat freak, or other more severe forms of OCD). ☐
I get the winter blues or have SAD (seasonal affective disorder). ☐
I tend to be irritable, easily angered, and/or impatient. ☐
I am shy and afraid of going out or have fear of heights, crowds,
flying, and/or speaking in public. ☐
I feel anxious or have panic attacks. ☐
I have PMS (premenstrual syndrome with moodiness, cravings,
breast tenderness, and bloating before my period). ☐
I have trouble falling asleep. ☐
I wake up in the middle of the night and have trouble getting back
to sleep, or wake up too early in the morning. ☐
I crave sweets or starchy carbs like bread and pasta. ☐
I feel better when I exercise. ☐
I have muscle aches, fibromyalgia, and/or jaw pain (TMJ). ☐
I have been treated with and felt better when taking SSRIs
(serotonin-boosting antidepressants). ☐

---

* For your convenience, this quiz has been reprinted in *The UltraMind Solution Companion Guide*. Simply go to www.ultramind.com/guide, download the guide, and print out the quiz.

Scoring Key–Serotonin

Score one point for each box you checked.

Score	Severity	Care Plan	Action to Take
0–4	You may have a slightly low level of serotonin.	*The UltraMind Solution*	Complete the six-week program in Part III.
5–7	You may have a moderately low level of serotonin.	Self-Care	Complete the six-week program in Part III and optimize your serotonin levels using the self-care options in chapter 22.
8 and above	You may have a severely low level of serotonin.	Medical Care	Do both of the steps above and see a physician for additional assistance. I have outlined some of the options you should discuss with your doctor in chapter 22.

Everyone knows about serotonin. It is the feel-good molecule we are all in short supply of in our overstressed society. A severe lack of it is what makes people feel depressed. We use drugs like Prozac and Zoloft to make it more available to us, but these create problems for us in the long run, as you now know.

Interestingly, one of the reasons most people eat refined carbohydrates or sugars is to boost serotonin levels temporarily (which is one of the effects of these sugars), then they crash, which sends them out hunting for something starchy or sugary. Unfortunately, this ultimately makes us feel more depressed and causes us to gain weight—not a very effective strategy.

We certainly know that serotonin is necessary for a happy mood, reducing anxiety and irritability, and helping us to sleep. But why are our serotonin levels so low, and how does the body naturally produce serotonin? If we know that, we can take away the things that reduce serotonin and provide the things that help the body make more. And we can do this with much greater effectiveness and fewer side effects than medication.

Why Your Serotonin Levels Are Low

In the daily activity of any neurotransmitter there are so many things that can go wrong and cause it to malfunction in some way. Here is why serotonin levels go south.

❖ A tryptophan-deficient or low-protein diet. Tryptophan is the primary amino acid out of which serotonin is created. No tryptophan equals no serotonin equals a very unhappy mood. In fact, studies show that if you feed a group of people a mixture of amino acids without tryptophan you can induce depression within *hours!*[16]

❖ Stress and high cortisol levels (the stress hormone). Cortisol increases the activity of enzymes that break down tryptophan. That leaves less around to make serotonin.

❖ Anything that causes inflammation (such as food allergies, infections, toxins, or a high-sugar diet). Inflammatory messenger molecules called *cytokines* such as interferon gamma (INF γ) stimulate the enzymes TDO and IDO, which break down tryptophan and force it into a pathway that makes the excitatory neurotransmitter *glutamate*, which kills brain cells.

❖ Simply not making enough serotonin. This happens for many reasons. You may not have enough of the building blocks (the amino-acid tryptophan) because you eat too much sugar and not enough protein as suggested above, or you may have genetic predispositions that make it more difficult for you to create the neurotransmitter in the first place.★

❖ Blood-sugar imbalances (insulin resistance or prediabetes). This condition (which you will learn more about in chapter 7) comes from eating a processed-food, high-sugar diet. It depletes your serotonin after a short spike, leading to mood swings.

❖ You may be deficient in vitamin B_6. B_6 is the helper or catalyst for the enzyme that converts tryptophan into serotonin. Deficiency in B_6 is often caused by stress, alcohol, and medications like birth-control pills.

❖ Magnesium deficiency. This is so common in our society because stress, caffeine, sugar, and alcohol all deplete magnesium, which in turn prevents the body from making serotonin.

★ Those who have an SNP (single nucleotide polymorphism) or genetic variation of the enzyme THP2 have an 80 percent reduction in ability to make serotonin.

The good news is that you can overcome this weakness by taking folate and the supplement 5-HTP (5-hydroxytryptophan), which is normally produced from 5-HTP dietary tryptophan, the molecule that is the next step in the process of making serotonin. If you take 5-HTP, you skip that weak step.

Those are just a few of the ways that the production of *one* neurotransmitter can be inhibited. And every one of them is similarly influenced by your diet and lifestyle. So let's see . . . what are your options here? Take Prozac, an SSRI, which helps to improve half the symptoms half the time with plenty of side effects, or try to cut out sugar in your diet, eliminate food allergies and toxins, learn how to manage stress, and take B$_6$, folate, magnesium, and amino acids, which have no side effects and correct the cause of your depleted serotonin production in the first place.

What would you choose?

When Prozac came on the market, most of the research on the use of tryptophan or its by-product, 5-HTP, to help the body naturally produce serotonin, slowed way down or was stopped.

But the evidence is strong that supplementing with the building blocks of serotonin, while at the same time addressing the other underlying reasons for low-serotonin production, is not only safer but more effective than just taking Prozac or other SSRIs.[17;18]

No one has committed suicide because he or she was taking vitamins or amino acids, but there is up to a 60 percent increased risk of suicide attempts in people taking some types of antidepressants and an overall 39 percent increase in suicide from all antidepressants.[19] You don't hear about nutritional treatments like these, because supplement manufacturers don't have billions to advertise on television or millions to fund large studies the way pharmaceutical companies do.

In chapter 22, you will learn how to fix low serotonin levels naturally, using the concepts I have discussed here.

GABA: Get Relaxed

Do you have low GABA levels? Take the following quiz to find out.

In the box on the right, place a check for each positive answer. Then find out how severe your problem is using the scoring key below.

GABA QUIZ*

It is hard for me to relax and kick back. ☐
I am easily stressed out or overwhelmed. ☐
It is common for me to feel overworked or pressured. ☐
My body is stiff or uptight. ☐
I sometimes feel weak and shaky. ☐
I am bothered by loud noises, lights, or too much activity. ☐

I feel more anxious or stressed if I skip meals. ☐
I use substances such as sugar, alcohol, and/or drugs
to help me relax. ☐

---

* For your convenience, this quiz has been reprinted in *The UltraMind Solution Companion Guide*. Simply go to www.ultramind.com/guide, download the guide, and print out the quiz.

Scoring Key—GABA

Score one point for each box you checked.

Score	Severity	Care Plan	Action to Take
0–2	You may have a slightly low level of GABA.	*The UltraMind Solution*	Complete the six-week program in Part III.
3–4	You may have a moderately low level of GABA.	Self-Care	Complete the six-week program in Part III and optimize your GABA levels using the self-care options in chapter 22.
5 and above	You may have a severely low level of GABA.	Medical Care	Do both of the steps above and see a physician for additional assistance. I have outlined some of the options you should discuss with your doctor in chapter 22.

We are a stressed-out society. And we push ourselves to burnout with habits like overworking, not enough sleep, too much coffee, too much sugar, refined foods, and junk food that we use to temporarily relieve our stress, as well as exposure to environmental toxins and silent infections.

Your adrenal glands produce powerful chemicals (cortisol, epinephrine, and norepinephrine) that help you respond to stress. These chemicals are excitatory hormones, neurotransmitters that get our bodies ready for dangerous situations (which was the original purpose of the anxiety response).

However, with your foot to the gas pedal like this all the time, you burn out and feel stressed, anxious, exhausted, can't sleep, and are either tired or wired constantly.

Thankfully, our brains have an antidote to these stress hormones.

It is called GABA (gamma-aminobutyric acid) and it calms the brain from too much of the neurotransmitters epinephrine and norepinephrine.

It is like a brake on overstimulation in the brain. When you have low levels of GABA, it is harder for you to relax after your body has released these excitatory neurotransmitters.

People with anxiety, panic attacks, insomnia, seizures, and schizophrenia all have low levels of GABA. Who likes the feeling of tense muscles, a pounding heart, dry mouth, sleeplessness, fatigue, and sweaty palms? No one. That's why so many self-medicate with the medications mentioned above.

Valium works by imitating GABA, our natural brain relaxant. Many use alcohol or marijuana to self-medicate for anxiety. These too act like GABA in the brain. But using alcohol, marijuana, or tranquilizers backfires because they are all addictive and produce diminishing returns over time so you need more and more to "relax."

Why not just take GABA supplements? Well, thankfully, you can. And you can use other natural substances to boost GABA levels to overcome the anxiety that millions of you experience every day.

One study showed that within sixty minutes of taking GABA, alpha brain waves (a sign of relaxation) were increased on EEG tests. Taking GABA also boosted the immune system, which functions best when you are relaxed.[20]

You can take GABA supplements directly, or supplement your diet with the raw materials out of which GABA is produced. For example, another key amino-acid helper called *taurine* boosts the production of GABA and helps relax the nervous system. It can even reduce seizures.[21]

Other helpful brain relaxants that boost GABA include theanine from green tea, inositol (a B vitamin), other B vitamins such as B_3, B_6, and B_{12}, and magnesium. Calming herbs such as kava, valerian, hops, and passion flower can also be helpful.

Later I will show you how to use these natural stress antidotes to balance your brain.

Acetylcholine: Remembering and Learning Things

In the box on the right, place a check for each positive answer. Then find out how severe your problem is using the scoring key below.

ACETYLCHOLINE QUIZ*

I find myself writing things down so I won't forget them.	☐
I find it hard to do math in my head.	☐
I have a hard time finding words or remembering what I was saying if interrupted during a conversation.	☐
I get nervous or anxious when I have to learn something new like new software at work.	☐
When reading a book or watching a movie I find it harder to follow the plot than it used to be.	☐
I misplace my keys, wallet, or glasses frequently.	☐
I have trouble focusing during long conversations or meetings.	☐
I feel like my brain is just not functioning at its peak.	☐

_____

* For your convenience, this quiz has been reprinted in _The UltraMind Solution Companion Guide_. Simply go to www.ultramind.com/guide, download the guide, and print out the quiz.

Scoring Key—Acetylcholine

Score one point for each box you checked.

Score	Severity	Care Plan	Action to Take
0–2	You may have a slightly low level of acetylcholine.	_The UltraMind Solution_	Complete the six-week program in Part III.
3–4	You may have a moderately low level of acetylcholine.	Self-Care	Complete the six-week program in Part III and optimize your acetylcholine levels using the self-care options in chapter 22.
5 and above	You may have a severely low level of acetylcholine.	Medical Care	Do both of the steps above and see a physician for additional assistance. I have outlined some of the options you should discuss with your doctor in chapter 22.

If you have trouble remembering and learning new things, chances are your levels of this very important neurotransmitter are depleted. Acetylcholine helps with sharpening your thinking process, memory, motivation, and concentration.

In fact, the cells that produce acetylcholine in the brain are damaged in people with Alzheimer's, which accounts for their dementia. Most of the drugs that treat dementia are designed to block the action of the enzyme that breaks down acetylcholine in the brain. In this way they are similar to SSRIs, which block the reuptake of serotonin after it has been used. But dementia drugs have even worse side effects and not much benefit.[22]

The real questions are why are your cells damaged in the first place, and how can you help your body naturally make more acetylcholine?

The good news is that we know what damages the brain—imbalances in the seven keys—and we can address the problem systemically. We can use natural substances to help boost acetylcholine just as we can with all the other neurotransmitters we have discussed in this section.

This neurotransmitter is made from the B vitamin choline (as you may remember from our discussion above about PC), with the help of another B vitamin called B_5 or pantothenic acid. Eggs and lecithin from soy are great dietary sources of choline. And supplementing with PC and PS helps the body make more of it as well.

Keep in mind that what I have just described covers only four of the major neurotransmitters that dictate how you feel, how clearly you think, how attentive you are, and how well you remember things.

There are dozens of others.

The UltraMind Solution allows you to get all of them back in balance. By doing so, you take one more step away from the mood, memory, and behavior problems that plague you—and one step closer to UltraWellness.

If you don't think this has the potential to help you heal your brain, let me tell you a story.

At thirty-six, Sarah was a doctor who had long suffered a low-grade depression. She found herself anxious, unable to fall asleep easily, and often woke up at 3 A.M. unable to sleep the rest of the night.

All her life she had been a perfectionist, impatient with her children, her husband, and herself.

Her premenstrual syndrome had been getting worse over the years, with bloating, sugar cravings, breast tenderness, and terrible mood swings.

The world had always seemed to have a dullness to it, and her ability to experience joy at seeing a sunset or pleasure from her daily life felt limited. The glass always seemed half empty.

She tried to live well—ate fresh whole foods, exercised regularly, and did yoga. But she just couldn't get the dark cloud to lift. Nothing in her outer world seemed to con-

tribute to her suffering. She had a great job, wonderful friends and family, no great stresses or losses—just no joy.

Upon testing, we found she had very depleted amino acids and very low levels of vitamin B_6, essential for making serotonin. It turned out she had chronic mercury toxicity, which depleted all her amino acids because they help the body get rid of toxins.

In the long run we got rid of her mercury, but in the short run, just by taking vitamin B_6 (along with its helper folate and B_{12}) and 5 HTP (5-hydroxytryptophan) to boost serotonin levels naturally, she felt the cloud lift, her sleep improve, her PMS diminish, and her ability to experience joy return.

Carbohydrates: Whole Food for a Whole Brain

Carbohydrates are the single most important food for long-term health and brain function.

This may be a shocking statement given the low-carb movement and "carbophobia" in America, but it's true.

Of course, I don't mean the overprocessed, refined, sugary white food we commonly think of as carbohydrates, such as doughnuts, bread, bagels, muffins, colas, juices, and most junk food.

And I don't mean the cheap, supersweet, government-subsidized high-fructose corn syrup that is driving our epidemic of obesity and disease and contributing to our epidemic of mental illness.

The carbohydrates I am talking about are the real, whole, nourishing plant foods that the human species has thrived on since the dawn of evolution.

In *UltraMetabolism: The Simple Plan for Automatic Weight Loss,* I explained that most of the foods consumed by humans over the years have been carbohydrates.

Plant foods are composed mostly of carbohydrates: *vegetables, fruits, beans, whole grains, nuts, seeds, herbs, and spices.*

These foods contain slowly released sources of sugar that prevent surges of blood sugar and insulin, toxic to the brain (see chapter 7).

The slowly released carbohydrates from whole, unprocessed plant foods also helps keep our serotonin levels even.

Carbohydrates also contain *all* the vitamins (except B_{12}) and minerals our bodies need to operate normally and optimally.

They also contain fiber, which helps normalize our digestive function and slows the absorption of sugar and fats into the body, which keeps us balanced.

The bonus factor in plant foods are *phytonutrients*—colorful healing compounds made by plants to protect themselves, but which also protect us against aging, obesity, brain damage, and more.

For example, broccoli and the rest of the cruciferous vegetable family contain powerful detoxifying compounds that protect us against environmental toxins. Green tea contains anti-inflammatory, antioxidant, and detoxifying properties. Resveratrol from red grapes boosts our energy production and protects our cells. These are just a few examples of the thousands of phytonutrients in the plant foods that should be the foundation of our diet.

Michael Pollan, the author of *The Omnivore's Dilemma,* summed up all nutritional research in three simple principles:

"Eat food. Not too much. Mostly plants."

In fact, you need know nothing else to be vibrantly healthy.

That's it. Eat real, whole food as it comes from the earth: fresh vegetables, fruits, beans, whole grains, nuts, seeds, herbs and spices, and lean animal protein like fish, chicken, and eggs. Imagine what your great-grandmother would recognize as food, or what might have been on her dinner table. Just food. There is really no such thing as junk food—there is just food, and then there is junk.

Vitamins and Minerals: Will They Give You a Metabolic Tune-Up or Just Make Expensive Urine?

✧

I don't think people need vitamins and they are a waste of money . . .

That is *only* if they eat wild, fresh, whole, organic, local, nongenetically modified food grown in virgin mineral- and nutrient-rich soils and not transported across vast distances and stored for months before being eaten. And if they work and live outside, breathe only fresh unpolluted air, drink only pure, clean water, sleep nine hours a night, move their bodies every day, and are free from chronic stressors and exposure to environmental toxins.

Then we don't need vitamins.

But, of course, I have described absolutely no one on the planet. In reality, we *all* need vitamins.

Most people don't understand the role of vitamins and minerals in our bodies. I certainly didn't when I finished medical training.

I thought if we just had enough to prevent us from some horrible deficiency state like scurvy (vitamin C deficiency), then we didn't have to worry about how much we were getting.

I also thought that if we ate "enriched food" like white flour with a few vitamins added back in, or milk with vitamin D added in, additional vitamin supplementation was a waste.

What most people don't realize is the same thing I was unaware of when I first started practicing medicine: the real reason our food supply must be "enriched" is because it is so processed that it is "impoverished" to start with.

So why can't you just eat "nutrient-rich" food, instead of eating "nutrient-poor" food?

Today, even with our "enriched food," more than 92 percent of Americans are deficient in one or more vitamins. That doesn't mean they are receiving less than the amount they need for optimal health. It means they receive less than the *minimum* amount necessary to prevent deficiency diseases.

In a study published in the *American Journal of Public Health,* researchers found that 6 percent of those tested had serious vitamin C deficiency and 30 percent were borderline low.[23] A report in the journal *Pediatrics* found obesity and malnutrition coexisting. Obese, overfed, and undernourished children with cognitive disorders were found to have scurvy and severe vitamin D deficiency or rickets. These deficiencies damaged their brains.[24] You never think of overweight people as malnourished, but they can be!

A USDA survey showed that 37 percent of Americans don't get enough vitamin C, 70 percent not enough vitamin E, almost 75 percent not enough zinc, and 40 percent not enough iron.[25]

I would say 100 percent of us don't have enough of the basic nutrients to create optimal health or give ourselves a metabolic tune-up.

There are many reasons the foods you eat no longer contain the nutrient levels you require for optimal health. Crops are raised in soil where nutrients have been depleted. Plants are treated with pesticides and other chemicals so they no longer have to fight to live, which further diminishes their nutrient levels and their phytonutrient content (not to mention the toxic exposure you receive from such chemicals). Animals are cooped-up in pens or giant feedlots instead of roaming free, eating the nutrient-rich wild grains and grasses they once consumed. Since cows' stomachs are adapted to grass instead of the corn they now eat, they must take antibiotics to prevent them from exploding.

To complicate this further, all of us are exposed to hazardous toxins and chemicals that poison our bodies, we live with too much stress, we don't sleep enough, we don't exercise enough, and we are inflamed, making the nutritional demands on our bodies even heavier.

In today's world *everyone* needs a basic multivitamin and mineral supplement. The research is overwhelming on this point.[26]

The question is not how much of a certain nutrient or vitamin do we need not to get sick, but how much do we need to be optimally healthy!★ In fact, lower amounts recommended by the government may *not* be high enough.

For most people, a high-quality multivitamin; a calcium–magnesium supplement; vitamin D; fish oil; and special B vitamin complex including folate, B_6, and B_{12} will take care of the basics. I will give you specific guidelines on this basic supplement program in Part III.

I have tested for vitamin and nutrient deficiencies in thousands of patients and found that by correcting them people feel better, improve their mood, mental sharpness, memory, and ability to focus, as well as have more energy, and even lose weight. Correcting deficiencies also helps prevent disease. I have seen depression, anxiety, bipolar disease, autism, ADHD, mood swings, Parkinson's, and dementia go away or dramatically improve.

The basic vitamin recommendations outlined above (which I will discuss in more detail in Part III) include nutrients that form the backbone for proper brain function, for mood, memory, behavior, and attention problems. They are needed to fix your broken brain.

Let's take a look at the way nutrient deficiencies affect our health and our brain function.

Nutrients: The Keys to Health and Brain Power

Nutrients are powerful in both sickness and in health. Imagine a world where hundreds of debilitating, severe, often life-threatening diseases could be cured within days by taking substances without any side effects; substances that are completely safe and cost only pennies a day. That is the power of vitamins and minerals.

★ Dr. Robert Heaney, one of the world's leading vitamin D researchers, in a recent groundbreaking editorial in *The American Journal of Clinical Nutrition* about the delayed (yet very serious) consequences of taking *less* than the optimal amounts of nutrients for life, said that "because the current [vitamin] recommendations are based on the prevention of [deficiency] disease only, they can no longer be said to be biologically defensible. The pre-agricultural human diet . . . may well be a better starting point for policy. The burden of proof should fall on those who say that these more natural conditions are not needed and that lower intakes [of nutrients] are safe."

Now imagine that very few people were being treated with these cost-effective, safe, extremely effective strategies.

Imagine what the medical ward might look like.

As you walked the halls you would see endless suffering: people with teeth falling out and bleeding gums, blindness, insanity, dementia, scaly bloody skin, uncontrollable diarrhea, severe depression, diabetes, and heart attacks. You would see people unable to walk because of lack of balance, children unable to talk and locked in their inner worlds, those whose bones bend under the weight of their bodies, people with loss of nerve function, severe infections that can't be cured with antibiotics, pale skin, hair falling all over the floor, and peeling or grossly deformed fingernails that take the shape of spoons.

These are the symptoms of vitamin and mineral deficiencies. Today we live in such a world. For some, symptoms of nutrient deficiency may be subtle. In fact, they are often invisible. But they cause no less suffering.

Many of the day-to-day complaints we think we have to live with as we age are the result of nutritional deficiencies.

These nutritional deficiencies range from problems like the epidemic of broken brains (which can be traced back to our nutrient-depleted toxic diet) to problems like reflux, allergies, and asthma to chronic diseases like heart disease, diabetes, and cancer.

Whether you are suffering from a bad mood, difficulty concentrating, or have a more serious condition such as depression or Alzheimer's disease, it is likely that nutritional deficiencies are one of the primary causes.

This is not a nutrition textbook, but I must focus on a few important nutrients for optimal brain function, how they affect your mind and body, and what happens if you don't get them. Essential nutrients are called "essential" because they are just that. Without them we cannot survive and thrive. That is why I recommend that *everyone* take a full complement of essential nutrients *every day*. I will explain which nutrients you need to take daily in Part III.

Some may need more or less of these nutrients, and some may need a special form. But we *all* need *all* of them. They work to run your biochemistry. Without them, the functions of your mind and body slow down or grind to a halt. These nutrients are the stuff of life.

Do you need a study to tell you that you need to drink water, breathe air, and sleep every night? You don't need a study to know you require these nutrients either (though there are literally hundreds of studies that prove you do).

These are the essential ingredients for being alive. It is that simple.

Essential Daily Vitamins and Minerals

Vitamins

Vitamin A
Carotenoids
Vitamin D
Vitamin E
Vitamin K
Vitamin C
Vitamin B_1 (thiamin)
Vitamin B_2 (riboflavin)

Vitamin B_3 (niacin)
Vitamin B_5 (pantothenic acid)
Vitamin B_6 (folic acid)
Vitamin B_{12}
Biotin
Choline
Inositol

Minerals

Macrominerals (needed in large amounts)

Calcium
Chloride
Magnesium
Phosphorus

Potassium
Sodium
Sulfur

Trace Minerals (needed in small or trace amounts)

Copper
Iodine
Iron
Manganese
Molybdenum
Selenium

Vanadium
Zinc
Boron
Chromium
Silicon

Essential Amino Acids

Tryptophan
Methionine
Phenylalanine
Threonine

Valine
Leucine
Isoleucine
Lysine

Essential Fatty Acids

Omega-6 Fats

Linoleic acid

Gamma linolenic acid (GLA)

Omega-3 Fats

Alpha linoleic acid (ALA)
Eicosapentanoic acid (EPA)

Docosahexaenoic acid (DHA)

SPECIAL NOTE ON CONDITIONALLY ESSENTIAL NUTRIENTS

Our bodies are resourceful and make most of what we need from a very few basic raw materials. However, under certain conditions, such as stress, toxicity, medication use, infection, genetic variations, or aging, we may need what are called "*conditionally essential*" nutrients. They are called that because they are needed under certain special conditions.

Many of the brain-supportive nutrients, including amino acids like tyrosine, special fats like phosphatidylserine, or parts of our normal biochemistry such as coenzyme Q10, acetyl-L-carnitine, alpha lipoic acid, and others, fall into this category.

While not everyone may need them, many of us do, particularly if we are in the category of the 162 million with chronic illness. They are very helpful in clearing up biochemical traffic jams and train wrecks and making things run the way they were designed so we can function optimally and thrive in every way—mentally, emotionally, physically, and spiritually.

A New Model of Nutrition: Turning "Minimum Daily Requirements" Upside Down

Doctors learn that vitamins are important to prevent deficiency diseases (diseases caused by a lack of specific vitamins or minerals) like scurvy or rickets. Too little vitamin C and you get scurvy. Too little vitamin D and you get rickets. That's it. That is the extent of our nutritional training.

However, there is a new concept emerging. Having enough of a nutrient to prevent one of these deficiency diseases, but *not enough to optimize cellular function,* will lead to "long-latency" deficiency diseases (diseases that take a long time to manifest themselves) like heart disease, cancer, depression, schizophrenia, attention–deficit disorder, or Alzheimer's disease.

For example, if you are severely deficient in folic acid, you will have anemia after a few months, or have a baby with birth defects. This is a deficiency disease. But if you don't have enough folic acid for optimal function over thirty to forty years, you will double your risk of Alzheimer's disease.[27] This is a long-latency deficiency disease. There are dozens of examples like this of diseases caused by long-term nutrient deficiency.

Let's examine our old model of nutrition, and how we need a radically different view if we are to effectively address, not only our broken brains but also all chronic illness.

The old model of nutrition is based on providing the minimum amount of nutrients, vitamins, and minerals to prevent deficiency diseases. The questions being asked are: how much vitamin C is needed to prevent scurvy? How much thiamine is needed to prevent beriberi? How much niacin is needed to prevent pellagra? How much vitamin D is needed to prevent rickets?

The answer is not very much.

Understanding the role of vitamins and minerals in health this way is based on the concept that individual nutrients have one physiological role: to prevent the deficiency diseases. Vitamin C prevents scurvy. Vitamin D prevents rickets. That's it. As long as you don't have those problems, you are getting enough of the vitamins and minerals you need.

The current dietary reference intakes (DRIs), or the amount of nutrients we are told is safe and desirable by the government, are based on this outdated concept. Oddly, the USDA, or United States Department of Agriculture, not the Health and Human Services Department, sets the DRIs. Unfortunately, our nutritional needs, agricultural policy, and government subsidies of our industrial food supply compete with each other. The subsidies are primarily for corn and soybeans, which are used to make high-fructose corn syrup, trans fats, and most of the raw materials for the fast food, junk food, and processed food industry. Policy often overrides science in the end.

The thinking that led us to believe the DRIs are suitable recommendations for what we need to operate optimally is no longer scientifically sound. Since the human genome has been deciphered, we now recognize that there is vast biochemical variability within the population.

We all have unique nutritional and biochemical needs.

Using a single baseline for determining the dietary reference intakes for different people in the population does not fit with our understanding of this biochemical diversity. Different people have different needs. Some need more of particular types of vitamins and minerals than others.

What's more, there is mounting evidence that taking just enough of a vitamin to avoid deficiency diseases doesn't give you *nearly* enough of that vitamin to achieve optimal health.

To understand this, we need to take a look at how your genetic makeup, the nutrients you consume, and special proteins called enzymes all work together to determine how healthy or ill you are mentally and physically.

This information is going to revolutionize the way you think about your health.

So how are genes and vitamins connected?

Vitamins, Genes, and Enzymes: Making Things Happen in Your Body

Humans have approximately thirty thousand genes. In that sense we are not that different from an earthworm.

What makes humans different from earthworms (and from each other) is the 1.5 to 3 million subtle differences in their genes called polymorphisms (single nucleotide polymorphisms, or SNPs). These slight alterations in your genetic structure determine everything—all the quirky, individual tendencies you have. They also create the unique biochemical needs within the population.

How?

The only function of your DNA is to make proteins, as I said earlier (page 95). Enzymes are one of thousands of proteins created from your DNA. However, these particular proteins are critically important, because they are the catalysts that help turn one molecule into another—they are the helpers that slow down or speed up all the trillions of chemical reactions that happen every second in your body.

Nutrients, in turn, control the function of these enzymes. They tell your enzymes what to do. They turn on or turn off the chemical reactions in your body.

Making Happy Mood Chemicals

Let's look at how we make serotonin as an example of how this works. Serotonin is a peptide (which is just a little protein) known as a neurotransmitter, which boosts our mood. You don't eat serotonin, but your body makes it. It builds serotonin from the amino-acid tryptophan that comes from the protein in our turkey sandwich.

The enzyme designed to convert tryptophan from turkey into serotonin needs vitamin B_6, or pyridoxine, to help it perform its chemical wizardry. No B_6, no enzyme reaction, no serotonin, no happy mood. The result? Depression—along with a host of other potential problems.

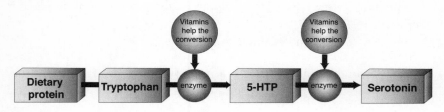

Figure 8: Conversion of dietary protein to serotonin

But the real critical element in this equation is *you*. You may need more B_6 to get your enzymes to turn tryptophan into serotonin than your next-door neighbor does. Your genes may not have created an enzyme that is as responsive to B_6 as your neighbor's enzymes are, or just runs a little more slowly. Hence you need *more* B_6 to do the job.

Why?

Because you are a genetically unique individual. As a result your enzymes are constructed differently and respond to nutrients differently than those of your neighbors. About one-third (or 1 million) of your SNPs (the variations in your genes) are dedicated solely to the job of determining how effectively your enzymes are controlled by the nutrients you consume!

Why is this critical to your health? If you understand that one-third of the *entire* variation in your genetic code affects the function of your enzymes, and that nutrients are the control switches for those enzymes, you will want to make sure you have all the right raw materials (nutrients) to make those enzymes function optimally.

Right?

What happens if you don't get the right nutrients to help your enzymes function optimally? It's simple: you get sick. If your enzymes run too slowly or too quickly your core systems get pushed out of balance. The results are mental disorders, illness, and weight gain. Controlling the function of your enzymes means controlling your health.

This is why nutrients are so essential. Without them, your biochemical wheels grind to a halt. Your enzymes don't get the messages they need to perform their critical functions. Of course, this isn't an all-or-nothing situation. It's not as though you either have nutrients or you don't. You have differing levels of nutrients and different enzymes that respond differently than other people's enzymes do to these nutrients.

This is why making sure you have the right amount of nutrients for *you* is so important. And one of the easiest ways to do that is by taking vitamins and minerals. Vitamins and minerals are the cofactors (or *coenzymes*) that make things runs smoothly. Vitamins and minerals help your enzymes do what they were intended to do.

It is for this reason that using a single baseline like the DRI to determine everyone's nutritional needs no longer makes sense. The overwhelming evidence that now exists indicates that giving *more* than the minimum amount of nutrients necessary to avoid deficiency diseases may be critical to healing disease.

Bruce Ames, Ph.D., professor of biochemistry and molecular biology, at the University of California, Berkeley, in his landmark review of over fifty enzymes controlled by nutrients that vary genetically from person to person, states that: "Our analysis of metabolic disease that affects cofactor binding [the joining of the vitamin or nutrient to the enzyme], particularly as a result of polymorphic mutations [person-to-person genetic variations], may present a novel rationale for high-dose vitamin therapy, perhaps *hundreds of times* the normal dietary reference intakes (DRI) in some cases."[28]

This means that genetically some of us may require much higher (and even mega) doses of certain vitamins for our enzymes and cells just to function normally. In fact, many of us are born with needs that may be two to one hundred times higher than someone else's.

Few Vitamins and Minerals, Many Jobs

Also absent from our current nutritional recommendations is the notion that each vitamin and mineral has many—and sometimes hundreds—of functions. The body uses the same nutrients for many different jobs. A single nutrient may catalyze hundreds of biochemical reactions and suboptimal levels may lead to cellular and molecular dysfunction that is not recognized as a "deficiency disease," yet still has a dramatic impact on our health.[29]

For example, just a little vitamin D[30;31] prevents rickets, but a higher dose may have a role in treating or preventing heart disease, osteoporosis, tuberculosis, multiple sclerosis, polycystic ovarian syndrome, depression, epilepsy, type 1 diabetes, and cancer. Folate not only prevents dementia, but also depression, colon and breast cancer, birth defects, Down syndrome, and more. Magnesium plays a role in over three hundred enzyme reactions.

That's only three vitamins and minerals! Imagine the havoc suboptimal levels of many or all of the nutrients I listed on pages 118–19 might wreak on your body.

Robert Heaney, M.D., professor of medicine at Creighton University,[32] admonishes us that this view overlooks two important facts.

First, living for a long time with suboptimal levels of nutrients may cause similar but more subtle effects as the regular deficiency diseases. For example, having soft, tender bones may result from low-grade vitamin D deficiency. Though this wouldn't be defined as rickets, the effects are similar.

Second, there may also be very different mechanisms for developing disease after many years of low-grade deficiency because nutrients are involved in so many body functions. That is how suboptimal levels of folate can lead to cancer, heart disease, depression, or dementia.

The bottom line: we need nutrients, they are essential, and without them our bodies and our brains don't function.

Now that we have established the critical role of nutrients as the building blocks of life, let's look more closely at the ones that are the most important for the brain and mind.

The Mighty Methylators for Mental Health: Folate, B$_6$, and B$_{12}$

If you have ever seen a map of the New York subway system you know it is an incredibly complex interconnected set of train tracks. Imagine what would happen if there were a break in those tracks. Worse, imagine what would happen if there were a break in the tracks at Penn Station or Grand Central Terminal. Much of the interconnected networks of trains would slow or shut down.

If you have ever seen a map of the biochemical pathways of a human being you know that it is thousands of times more complex than the New York subway. This map would fill an entire wall, and the words would be so small you could barely read them.

The most important set of biochemical pathways in your body, perhaps the central switching station for the whole operation, are the "train tracks" responsible for keeping two specific trains (or biochemical processes) running smoothly. They are the "*methylation*" train and the "*sulfation*" train.

Many critical steps of our biology depend on these trains running smoothly and constantly. A break in the tracks on which these critical, interconnected processes depend causes *many* illnesses.

Problems with methylation and sulfation are involved in all mental illness and neurological dysfunction, especially depression, autism, attention deficit disorder, Alzheimer's, Parkinson's, and more. They are also responsible for heart disease and cancer.

There are a few processes so central to health and biology that they explain much of what goes wrong with our brains, and how disease is created in general. Methylation and sulfation are two such processes. Think of these as natural laws—like the laws of physics—that explain all the phenomena we see with a few basic principles. Think of these interconnected biochemical pathways as part of the basic laws of biology.

In fact, breaks in the methylation and sulfation tracks are the deep roots of nearly all illness and can explain what goes wrong in nearly *all* the other keys of UltraWellness.

Why Are "Methylation" and "Sulfation" So Important?

Every important function in our bodies is regulated by or depends on these simple processes.

Our genes and our nutritional state control whether the methylation and sulfation trains run slowly or quickly, and whether or not they are likely to run off the tracks. Good genes and good nutrition lead to on-time express trains. Bad genes, poor diet, and toxins lead to train wrecks.

The good news is that these processes can be almost completely fixed through diet, detoxification, and special nutritional supplements, even if you have "bad" genes.

For methylation and sulfation to stay on track, your body needs a daily source of three special vitamins—B_{12}, B_6, *and folate*—to help keep the process of *methylation* running.

Beside B_{12}, B_6, and folate the body also needs a continual source of *sulfur* for the *sulfation* train specifically. This comes from foods like broccoli and garlic as well as fish, eggs, sunflower seeds, and poultry, which are high in methionine, and can be boosted by special nutrients such as NAC (n-acetylcysteine) and alpha lipoic acid and an herb like milk thistle.

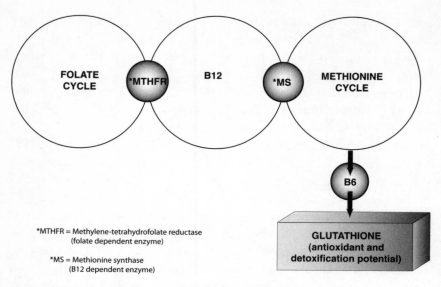

Figure 9: Methylation cycle (control of DNA, creation of cell membrane, and production of cellular energy), detoxification, and antioxidant protection

A lack of these important nutrients is what causes the methylation and sulfation trains to break down. The tracks break, and the trains grind to a halt. And that prevents your brain from functioning the way it was designed, leading to depression, autism, ADHD, dementia, and almost all variations of broken brains.

Because sulfation is a critical part of detoxification, I will focus on that process more in chapter 10. For now, let's look more closely at methylation.

Do you have problems with methylation? Take the following quiz to find out.

In the box on the right, place a check for each positive answer. Then find out how severe your problem is using the scoring key below.

METHYLATION QUIZ*

I eat animal protein (meat of any kind, chicken, dairy, cheese, eggs) more than five times a week. ☐

I eat more than one to two foods a week with hydrogenated fats (margarine, shortening, processed or packaged foods) a week. ☐

I have servings of animal protein greater than four to six ounces (the size of the palm of your hand) at a meal. ☐

I eat less than one cup of dark green leafy vegetables a day. ☐

I eat fewer than five to nine servings (one-half cup = one serving) of fruits and vegetables a day. ☐

I have more than three alcoholic drinks a week. ☐

I have depression or depressed mood or other mood or behavioral disorders. ☐

I have a history of heart attack or other heart disease. ☐

I have a history of stroke.

I have a history of cancer (especially colon, cervix, breast). ☐

I have a history of abnormal PAP tests (cervical dysplasia). ☐

I have a history of birth defects in offspring (spina bifida, neural tube defects, or Down syndrome). ☐

I have a history of dementia. ☐

I have a loss of balance or sensation in the feet.

I have a history of multiple sclerosis or other diseases with nerve damage. ☐

I have a history of carpal tunnel syndrome. ☐

I do not take a multivitamin.

I am over sixty-five years old. ☐

---

* For your convenience, this quiz has been reprinted in *The UltraMind Solution Companion Guide*. Simply go to www.ultramind.com/guide, download the guide, and print out the quiz.

Scoring Key—Methylation*

Score one point for each box you checked.

Score	Severity	Care Plan	Action To Take
0–8	You may have a low-level problem with methylation.	*The UltraMind Solution*	Complete the six-week program in Part III.
9 and above	You may have a severe problem with methylation.	Medical Care	Complete the six-week program in Part III and see a physician for additional assistance. I have outlined some of the options you should discuss with your doctor in chapter 22.

---

* Note that for this quiz there are only two scores. Low-level problems are treated on the six-week program. If you have severe problems, I strongly encourage you to seek the assistance of a physician trained in Functional Medicine.

Why the Methylation Train Needs to Run on Time

Almost every mental disorder and neurodegenerative disease from depression to Alzheimer's,[33] from ADHD to autism,[34] from Parkinson's[35] to bipolar disease[36] can be improved by fixing problems with methylation and sulfation trains. It is one of the most exciting areas of research in medicine today.

Fixing these biochemical trains also prevents heart disease, osteoporosis, strokes, cancer, Down syndrome, spina bifida, and more.

Methylation is the center of our biochemistry and brain function because it:

- ✤ Keeps Our DNA Working
  - ✤ Protects our DNA: it repairs damaged DNA.
  - ✤ Switches DNA on and off at the right time to keep us healthy.
- ✤ Helps Neurotransmitters Work
  - ✤ It is necessary for the production and removal of neurotransmitters including dopamine, serotonin, and norepinephrine to keep things in balance.
  - ✤ It helps the receptors on cells get ready to receive messages from neurotransmitters.
  - ✤ It makes cell membranes more fluid, and less stiff and more receptive to brain messenger chemicals.
  - ✤ It helps produce PC, the major fatty fluid component of cell membranes.
- ✤ Is the Major Antioxidant System
  - ✤ It lowers homocysteine (an unhealthy compound that can damage blood vessels and brain cells through oxidation).
  - ✤ It is critical in controlling oxidative stress or the rusting process common to almost every disease through the production of glutathione (see page 238)
- ✤ Is the Key to Detoxification
  - ✤ It helps recycle molecules needed for detoxification (namely, the body's major detoxifier, or glutathione—see page 238).
- ✤ Cools Inflammation
  - ✤ It controls and reduces inflammation by producing glutathione and reducing oxidative stress (which triggers inflammation).
- ✤ Is the Link to All Chronic Disease
  - ✤ It prevents dementia, cancer, heart disease, and almost every known age-related disease.

It's easy to see why breaks in the tracks on which the methylation train runs lead to many of the mental and physical health problems people suffer with every day. Let's look at some of the research on how this process is linked to so many mental illnesses and brain disorders specifically. This is only the tip of the iceberg, but it gives you a sense of how huge this problem is.

Depression and Mood Disorders

Overwhelming evidence links low folate, B_{12}, and B_6 levels to depression and mood disorders. Deficiency or insufficiency of these vitamins is very common. And remember, it is these deficiencies that cause the methylation train to slow down. These special nutrients keep the enzymes going that run the methylation train.

Victor Herbert first discovered the consequences of this deficiency in 1962.[37] He used himself as a study subject, consumed a folate-deficient diet for four and a half months, and experienced progressive insomnia, forgetfulness, and irritability. All these symptoms disappeared within two days of taking folate. In another study of 2,682 middle-aged men in Finland,[38] those with the lowest dietary folate intake had a 67 percent greater risk of depression.

One remarkable study in the *American Journal of Psychiatry*[39] found that 27 percent of severely depressed women over sixty-five years old were B_{12} deficient. This was found *not* by blood levels of B_{12}, but by the functional indicator of whether B_{12} was doing its job—*methylmalonic acid*. If you think about it, this suggests that more than one-quarter of all severe depression can be cured with B_{12} shots!

Doctors are now using a "prescription" folate called Deplin to treat depression and to improve the effectiveness of antidepressants.[40] In fact, if you have folate deficiency, it is unlikely that antidepressants will even work.

What's remarkable is how backward the thinking about depression is. Doctors tend to only use vitamins *if* the antidepressants don't work.[41] They should be prescribing the vitamins in the first place and then supplementing with antidepressants only *if* vitamins and lifestyle changes don't work.

People with a low folate level have only a 7 percent response to treatment with antidepressants. Those with a high folate have a response rate of 44 percent. That's six times better. In medicine, if we get a 15 to 30 percent improvement we are happy; but a 600 percent improvement should be headline news.

Supplementing with methylation vitamins is part of the miracle cure that turned lifelong depression around for my patient Joe.

*N*o matter what he did Joe could not get out from under his dark cloud of depression. He came to see me at fifty-one years old, after a parade of psychiatrists and psychiatric medication for bipolar disease—mood stabilizers like Lithium, Depakote, and Abilify; antipsychotics like Zyprexa and Clozaril; antiseizure medication like Lamictal and Neurontin, and stimulants like Provigil, Adderall, and Ritalin; and even Parkinson's drugs like Requip to raise his dopamine.

Even with a multidrug cocktail he couldn't overcome his depression. He complained that his depression stole his life. Many days he could not get out of bed, go to work, or focus. He had no energy and needed daily naps. The depression also affected his marriage—he could not make plans or go out.

The symptoms lasted for years and years and years. During the previous five years he had gained fifty pounds (often a side effect of the medication), and developed high blood pressure and high cholesterol. He could sleep only a few hours a night and had uncontrollable food cravings at night for bread, pasta, and sugar. He also had psoriasis and terrible stomach bloating after eating.

After testing we found he had many, many things out of balance—his blood sugar, low testosterone levels, low levels of serotonin and dopamine, and dairy allergies. He hated fish and had very low omega-3 fats. But the most dramatic finding was severe B_{12}, folate, and B_6 deficiency. His methylation train was stuck.

After cleaning up his diet, balancing his blood sugar and testosterone, giving him fish oil, and fixing his digestion, we gave him doses of folic acid, B_6, and B_{12} shots.

Subsequently his sleep improved, he was able to work out with a trainer, and for the first time in a few decades, he felt his depression lift. And it did not return!

After a year, he called me to thank me for giving him his life back. While he wasn't able to get off all his medications, he was able to feel joy again, didn't need any more naps, and lost thirty pounds.

Dementia

The Baltimore Longitudinal Study of Aging found that 35 percent of people were deficient in folate and that the risk of getting Alzheimer's was increased 60 percent in those who were deficient in folate.[42] In one double-blind, placebo-controlled study of elderly patients with memory complaints, giving 15 mg of folate a day showed significant improvements in memory.

In another ten-year study in the *American Journal of Clinical Nutrition*,[43] doctors found that in those over sixty-five years old, low-vitamin-B_{12} status was associated with more rapid cognitive decline.

I see cases like this over and over again in my practice—get the methylation train running smoothly again and memory improves almost overnight. That is what happened for Eleanor.

*E*leanor was a seventy-two-year-old patient of mine who noticed a progressive decline in her memory and mood and believed it was just normal aging. She couldn't remember names well, would forget why she came into a room, and felt like she was slipping away.

She also took acid-blocking medication for reflux, which prevents B_{12} absorption. Even with adequate dietary B_{12} we don't absorb B_{12} as well as we age, so the medication turned a small problem into a big one. This led to a severe B_{12} deficiency, which not only made her lose her memory, but also led to increasing fatigue and depression.

Eleanor was way off the methylation tracks. Just giving her special B_{12} shots (methyl B_{12}) and special forms of folate (5 MTHF) improved her mood, memory, and energy almost overnight.

ADHD and Autism

Some of the most interesting studies regarding trouble with the methylation and sulfation trains come from the world of autism and ADHD.

Dr. Richard Deth of Northeastern University has discovered that the brain receptors for dopamine, the neurotransmitter that is essential for focus and attention (two things notably lacking in ADHD and autism), require methylation to work properly.

In fact, children with ADHD and autism tend to have slightly quirky dopamine receptors that are easily disturbed by anything that messes up methylation.

To be turned on, these dopamine receptors need vitamin B_{12} acting as a helper to specific enzymes. Unfortunately toxins, especially mercury, poison a particular enzyme (MS or methionine synthase). This can lead to a biochemical traffic jam.[44]

Getting the traffic flowing with methyl B_{12} often has miraculous effects on these children. The special form of B_{12} helps synchronize neuronal or brain activity. In one of my autistic patients, the school knows exactly which day he gets his B_{12} shots: he is focused, happy, and engaged.

Wow! That's a rather long list of problems that are caused by improper methylation. So let's take a look at what causes the methylation and sulfation trains to come off the tracks. That will lead us to better understand how we can repair the problem.

What Causes the Train Wrecks?

Unfortunately, many things can affect optimal methylation and sulfation. But it can be boiled down to two main issues—your genes and your environment.

Genes load the metabolic gun and the environment pulls the trigger. And often a combination of genes sets the stage for problems. There is no one gene for Alzheimer's or autism—there are multiple genes that interact with a complex and often toxic environment.

That's how the gun gets loaded.

But whether we pull the trigger or not is largely dependent on us. You may have genetic predispositions to certain diseases, but that doesn't mean you *have* to get sick.

What Makes Us Sick: Our Nutrient-Poor, SAD Diet and Toxins

Our toxic, nutrient-poor "dietary" environment undersupplies the raw materials for proper biochemical and metabolic functioning, namely nutrients, and oversupplies a load of chemicals, additives, pollutants, and allergens. This sends the train right off the tracks.

The single biggest environmental influence you can control is what you eat. Remember, food is not just calories; it is information. It tells our genes what to do.

You see, the real cause of the epidemics of mental and physical illness in this country is our SAD diet—the Standard American Diet—which is nutrient-deficient and packed with chemicals that poison our bodies.

Remember the only reason we need to "enrich" our food with nutrients is that it's "impoverished" in the first place.[45] It is grown in nutrient-depleted soils,[46] artificially supported with petrochemical fertilizers, protected by pesticides and herbicides, and is genetically designed to fit in boxes, be transported over long distances, and stay "fresh" for a long time.[47]

The highly processed, nutrient-poor foods that are sold to us do exactly the opposite of enriching us. They turn off the right genes, turn on the wrong ones, and send your system into chaos.

They are literally a trigger for the loaded gun.

Other Environmental Factors Interfere with Methylation

There are many other things that interfere with methylation in the body besides our SAD diet. Excess animal protein, sugar, saturated fat, coffee, alcohol, milk allergy, zinc deficiency, irradiation of food, the measles virus, smoking, poor digestion, certain medications (acid blockers, contraceptives, diuretics), and environmental toxins—especially mercury and organophosphate pesticides—all interfere with normal methylation and/or disrupt normal vitamin status.

Keeping the Trains Running

Whew! That was like going to medical school! But now you know some critical things to help your mood, behavior, memory, and attention (as well as almost all chronic disease), which are connected to these twin trains of methylation and sulfation.

You also learned that genes set the stage for trouble, and that a poor diet and environmental toxins push you into a biochemical train wreck, which you experience as ADHD, depression, bipolar disease, autism, dementia, and other chronic illnesses.

The good news is that we now know how to fix these breaks in the tracks, and correct the collateral damage known as "disease" with a few simple tricks. Clean up your diet, get rid of toxins, and take a few supplements. That's it!

Vitamin D: D for Depression and Dementia

Are you deficient in vitamin D? Take the following quiz to find out.

In the box on the right, place a check for each positive answer. Then find out how severe your problem is using the scoring key below.

VITAMIN D QUIZ*

I have seasonal affective disorder. ☐
I experience a loss of mental sharpness or memory. ☐
I have sore or weak muscles. ☐
I have tender bones (press on your shin bone—if it hurts you are vitamin D deficient). ☐
I work indoors. ☐
I avoid the sun. ☐
I wear sunblock most of the time. ☐
I live north of Florida. ☐
I don't eat small fatty fish such as mackerel, herring, sardines (the main sources of dietary vitamin D). ☐

(continued)

I have osteoporosis. ☐
I have broken more than two bones or had a hip fracture. ☐
I have autoimmune disease (i.e., multiple sclerosis). ☐
I have osteoarthritis (vitamin D deficiency weakens bones and
leads to deterioration). ☐
I have frequent infections. ☐
I have prostate cancer. ☐
I have dark skin (any race other than Caucasian). ☐
I am sixty years old or older. ☐

---

* For your convenience, this quiz has been reprinted in *The UltraMind Solution Companion Guide*. Simply go to www.ultramind.com/guide, download the guide, and print out the quiz.

Scoring Key—Vitamin D *

Score one point for each box you checked.

Score	Severity	Care Plan	Action to Take
0–8	You may have a slightly low level of vitamin D.	*The UltraMind Solution*	Complete the six-week program in Part III.
9 and above	You may have a severely low level of vitamin D.	Medical Care	Complete the six-week program in Part III and see a physician for additional assistance. I have outlined some of the options you should discuss with your doctor in chapter 22.

---

* Note that for this quiz there are only two scores. Low-level problems are treated on the six-week program. If you have severe problems, I strongly encourage you to seek the assistance of a physician trained in Functional Medicine.

What vitamin deficiency affects over half of the population, is almost never diagnosed, and has been linked to depression, dementia, many cancers, autoimmune diseases like multiple sclerosis and fibromyalgia, high blood pressure, heart disease, diabetes, chronic muscle pain, and bone loss?

What vitamin is almost totally absent from our food supply? What vitamin do we need up to twenty-five times more of than the government recommends for us to be healthy? What vitamin is the hidden cause of so much suffering that is so easy to treat?

If you guessed vitamin D, you are correct.

For the last fifteen years of my practice, my focus has been to discover what the body needs to function optimally. And I have become more interested in the role of specific nutrients as the years have passed. In the past five years I have tested almost every patient in my practice for vitamin D deficiency, and I am shocked by what I see. I am also amazed by what happens when their vitamin D status reaches an optimal level.

Each nutrient has its role, but vitamin D deficiency is a major epidemic that is under the radar of most doctors and public health officials. It has been linked to depression, dementia, an increased risk of death, and even autism. Consider the following:

- In one study of elderly patients the average level of vitamin D was 18 ng/ml (nanograms per milliliter) when normal is between 50 and 80. Almost 60 percent of them were under 20 ng/ml. Those with the lowest vitamin D levels had the most depression and the worst performance on objective tests for dementia and cognitive function.[48]
- We know that vitamin D levels drop precipitously in winter, that this is associated with seasonal affective disorder, and that giving vitamin D supplements can prevent this.[49]
- New insights into brain development in the womb link vitamin D deficiency with autism. Vitamin D is necessary for the normal development of the brain and reduces brain inflammation that is characteristic in autism.[50]
- A review in the *The Archives of Internal Medicine* of all randomized trials on vitamin D supplementation found a reduction in death of 7 percent from all causes.[51] This should have been headline news, and would have been if it was a drug.

Most doctors think that if you don't have rickets you don't have vitamin D deficiency. They couldn't be more wrong. The real question is not how *little* we need not to get rickets (400 IU a day), but how much we need to be optimally healthy and how much we were designed to have (approximately 5,000 to 10,000 IU a day).

We are not living in the environment in which we were designed to thrive. People who live in northern climates no longer eat a diet of fatty wild fish like mackerel and herring and cod liver oil—which are among the few natural dietary sources of vitamin D.

For the rest of us, the key is sunlight. Most of us live and work indoors, but 80 to 100 percent of our vitamin D requirement comes from our exposure to sunlight. And concerns about skin cancer encourage use of sunblock, which stops 97 percent of the skin's production of vitamin D. Use of sunscreen, dark skin color, increase in latitude, changes in seasonal sun exposure, aging, and wearing clothes that cover most of our body all affect our risk of vitamin D deficiency.

Newer research by Dr. Michael Holick,[52] a vitamin D pioneer and professor of medicine, physiology, and dermatology at Boston University School of Medicine, recommends intakes of up to 2,000 IU a day,[53] or enough to keep blood levels of 25-hydroxy vitamin D at between 40 to 60 ng/ml. Lifeguards have levels of over 100 ng/ml without toxicity.

So supplementation is essential unless we are spending all our time at the beach, eating thirty ounces of wild salmon a day, or downing ten tablespoons of cod liver oil a day! The exact amount needed to get your blood levels to the optimal range (50 to 80 ng/ml) will vary depending on your age, genetics, how far north you live, how much time you spend in the sun, and even the time of the year.

We are scared into thinking that high doses are toxic, but one study of healthy young men receiving 10,000 IU of vitamin D for twenty weeks showed no toxicity (I wouldn't try that, though, without a doctor's supervision).

Here is a story of one of my patients to show just how powerful supplementing with vitamin D can be.

Norah, a fifty-two-year-old woman, worked and lived in Boston. She spent her time as a software programmer in the basement of an old building. Every winter she would sink into a deep, dark slump. She dreaded the shortening of the days.

Like most women, she kept out of the sun to prevent skin cancer and wrinkles and always wore sunblock and a hat when out in the sun.

She also found her muscles ached worse in the winter, and her doctor told her that she had osteoporosis. She was told she had seasonal affective disorder—which just meant she was getting depressed in the winter!

We found she had extremely low vitamin D levels. By giving her high doses over a few months we were able to get her vitamin D up to normal—and with that her depression lifted and her achy muscles resolved.

Mental Minerals: Essential Ingredients for the Nervous System

More than eighteen minerals are essential for human nutrition. They work in similar ways to vitamins, as helpers for the body's enzymes. They are needed to make our bones (calcium) and our blood cells (iron) and for our nervous system. While all are important, there are a few that are key players in optimal brain function: magnesium, zinc, and selenium.

Magnesium: The Relaxation Mineral

Are you missing this MAGnificent mineral? Take the following quiz to find out.

In the box on the right, place a check for each positive answer. Then find out how severe your problem is using the scoring key below.

MAGNESIUM QUIZ*

I have depression. ☐
I feel irritable. ☐
I have attention deficit disorder (ADHD). ☐
I have autism. ☐
I am anxious. ☐
I have insomnia or trouble falling asleep. ☐
I have muscle twitching. ☐
I have premenstrual syndrome. ☐
I have leg or hand cramps. ☐
I have restless leg syndrome. ☐
I have heart flutters, skipped beats, or palpitations. ☐
I get frequent headaches or migraines. ☐
I have trouble swallowing. ☐
I have reflux. ☐
I am sensitive to loud noises. ☐
I feel fatigued. ☐
I have asthma. ☐
I have constipation (fewer than two bowel movements a day). ☐
I have excess stress. ☐
I have kidney stones. ☐
I have heart disease or heart failure. ☐

(continued)

I have mitral valve prolapse. ☐
I have diabetes. ☐
I have a low intake of kelp, wheat bran or germ, almonds, cashews, buckwheat, and dark green leafy vegetables. ☐

* For your convenience, this quiz has been reprinted in *The UltraMind Solution Companion Guide.* Simply go to www.ultramind.com/guide download the guide, and print out the quiz.

Scoring Key—Magnesium*

Score	Severity	Care Plan	Action to Take
0–12	You may have a slightly low level of magnesium.	*The UltraMind Solution*	Complete the six-week program in Part III.
13 and above	You may have a severely low level of magnesium.	Medical Care	Complete the six-week program in Part III and see a physician for additional assistance. I have outlined some of the options you should discuss with your doctor in chapter 22.

* Note that for this quiz there are only two scores. Low-level problems are treated on the six-week program. If you have severe problems, I strongly encourage you to seek the assistance of a physician trained in Functional Medicine.

If you are deficient in this critical nutrient you are twice as likely to die. This is reported from a study of hospitalized patients in the *Journal of Intensive Care Medicine.*[54]

Up to half of Americans are deficient in this nutrient and don't know it. And normal blood tests may miss it.

It accounts for a long list of symptoms and diseases, which are easily helped and often cured by adding this nutrient.

In fact, in my practice, this nutrient is one of my secret weapons against illness, particularly anxiety, insomnia, ADHD, and autism.

What is it?

It is magnesium. It is the stress antidote and the most powerful *relaxation mineral* that exists.

Now I find it very funny that more doctors aren't clued into this nutrient because we *use* it all the time in conventional medicine but *never* stop to think about why or how important it is to our general health or why it helps our body function better.

I remember using it when I worked in the emergency room. It was a critical "medication" on the crash cart. If someone was dying of a life-threatening arrhythmia (an irregular heartbeat), we used intravenous magnesium.

If someone was constipated or needed to prepare for a colonoscopy, we gave them milk of magnesia or a green bottle of liquid magnesium citrate, which emptied their bowels.

But you don't have to be in the hospital to benefit from treating magnesium deficiency. You can treat yourself now, and chances are you *are* deficient, because as I said above, up to half of all Americans don't get enough magnesium.

Think of magnesium as the *relaxation* mineral. Anything that is tight, irritable, crampy, stiff—whether it is a body part or even a *mood*—is a sign of magnesium deficiency. If you suffer these kinds of symptoms it's likely you don't get enough magnesium.

This critical mineral is responsible for more than three hundred enzyme reactions in the body and is found in all your tissues, but mainly in your brain, bones, and muscles. It is necessary for your cells to make energy, for many different chemical pumps to work, to stabilize membranes, and to help muscles relax.

The list of conditions that are related to magnesium deficiency is very long. There are more than 3,500 medical references on magnesium deficiency.

But it is mostly ignored because it is not a drug, even though it is *more* powerful in many cases than drugs, which is why we use it in life-threatening and emergency situations like seizures and heart failure in the hospital.

You might be suffering from magnesium deficiency if you experience any of the following things:

❖ Anxiety, autism, ADHD, headaches, migraines, chronic fatigue, irritability, muscle cramps or twitches, insomnia, sensitivity to loud noises, palpitations, angina, constipation, anal spasms, fibromyalgia, asthma, kidney stones, diabetes, obesity, osteoporosis, high blood pressure, PMS, menstrual cramps, irritable bladder, irritable bowel syndrome, reflux, trouble swallowing, and more.

We eat a diet that has practically no magnesium—a highly processed, refined diet that is based mostly on white flour, meat, and dairy, none of which contain magnesium.

We are under chronic stress and this also decreases our magnesium levels. In fact, one study in Kosovo found that those under chronic war stress lost large amounts of magnesium in their urine.

Magnesium levels are also decreased by excess alcohol, salt, coffee, sugar, phosphoric acid in colas, profuse sweating, chronic diarrhea, excessive menstruation, diuretics (water pills), antibiotics, other drugs, and some intestinal parasites.

We live lifestyles that cause us to lose whatever magnesium we have in our bodies, and we never replace it.

When was the last time you had a good dose of sea vegetables (seaweed), nuts, greens, and beans? If you are like most Americans, your nut consumption mostly comes from peanut butter, and mostly in chocolate peanut butter cups. As for seaweed, greens, and beans . . . well, most Americans don't eat much of these at all.

So if you suffer from any of the symptoms I mentioned or have any of the diseases I noted—it is an easy fix!

But how do you fix it? Simply increase beans, greens, and seaweed in your diet. Get rid of the magnesium suckers like stress, coffee, alcohol, and sugar. And take an extra magnesium supplement.

In other words, follow the UltraMind Solution. (I will explain how you can do it in more detail in Part III.)

Magnesium supplementation had magnificent effects on my patient Mary. Let me tell you her story.

Many of my patients are doctors—and usually they have run the gamut of specialists and experts to find a solution to their ills. Mary, a thirty-six-year-old physician, was no exception.

For years she suffered intractable migraines, finding only marginal relief in the strongest narcotic pain medication and antinausea pills. She had been to every headache clinic and tried every medication to prevent or treat her migraines without any relief. After listening to her story, the solution was obvious to me . . .

Besides the migraines, she suffered from panic attacks, anxiety, insomnia, and palpitations, as well as muscle cramps and severe constipation—she went to the bathroom only once a week.

Every symptom she had pointed to everything in her body being tight or twitchy—tight emotions, tight head, twitchy heart, tight muscles, really tight bowels.

Mary was so depleted in magnesium she needed nearly ten times the amount I usually give people. Once her levels normalized we reduced the dose, and within days her anxiety, insomnia, palpitations, muscle cramps, constipation, and, most important, the migraines she had for years were gone.

Minerals and the Brain: Zinc and Selenium

We, of course, need all the essential minerals. That's why they call them essential!

We have already talked about the most important one—magnesium. But a few more stand out as critical for brain function and health. Zinc and selenium are specifically important for your brain, so we need to review them before we close.

Zinc

In the box on the right, place a check for each positive answer. Then find out how severe your problem is using the scoring key below.

ZINC QUIZ*

I have impaired taste. ☐
I have impaired smell. ☐
I have weak nails (thin, brittle, or peeling). ☐
I have white spots on my nails. ☐
I have frequent colds or respiratory infections. ☐
I have diarrhea. ☐
I have eczema or other skin rashes. ☐
I have acne. ☐
My wounds heal poorly. ☐
I have allergies. ☐
I am losing my hair. ☐
I have dandruff. ☐
I have erectile dysfunction. ☐
I have an enlarged or inflamed prostate. ☐
I have inflammatory bowel disease (ulcerative colitis,
Crohn's disease). ☐
I have rheumatoid arthritis. ☐
I consume hard water (which depletes zinc). ☐
I consume more than three alcoholic beverages per week. ☐
I sweat excessively. ☐
I have kidney or liver disease. ☐
I am over age sixty-five. ☐
I use diuretics (water pills). ☐

(continued)

I have a low intake of dulse (seaweed), fresh gingerroot, egg yolks, fish, kelp, lamb, legumes, pumpkin seeds.   ☐

---

* For your convenience, this quiz has been reprinted in *The UltraMind Solution Companion Guide*. Simply go to www.ultramind.com/guide download the guide, and print out the quiz.

Scoring Key—Zinc*

Score one point for each box you checked.

Score	Severity	Care Plan	Action to Take
0–12	You may have a slightly low level of zinc.	*The UltraMind Solution*	Complete the six-week program in Part III.
13 and above	You may have a severely low level of zinc.	Medical Care	Complete the six-week program in Part III and see a physician for additional assistance. I have outlined some of the options you should discuss with your doctor in chapter 22.

---

* Note that for this quiz there are only two scores. Low-level problems are treated on the six-week program. If you have severe problems, I strongly encourage you to seek the assistance of a physician trained in Functional Medicine.

We are in a global zinc deficiency epidemic. More than one third of the world's population is zinc-deficient and in some populations up to 73 percent are deficient.[55] This is a *huge* problem because zinc is used by more enzymes (over three hundred) than any other mineral, including those that help your DNA repair, replicate, and synthesize proteins.

Think back to the beginning of this chapter to understand why that's so important. Your DNA's job is to build protein. If that stops, your system breaks down from its roots.

Zinc is important in immunity and controlling inflammation, a critical factor in brain dysfunction. It is also extremely important for activating your digestive enzymes; this helps you break down and digest food better and aids in preventing food allergies—one of the chief causes of inflammation (and consequently brain diseases in so many). I will discuss the critical importance of inflammation in brain health in chapter 8.

Zinc also helps rid the body of heavy metal toxins like mercury by helping a key enzyme called metallothionein. Problems with metallothionein have been linked to many neurobehavioral problems, including ADHD and autism. In fact, the highest concentration of metallothionein is in the brain, especially in the memory center, or hippocampus.

Low zinc levels have been linked to depression[56] as well as changes in behavior, learning, mental function, and susceptibility to convulsions. Zinc is also needed for the enzyme dopamine hydroxylase that makes the happy hormone noradrenaline from dopamine. This is, perhaps, one of the primary reasons zinc deficiency is associated with depression.

There have also been links between zinc deficiency and schizophrenia. It seems that up to 50 percent of schizophrenics have a biochemical quirk called the mauve factor (a chemical by-product from oxidation injury to our fats and proteins).[57] These odd compounds can bind to zinc and vitamin B_6, leading to a functional zinc deficiency.

One of my patients told me the story of her schizophrenic brother who woke up from his madness by simply taking high doses of zinc, B_6, and niacin.

Dr. Abram Hoffer, the father of orthomolecular psychiatry, has successfully treated thousands of schizophrenic patients using this approach.[58] An extensive review of the mauve factor in many diseases by Woody McGinnis[59] and his group documents how the neurotoxin influences mood, brain, and behavior. Mauve factor can be measured in the urine. Taking zinc, B_6, and niacin can correct this problem.

Low zinc also affects taste and appetite and is linked to eating disorders. If you can't taste your food, you either become anorexic or you overeat!

Adequate zinc is absolutely critical for a healthy brain and body. And many of us are deficient and don't know it. So eat pumpkin seeds and take zinc.

Selenium

Selenium is worth mentioning when it comes to the health of the brain and mood because it functions in a number of key systems in the body.

It helps you make thyroid hormone, so necessary for proper mood and brain function.

It helps your body make more glutathione, and supports your body's main detoxification and antioxidant system. (We will discuss this more in chapter 10.)

And it is important in helping your body make some of the essential fatty acids which we know have a huge impact on mood, autism, ADHD, dementia, and just about everything else to do with the brain.

No wonder studies have found that selenium supplementation boosts mood![60]

Optimize Your Nutrition

This journey through the world of nutrients and the brain is just a glimpse of the astounding world of scientific literature on this subject. I have highlighted just a few of the most important considerations and the implications for treatment of our epidemic of mental and brain disorders.

By using this approach, we go to the roots of the problem. We focus on how the body works, why it breaks down, and how to fix it using some very simple principles.

As you move toward UltraWellness and an UltraMind, remember what we learned in this chapter:

1. You must have the essential fats—DHA, EPA, PC, and PS—for your brain and every one of your 100 trillion cells to function well.
2. Amino acids are the building blocks of moods, thought, and memory—get them tuned up. They help produce all the neurotransmitters needed for optimal brain function.
3. Carbohydrates from whole unprocessed plant foods full of phytonutrients, vitamins, minerals, and fiber are essential for your health and your brain.
4. Keep the methylation and sulfation trains running with the right types and amounts of folate, B_{12}, B_6, and sources of sulfur in the diet and supplements. (See chapter 10 for more information about the sulfation train specifically.)
5. Most of us have a vitamin D deficiency. Getting enough on board will help your brain and prevent many diseases.
6. Magnesium is the major relaxation mineral.
7. Zinc and selenium are absolutely critical for a happy, healthy brain and body.

Nutrition is of fundamental importance. It is the foundation on which your body runs, the source for all the raw materials you need to thrive. What you have learned in this chapter should form the basis for a whole new understanding of how your mind and your body function.

But this is still only one of the keys to UltraWellness.

Now let's look at how hormonal imbalances affect your thoughts, mood, memory, and behavior.

CHAPTER 7

KEY #2: BALANCE YOUR HORMONES

M any of us are living a life out of balance but don't recognize it.

- Do you feel your life is a song played badly out of tune?
- Does your mood and energy swing up and down, making your life crazy?
- Do you crave sugar or salt?
- Are you overweight and putting on more and more belly fat?
- If you are a woman, do you have premenstrual syndrome or painful or heavy periods?
- Are you depressed?
- Do you sleep poorly?
- Are you less interested in sex?
- Do you have thinning hair, dry skin; do you feel sluggish in the mornings?
- Do you feel tired but wired?
- Do you have to live on coffee in the morning and a few glasses of wine at night just to wake up, and then calm down every day?

If you do, you are not alone. In fact, this is how most Americans feel, because we are living out of harmony with our natural biological rhythms. Small molecules in our body that we depend on to keep us in balance are running haywire.

These messenger molecules are involved in almost every function of the body in one way or another, and they are critical to our well-being.

There are three main communications systems in your body. They direct all the traffic and messages from your nervous system (including the gut, the site of your second brain), your endocrine or hormonal system, and your immune system. Each of these systems is part of a larger integrated system called the "psycho-neuro-endocrine-immune" system, or PNEI.

The three main communication systems are:

1. Neurotransmitters—Messengers of the Nervous System (The most important are dopamine, epinephrine, norepinephrine, serotonin, GABA, and acetylcholine. I discussed these in chapter 6.)
2. Hormones—Messengers of the Endocrine System (This chapter will focus on these important molecules.)
3. Cytokines—Messengers of the Immune System (I will discuss these in the next chapter, when we talk about inflammation.)

All of your hormones and your brain and immune messenger chemicals work together in a symphony. Understand how and why these three systems get out of balance and you will go a long way toward understanding why Americans run around tired, depressed, stressed, forgetful, unfocused, and overweight!

In this chapter, we will focus specifically on hormones. To adequately explore the role of hormones in your mood and brain function would require a textbook. Here, I want to give you a road map that will help you understand how key hormones play a role in your health, why they get out of balance, and how to get them back in balance.

The Command and Control Center for Your Whole Body

Health is good communication. All your cells talk to each other. They do so through many different messengers and "languages." There is the endocrine language, or hormones; the immune language, or cytokines (see page 175 for more on these); and the nervous system language, or neurotransmitters.

Your hormones are produced and controlled by your endocrine glands. And the conductors or the command and control centers for all your endocrine glands happen to be located in your brain. They are the *hypothalamus* and the *pituitary* gland.

These glands send signals to distant parts of the body to control:

+ Your stress response through your adrenal glands.
+ Your blood-sugar balance through your pancreas.
+ Your thyroid hormone via your thyroid gland.
+ Your sexual behavior, which functions through your reproductive organs.
+ Your growth, sleep, mood, and much more.

This network of glands (the hypothalamus, pituitary, pineal, adrenal, thyroid, parathyroid, pancreas, ovaries, and testes) both send and receive messages in a finely orchestrated symphony and have their effects through the whole body.

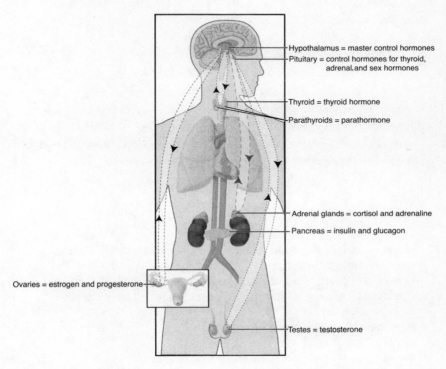

Figure 10: The hormone system: bidirectional communication between your brain and your endocrine glands

There are three big epidemics of hormonal problems in America today—too much *insulin* (from sugar), too much *cortisol and adrenalin* (from stress), and not enough *thyroid hormone.*

These all interconnect with and affect the other major category of hormones—*our sex hormones.*

Imbalances or disturbances in any one of these interconnected systems can influence the way our brain functions and lead to everything from depression to dementia, from anxiety to ADHD, and, of course, are linked to the other major epidemic we face in the twenty-first century—overweight and obesity.

For now we will look at the role that insulin, thyroid, and sex hormones play in your mood and brain function. We will also briefly look at the role of melatonin and growth hormone, which are also important. We will leave cortisol and DHEA to chapter 12, because they are intertwined with stress and your experience of the world.

If you focus on just these few—insulin, thyroid, sex hormones, melatonin, growth hormone, and cortisol (the stress hormone)—all the rest come into balance.

Don't Panic, It's Just Your Blood Sugar: Insulin and Your Brain

Do you have problems with unstable blood sugar and are you at risk for insulin resistance? Take the following quiz to find out.

In the box on the right, place a check for each positive answer. Then find out how severe your problem is using the scoring key below.

INSULIN QUIZ*

I crave sweets, eat them, and though I get a temporary boost of energy and mood, I later crash. ☐

I have a family history of diabetes, hypoglycemia, or alcoholism. ☐

I get irritable, anxious, tired, and jittery or get headaches intermittently throughout the day but feel better temporarily after meals. ☐

I feel shaky two to three hours after a meal. ☐

I eat a low-fat diet and can't seem to lose weight. ☐

If I miss a meal, I feel cranky and irritable, weak, or tired. ☐

If I eat a carbohydrate breakfast (muffin, bagel, cereal, pancakes, etc.), I can't seem to control my eating for the rest of the day. ☐

Once I start eating sweets or carbohydrates, I can't seem to stop. ☐

If I eat fish or meat and vegetables, I feel good, but seem to get sleepy or feel "drugged" after eating a meal full of pasta, bread, potatoes, and dessert. ☐

I go for the bread basket at the restaurant. ☐

I get heart palpitations after eating sweets. ☐

I seem salt sensitive (I tend to retain water). ☐

I get panic attacks in the afternoon if I skip breakfast. ☐

I am often moody, impatient, or anxious. ☐

My memory and concentration are poor. ☐

Eating makes me calm. ☐

I get tired a few hours after eating. ☐

I get night sweats. ☐

I am tired most of the time. ☐

I have extra weight around the middle (waist-to-hip ratio >
0.8—measure around the belly button and around the bony
prominence at the front of the top of the hip). ☐
My hair thins in the places I don't want it to (if a woman, my body;
if a man, my head) and it grows in the places it shouldn't (my face
if I am a woman). ☐
I have polycystic ovarian syndrome or am infertile. ☐
I have high blood pressure. ☐
I have heart disease. ☐
I have type 2 diabetes (what used to be known as adult onset). ☐
I have chronic fungal infections (jock itch, vaginal yeast infections,
or dry scaly patches on my skin). ☐

* For your convenience, this quiz has been reprinted in *The UltraMind Solution Companion Guide*. Simply go to www.ultramind.com/guide, download the guide, and print out the quiz.

Scoring Key—Insulin

Score one point for each box you checked.

Score	Severity	Care Plan	Action to Take
0–7	You may have a mild insulin imbalance.	*The UltraMind Solution*	Complete the six-week program in Part III.
8–12	You may have a moderate insulin imbalance	Self-Care	Complete the six-week program in Part III and optimize your insulin levels using the self-care options in chapter 23.
13 and above	You may have a severe insulin imbalance.	Medical Care	Do both of the steps above and see a physician for additional assistance. I have outlined some of the options you should discuss with your doctor in chapter 23.

If you want to be depressed, tired, anxious, hyperactive but unfocused, and lose your memory, not to mention pack on belly fat, clog your arteries, fuel cancer cells, and get dementia, then keep eating the way you do (if you are one of the average Americans who eats 158 pounds of sugar a year).

Sugar promotes high levels of insulin (I'll tell you how in a moment). And too much insulin is the number-one cause of our chronic disease epidemic and a major unrecognized factor in mood disorders and dementia.

Let me tell you a story of a man who came to me. His story may be all too familiar to you . . . but it can have a happy ending for you, as it did for him.

James was a forty-six-year-old Wall Street executive who came to me for a cardiac stress test. He was a hard-driving, don't-look-up type of guy who was convinced he was dying of heart disease.

Every day, sometime in the late afternoon, he would experience the sudden onset of sweating, a racing heart, anxiety, and shortness of breath. In other words, he thought he was going to die!

In reality, he was just having panic attacks—severe onsets of anxiety that make some people feel like they are going to have a heart attack.

He was thick around the middle and after listening to his story and taking one look at him, I said, "You don't eat breakfast, do you?

"And you feel tired after eating so that is why you skip food during the day—to keep sharp for work—and when you feel like that you go for the vending machine or a soda and get a quick sugar fix and in a few minutes you feel better."

Shocked, he said, "How did you know?"

I explained to him that he was fighting with his genes and was insulin-resistant. This caused his insulin levels to rise, pushing his blood sugar very low, leading to wide swings in blood sugar and, ultimately, overall low blood sugar (hypoglycemia). That was responsible for his symptoms.

In other words, his hormones were severely out of balance and he was having panic attacks because of it.

He couldn't control his metabolism of carbohydrates because he had too much insulin in his blood. As a result his blood sugar was out of balance, leading to all his symptoms of anxiety, and taking him down the slippery slope toward brain aging, dementia, high blood pressure, heart disease, obesity, cancer, and more.

James is not alone.

Over 100 million Americans suffer from this condition we call *insulin resistance*. It affects many varieties of people and is not exactly the same in everyone, but the ultimate consequences are the same: depression, dementia, fatigue, weight gain, heart disease, and cancer.

Most afflicted have extra fat around the middle. (To find out if this applies to you, check your waist-to-hip ratio. This is the measurement around your belly button divided by the measurement around the hips. If it is greater than 0.8, you likely have insulin resistance.)

You may be tall or thin, short or fat, or any combination and still have insulin resistance.

While waist-to-hip ratio is a good indicator, the only sure way to know if you suffer from this condition is with an insulin-response test. This is done by measuring both your fasting blood sugar *and* your insulin levels, then measuring them again one or two hours later, after taking a 75 gm sugar drink. Your doctor can give you this test. (You will find some information on insulin testing in Part IV. I have also included an extensive section on testing in *The UltraMind Solution Companion Guide*. Go to www.ultra mind.com/guide and download the guide to access that information.)

Insulin resistance is not a genetic defect, an error in our development, or a mistake by God. It is simply a result of the fact that we have strayed from eating in harmony with our genes.

SWAMPED WITH SUGAR
THE MANY NAMES OF INSULIN RESISTANCE

When we eat too much sugar or refined carbohydrates, don't exercise, and are too stressed, our bodies change. At first we pump out more insulin to keep our blood sugar even. Then our cells must have more and more insulin to keep our blood sugar even. That is called insulin resistance, and it is a condition I will discuss more in a moment.

Keep eating sugar and over time you develop a collection of other problems—a fat belly, slightly high blood sugar levels (over 90), high triglycerides (over 100), low HDL (less than 60), high blood pressure (higher than 115/75), and inflammation in your blood. This is then called a "syndrome," specifically, "metabolic syndrome."

This syndrome is also known as "prediabetes," because it doesn't meet the strict criteria for diabetes, which is a blood sugar over 126. But damage occurs to your brain and your blood vessels even *before* you get diabetes. The name "prediabetes" gives the impression that you are not quite in trouble yet. Nothing could be further from the truth.

All of these different "conditions," or "illnesses," are actually the result of one simple problem—eating too much sugar (or anything that quickly turns to sugar, like processed foods or products made from flour).

Forget the fancy terms. Eating too much sugar and refined carbohydrates in any form is bad for your brain and your body. Period.

Historically, we ate the equivalent of only 20 teaspoons of sugar a year as a hunter/gatherer species.[1] Now we eat 158 pounds per person per year, or about 50 teaspoons or half a pound each day.[2] The average schoolboy has 34 teaspoons of sugar a day.

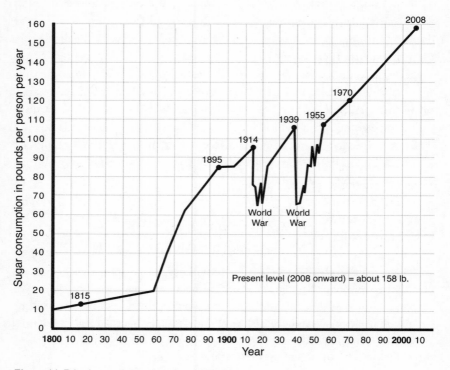

Figure 11: Rise in sugar consumption 1800–2008

We evolved in a world without supermarkets, convenience stores, and fast-food restaurants. We had to work for our food and had limited access to refined foods or excess calories.

Now we spend more money on processed and junk food in convenience stores at gas stations than on gas. We spend more on fast food than on new cars, new computers, and higher education *combined*!

In fact, our genes are preagricultural. We started farming only ten thousand years ago and started refining flour only about two hundred years ago with the discovery of the steam engine–powered flour mill. The food industry has "progressed" a great deal in the last hundred years.

Our genes have not kept up with these technological innovations.

Yet fifteen thousand low-fat foods (a.k.a. high-sugar, high-calorie foods) that we are not genetically designed to properly metabolize came onto the marketplace over the last fifteen to twenty years. The consequence? We have created an epidemic of increasing obesity, diabetes, heart disease, and brain disorders.

The scientific foundation for the low-fat movement was shaky from the start. Unfortunately, Madison Avenue marketing companies overpowered medical science to the detriment of us all.

Our bodies normally produce insulin in response to food in our stomach, particularly sugar. Our genetic code evolved at a time when we were eating twenty teaspoons of sugar a year. That means our insulin response is designed to handle *vastly* lower levels of sugar than what we consume today.

Our poor bodies respond to our new diet of low-fat, highly processed, and refined foods the only way they know how: they keep pumping out insulin in response to this overload of sugars.

Eventually we become resistant to all this insulin in our blood, just as we would become resistant to a drug. The body needs more and more of it to do the same job it once did with far less. So our insulin production system spirals out of control, pumping ever more into our bodies.

All this insulin tells us we are starving (that's literally the message our bodies get), so we crave foods with high-sugar content—the very same foods that caused the problem in the first place.

Perhaps this wouldn't be so bad if insulin metabolized only sugar. We once thought that was insulin's only role—to help sugar enter your cells to be metabolized, transforming the stored energy of the sun (in plant foods) with the oxygen we breathe into the energy we use every day to run our bodies.

Here is what too much insulin *really* does to your brain, your body, and your health:

- Now we recognize insulin as a major switching station, or control hormone, for many bodily processes. It is a major storage hormone—fat storage, that is.
- It also leads to mood and behavior disturbances such as depression, panic attacks, anxiety, insomnia, and ADHD.
- Try as you may, as long as your insulin levels are high you may fight a losing battle for weight loss. It acts on your brain to increase appetite—specifically an appetite for sugar.
- It increases LDL or "bad" cholesterol, lowers HDL or "good" cholesterol, raises triglycerides, and increases your blood pressure. Insulin resistance causes 50 percent of all reported cases of high blood pressure.

✢ It makes your blood sticky and more likely to clot, leading to heart attacks and strokes.

✢ It stimulates the growth of cancer cells.

✢ It increases inflammation and oxidative stress and ages your brain, leading to what is being called type 3 diabetes (also known as Alzheimer's disease).

✢ It increases homocysteine because sugar consumption decreases B$_6$ and folate. That takes the methylation train off the tracks, making it hard for your brain to function and leading to more brain injury.

✢ It also causes sex hormone problems and can lead to infertility; hair growth where you don't want it (your face if you're a woman); hair loss where you don't want to lose it (your head); acne in women; low testosterone, loss of chest, leg, and arm hair, and breast growth in men; and more.

What's the Research on Insulin and How It Damages Your Brain?

Pioneering new work out of Harvard and Brown universities from Drs. Denis Selkoe and Suzanne de la Monte has proved that insulin resistance (also known as prediabetes) is a major factor in starting the cascade of brain damage that steals the memory of over half of people in their eighties, leading to a diagnosis of Alzheimer's disease.

The reason is that insulin resistance leads to a cascade of damage,[3] which produces the inflammation so characteristic of brain problems, especially dementia. (I will discuss why inflammation affects the brain this way in the next chapter.)

Do You Have Predementia?

You don't even have to wait until your eighties to start feeling the effects insulin resistance has on your memory. Many people now have what we call *"predementia."*

In fact, you may notice that you have trouble remembering names and numbers. This may be a sign of predementia. While this memory loss could be the effect of stress (we know that the stress hormone, cortisol, destroys and kills the brain cells in the hippocampus responsible for memory), it may also be because of that little extra fat around your middle.

One study of 2,632 men and women over five years published in the *Journal of the American Medical Association*[4] found that those with metabolic syndrome (or insulin resistance) and inflammation had dramatic declines in cognitive function.

This is more serious than just forgetting your keys. It is called mild cognitive impairment (MCI). Think of it as a prelude to dementia. What are the personal, social, and medical costs of this silent epidemic?

A *New York Times* report on Alzheimer's echoed research that makes it clear how powerfully our lifestyle impacts brain aging and how much we can do to reverse it:

> *For years, the prevailing notion was that Alzheimer's was a disease of brain-cell death. . . . But now, many researchers are asking if that old hypothesis is correct. If they are right, it may be possible to stop Alzheimer's, and reverse the memory loss, if treatments begin before brain cells die.*[5]

In fact, new brain imaging techniques called PET scans (positron emission tomography), which look not at brain structure like a CT scan or regular MRI but at brain metabolism (cellular function and activity), have found altered and damaged brain function that occurs far in advance of the diagnosis of dementia.[6] Some experts say that changes can be identified decades before diagnosis.

This process of decline, which is related to insulin resistance in particular, starts in childhood and adolescence. Given the epidemic of childhood obesity and the fact that we are seeing heart disease in twenty-year-olds, will we soon see an epidemic of Alzheimer's when (or if) these kids turn forty?

However, insulin resistance doesn't lead only to cognitive decline, memory impairment, dementia, and Alzheimer's.

Other Problems Created by Insulin Resistance

It is well known that depression is more common in diabetics, but a Finnish study of young men found that those who had the worst insulin resistance had an almost threefold risk of having severe depression.[7]

One of my patients, a physician, was morbidly obese and had tried everything from liquid diets to gastric bypass, all of which failed. It wasn't until he got his insulin under control that he was successful in losing a hundred pounds, but what was more remarkable was the transformation in his mood and his cravings.

We often think cravings are psychological in nature, but just the way a child who is iron deficient may eat dirt, if we are overfed and undernourished with too many empty calories and not enough nutrients, our brains may search for more nutrients.

Food cravings go away almost instantly when the body is back in balance. It is your hormones and nutritional deficiencies that drive your hunger.[8]

The doctor mentioned above told me that for the first time in his life he was not hungry twenty-four hours a day after we got his body (and specifically his insulin levels) back in balance.

The good news is that all these problems from depression to dementia can be stopped and even reversed if intervention occurs early enough.

Some simple dietary changes, a little exercise, relaxation, and a few supplements can completely correct and reverse insulin resistance and the catastrophic effects it has on the body and the brain.

Balancing blood sugar and correcting insulin resistance are well within our reach, and the effects are dramatic. Major studies have shown that just regular walking is enough to prevent cognitive decline and dementia.[9]

Scientific advances over the last few decades have given us the tools to prevent, stop, and even reverse cognitive decline and address all the mood disturbances that come with swings in blood sugar and insulin.

While there are some new medications that can help, such as Glucophage and Actos, they have side effects and are only a Band-Aid unless used with a comprehensive nutritional, exercise, and stress management plan that is the foundation of the UltraMind Solution I provide in Part III.

My goal is to make your metabolism more efficient, to make your cells more intelligent and cooperative, not resistant. In other words, you may need much less insulin to accomplish the task of balancing your blood sugar. And your mood and memory may be protected from the mind-robbing effects of insulin and sugar.

Now let's look at the next hormone on our list—the thyroid.

Thyroid Gland: A Yellow Canary in a Coal Mine of Environmental Toxins

Do you suffer from a slugglish, low-functioning thyroid? Take the following quiz and find out.

In the box on the right, place a check for each positive answer. Then find out how severe your problem is using the scoring key below.

THYROID QUIZ*

I have thick skin and fingernails. ☐
I have dry skin. ☐
My hair is thinning, I lose hair, or have coarse hair. ☐
I am sensitive to cold. ☐
I have cold hands and feet. ☐
I have muscle fatigue, pain, or weakness. ☐
I have heavy menstrual bleeding, worsening of premenstrual
syndrome, other menstrual problems, or infertility. ☐
My sex drive has decreased. ☐
I retain fluid (swelling of hands and feet). ☐
I feel fatigued (especially in the morning). ☐
I have low blood pressure and heart rate. ☐
I have trouble with memory and concentration. ☐
The outer third of my eyebrows are thinning. ☐
I have trouble losing weight or recent weight gain. ☐
I have constipation. ☐
I am depressed and apathetic. ☐
I have an autoimmune disease (rheumatoid arthritis, multiple
sclerosis, or lupus are examples). ☐
I have celiac disease or am gluten-sensitive. ☐
I have been exposed to radiation treatments. ☐
I have been exposed to environmental toxins. ☐
I consume a lot of tuna, sushi, and/or have multiple dental
silver fillings. ☐
I have a family history of thyroid problems. ☐
I drink chlorinated or fluoridated water. ☐

* For your convenience, this quiz has been reprinted in *The UltraMind Solution Companion Guide.* Simply go to www.ultramind.com/guide, download the guide, and print out the quiz.

Scoring Key—Thyroid

Score one point for each box you checked.

Score	Severity	Care Plan	Action to Take
0–7	You may have slightly low thyroid function.	*The UltraMind Solution*	Complete the six-week program in Part III.
8–11	You may have moderately low thyroid function.	Self-Care	Complete the six-week program in Part III and optimize your thyroid using the self-care options in chapter 23.
12 and above	You may have severely low thyroid function.	Medical Care	Do both of the steps above and see a physician for additional assistance. I have outlined some of the options you should discuss with your doctor in chapter 23.

In my twenty years of medical practice I have seen an increasing amount of thyroid disease. The question is why. In my practice and my review of the research I have discovered the thyroid gland is the yellow canary in the body. It is sensitive to multiple influences from our diet, our lifestyle, and the environment, all of which influence its function.

As our food environment has become more toxic and our exposure to pollution, petrochemical and industrial wastes, and heavy metals toxins have increased, our thyroid problems have also increased.

Most people are unaware of the connection between the environment, their diet, and their thyroid health. Yet these are increasingly important factors that need to be considered in order to help people resolve thyroid problems.

More than 20 percent of women and 10 percent of men have low-thyroid function. Half of them are undiagnosed.[10] Most people with thyroid problems are flying under the radar. As a result, many chronic symptoms go untreated, which causes people unnecessary suffering.

These are the most common symptoms of poor thyroid function:

+ Fatigue
+ Sluggishness
+ Trouble getting up in the morning
+ Depression

- Memory loss
- Insomnia
- Dry skin and dry hair
- Constipation
- Fluid retention
- Menstrual problems
- Premenstrual syndrome
- Hair loss
- Cracked, chipped fingernails
- Low sex drive
- Weight gain
- Muscle aches and cramps
- And more vague common symptoms that often are not effectively treated by modern medicine.

I remember the story of one patient who was seventy-three years old. This woman came to see me because when she went to her doctor with complaints of fatigue, sluggishness, poor memory, slight depression, dry skin, constipation, and a little fluid retention, her doctor said, "Well, what do you expect? You're seventy-three and this is what seventy-three is supposed to feel like."

I don't believe that is true. I believe that most of the symptoms of aging we see are really symptoms of abnormal aging or dysfunction that are related to imbalances in our core body systems.

We tested this woman for a number of things and found she had a sluggish thyroid. She did not quite meet all the criteria for a conventional diagnosis of hypothyroidism, but had an autoimmune reaction to her thyroid that led it to function poorly.

After we simply replaced her missing thyroid hormone, supported her nutritionally, and implemented some simple lifestyle changes, she went from feeling old to feeling alert, energetic, and youthful and all of her other symptoms cleared up.

The research on how thyroid affects mood and cognitive function is clear. In one study of the elderly, "subclinical" hypothyroidism increased the risk of depression four times.[11] Yet many doctors prescribe Prozac before taking a good hard look at the thyroid and treating those who don't yet have full-blown hypothyroidism.

It seems that the thyroid hormone is critical for helping the brain make new brain cells (neurogenesis), particularly in the hippocampus, which is responsible for mood and memory.[12]

In fact, mood disorders in general, including bipolar disorder, are increased in people with altered thyroid function.[13] Research shows that low-thyroid hormone levels reduce the function of serotonin receptors (remember our discussion of these happy mood neurotransmitters and their receptors from chapter 6), which leads to depression.[14]

Aside from the clear effect thyroid has on mood, it is also clear that low thyroid affects cognitive function, memory, and other indicators of slowed mental processing,[15] and that treating the thyroid improves all areas of mental functioning, including mood, mental processing, memory, and general cognitive function.[16]

Unfortunately, even those doctors who do treat for thyroid conditions usually use just the inactive thyroid hormone or T4 (Synthroid, Levoxyl), hoping your body converts it to the active form or T3, which is the form of the hormone that actually works to boost your metabolism and improve your mood and brain power. But it is often necessary to give T3 itself to correct the mood and memory problems associated with low-thyroid function.[17;18]

In fact, psychiatrists have proven that the use of T3 as a treatment for depression is more effective than just using SSRIs,[19;20] even though most other types of doctors generally think this is unnecessary or harmful. This is just one more example of the absolute segregation of medical specialties and lack of communication about important and effective treatments.

Why Is There an Epidemic of Thyroid Problems?

It is clear from the research that environmental chemicals have a direct impact on the thyroid gland.[21] The thyroid produces hormones that run our metabolism and influence almost every function of the body; therefore, the effect of these environmental chemicals on the thyroid gland has wide-ranging effects on our system.

For example, PCBs and other industrial petrochemical toxins lower thyroid function.[22] Other pollutants such as chlorine, fluoride, and bromine negatively influence thyroid function.[23] These toxins increase the elimination of thyroid hormone, leaving us with less of it to facilitate our metabolism and brain function.

Another important factor in thyroid function is food allergy. Food allergies, like those to gluten, and other food sensitivities also negatively affect thyroid function and are frequently undiagnosed. I will discuss food allergies and how they relate to inflammation in chapter 8. However, you should keep in mind they can also impact your thyroid.

It is important to understand the role of the environment and our nutritional status, food allergens, and nutritional deficiencies—such as selenium, zinc, fish oil, iodine, and tyrosine (all of which are important for thyroid function)—if we are going to overcome this problem that has now reached epidemic proportions.

Unfortunately, many of the common diagnostic tests used to assess our problems are often inadequate or incomplete. Therefore, many people who need treatment go untreated. You may have a low-functioning thyroid, yet not be diagnosed with "hypothyroidism" (yet another name for a "disease" that isn't really a disease), because the current diagnostic criteria are outdated and don't pick up more subtle problems with your thyroid.

It is also important to understand that the current treatments for thyroid problems, including Synthroid, are often less than adequate for many people. Some require a more personalized approach that combines both the inactive, T4 hormone found in Synthroid and the active, T3 hormone found in other medications.

The thyroid also plays a huge role in weight control (and blood-sugar control) and, in fact, in determining your metabolic rate. I have seen so many patients struggle with their weight, only to have the pounds melt off and their mood and brain function improve when we addressed their thyroid problems.

Sex Hormones: Puberty, PMS, Perimenopause, and Andropause

"Seventy-five percent of women are found to have a mutant gene that threatens their relationships, work, and well-being."

"Over half of aging men will lose their sexual function, their testosterone levels will drop, and their estrogen levels will rise, making men more like women."

These are the beliefs that most of us unconsciously accept.

Women are defective, flawed, broken, and destined to suffer throughout their reproductive life from the curse of mood and behavior swings that are the result of the three Ps: Puberty, PMS or premenstrual syndrome, and perimenopause (the years leading up to and just after your final period). This is the "genetic flaw" that supposedly threatens them.

As they age, men, if you believe all the television commercials, supposedly need the little blue pill (Viagra) just to be men again.

Is this just a "normal" part of being a woman or a man? Is it the product of some defective, mutant gene?

Why do sex hormone levels drop up to 90 percent through the aging process?

Are we destined to suffer from impaired mood, muscle loss, poor sleep, memory loss, and sexual problems?

Of course not!

This suffering related to your reproductive life cycle is unnecessary. It is not bad luck, but bad habits such as drinking and smoking, our high-sugar and refined-carbohydrate diet, environmental toxins, and chronic stress that deplete our adrenal glands.

These glands are the ones that produce most of the sex hormones later in life. Beat them to death with chronic stress and poor diet and lifestyle habits and your sex hormones may suffer. Let's look at the result of these bad habits.

But before we do . . .

Are your sexual hormones out of balance? Take the following quiz to find out.

(Note: There is one quiz for women and one for men.)

In the box on the right, place a check for each positive answer. Then find out how severe your problem is using the scoring key below.

SEXUAL HORMONES QUIZ FOR WOMEN*

I have premenstrual syndrome. ☐
I have monthly weight fluctuation. ☐
I have edema, swelling, puffiness, or water retention. ☐
I feel bloated. ☐
I have headaches. ☐
I have mood swings. ☐
I have tender, enlarged breasts. ☐
I am depressed. ☐
I feel unable to cope with ordinary demands. ☐
I have backaches, joint, or muscle pain. ☐
I have premenstrual food cravings (especially sugar or salt). ☐
I have irregular cycles, heavy bleeding, or light bleeding. ☐
I am infertile. ☐
I use birth-control pills or other hormones. ☐
I have premenstrual migraines. ☐
I have breast cysts or lumps or fibrocystic breasts. ☐
I have a family history of breast, ovarian, or uterine cancer. ☐
I have uterine fibroids. ☐

I have perimenopausal symptoms (hot flashes, mood swings, headaches, irregular cycles, heavy bleeding, fluid retention, breast tenderness, vaginal dryness, brain fog, muscle and joint pain, low sex drive, weight gain). ☐
I have hot flashes. ☐
I feel anxious. ☐
I have night sweats. ☐
I have insomnia. ☐
I have lost my sex drive. ☐
I have dry skin, hair, and/or vagina. ☐
I have heart palpitations. ☐
I have trouble with memory or concentration. ☐
I have bloating or weight gain around the middle. ☐
I have facial hair. ☐
I have been exposed to pesticides or heavy metals (in the food, water, and/or air). ☐

* For your convenience, this quiz has been reprinted in *The UltraMind Solution Companion Guide*. Simply go to www.ultramind.com/guide, download the guide, and print out the quiz.

Scoring Key—Sexual Hormones for Women

Score one point for each box you checked.

Score	Severity	Care Plan	Action to Take
0–9	You may have a mild sexual hormone imbalance.	*The UltraMind Solution*	Complete the six-week program in Part III.
10–14	You may have a moderate sexual hormone imbalance.	Self-Care	Complete the six-week program in Part III and optimize your sexual hormones using the self-care options in chapter 23.
15 and above	You may have a severe sexual hormone imbalance.	Medical Care	Do both of the steps above and see a physician for additional assistance. I have outlined some of the options you should discuss with your doctor in chapter 23.

SEXUAL HORMONES QUIZ FOR MEN*

I have a reduced sex drive and have lost my vitality. ☐
I have trouble achieving or maintaining an erection. ☐
I am infertile or have low sperm counts. ☐
I have loss of muscle. ☐
I have increased abdominal fat. ☐
I am fatigued or have low energy. ☐
I feel a loss of direction and purpose or a sense of apathy. ☐
I have bone loss or bone fractures. ☐
I have increasing cholesterol. ☐
I have increased insulin and blood sugar. ☐
I feel weak. ☐
I feel depressed. ☐
I have been exposed to pesticides or heavy metals (in the food, water, and/or air). ☐

* For your convenience, this quiz has been reprinted in *The UltraMind Solution Companion Guide*. Simply go to www.ultramind.com/guide, download the guide, and print out the quiz.

Scoring Key—Sexual Hormones for Men

Score one point for each box you checked.

Score	Severity	Care Plan	Action to Take
0–4	You may have a mild sexual hormone imbalance.	*The UltraMind Solution*	Complete the six-week program in Part III.
5–6	You may have a moderate sexual hormone imbalance.	Self-Care	Complete the six-week program in Part III and optimize your fatty acids using the self-care options in chapter 23.
7 and above	You may have a severe sexual hormone imbalance.	Medical Care	Do both of the steps above and see a physician for additional assistance. I have outlined some of the options you should discuss with your doctor in chapter 23.

PMS is a condition that causes mood swings, irritability, depression, anxiety, fluid retention, bloating, breast tenderness, sugar cravings, headaches, and sleep disturbances. It affects 75 percent of women.

In 20 percent, it is so severe it requires medical treatment, and about 8 percent have extreme symptoms that have been given a new name: premenstrual dysphoric disorder (PMDD). Of course, a new drug called Sarafem has been "discovered" to cure it (it is only Prozac with a different label). This was a great sleight of hand by the pharmaceutical industry, skilled at producing new diseases to match its drugs.

What about *menopause*? The brain fog, memory loss, mood swings, sleepless nights, vaginal dryness, low sex drive, palpitations, and anxiety common in menopause are simply signs of hormonal imbalances (estrogen, progesterone, and testosterone). But are you truly destined to suffer?

And how about *andropause*? Although men experience a more gradual drop off in hormones, they too experience "andropause"—the slow decline in male (testosterone) and energy (DHEA) hormones, which leads to depression, fatigue, and loss of mental sharpness, not to mention loss of sexual desire and function.

What's wrong with this picture?

It is based on the assumption that these symptoms are an inevitable part of aging and require "medical intervention" with serious medication to correct.

Which is simply untrue.

To think that 75 percent of women have a design flaw that gives them PMS and requires medical treatment to live a normal life is just absurd. To think that we all have to dwindle, shrivel, and lose our emotional, physical, and sexual vitality is a burdensome self-fulfilling prophecy.

We now have endless examples of balance and thriving at any age. One of my eighty-one-year-old female patients with a twinkle in her eye recently told me about her new boyfriend and their wonderful love life.

PMS, menopausal symptoms, and andropause are signs of imbalances in your sex hormones. They are not the result of mutant genes that destroy our sexual vitality as we age. Instead, they are treatable symptoms of underlying imbalance in one of the core systems in your body. Get the sex hormones back in balance, and these problems usually disappear.

The emotional strain that comes with these conditions is a telling way to understand the connection these hormones have to your mind, your body, and your reproductive cycle. It is yet another example of the way the body affects the brain.

Depression or Hormonal Imbalance?

Let me tell you the story of a patient of mine with PMDD. She was barely able to function. She suffered three weeks out of every month with severe physical symptoms and debilitating depression. Was she Prozac-deficient? I think not.

*M*aureen *was thirty-seven years old. Many women feel worsening PMS symptoms as they get into their later reproductive years because of changes in hormonal cycles. Part of what Maureen experienced was severe depression, fatigue, anxiety, and food and sugar cravings that led to overeating and weight gain.*

She also had joint pains, breast tenderness, heavy bleeding, hot flashes, dry skin, acne, hair loss, trouble with memory, poor sleep, and no sex drive.

Maureen didn't drink alcohol, but was a big coffee drinker. She started the day with a bagel and cheese, had a cafeteria lunch, chocolates in the afternoon, and a healthy dinner followed by binging on ice cream, potato chips, and Cheerios.

She also complained of gas and bloating.

She also ate a lot of dairy, which a lot of people (this woman included) are sensitive to.

This is a story I hear all too often. The good news is that there was a simple solution for Maureen that didn't involve taking medication.

We know that sugar, caffeine, alcohol, stress, and lack of exercise all contribute to worsening PMS[24] and hormonal imbalances, including menopause and andropause.[25]

It is also true that dairy consumption can worsen hormonal imbalances because of all the hormones in milk.[26; 27] Even organic milk can come from pregnant cows— jacking up hormone levels.[28]

I helped Maureen change her diet, cut out the sugar and caffeine, eliminate her food allergens, take a few supplements and herbs, do a little exercise, and within one menstrual cycle her life changed.

All her symptoms resolved, she lost weight and dramatically increased her energy. Her mood stabilized (meaning her depression evaporated), and her acne and dry skin went away. All without medication.

The approach I take to this problem is part of the overall approach of Functional Medicine. Define the imbalance (in Maureen's case severe hormonal imbalances), address the causes first (namely diet/lifestyle in this case), and then help the body repair and regain balance. The body's natural intelligence takes care of the rest.

When you use this method to rebalance the hormones, not only do the physical symptoms of PMS, menopause, or andropause disappear, but the mental symptoms usually go away as well. That's because sex hormones act on various parts of your brain that influence your mood and behavior.

How Sex Hormones Act on the Brain

What many people don't know (although they experience this all the time) is that sex hormones act on the brain directly to affect mood and cognition.

For example, estrogen promotes the production of neurotransmitters, especially serotonin, making it a wonderful antidepressant (not to mention a great sleep aid).

In fact, there are receptors for all hormones, including estrogen, in the brain. And estrogen in the brain seems to be neuroprotective, potentially reducing the risk of dementia.[29] But a little too much can cause breast, uterine, and cervical cancer. Getting the balance right is essential.

Progesterone is another important sex hormone. Levels drop in PMS and in perimenopause, leading to increased anxiety and insomnia. There is evidence that natural, bioidentical (hormones identical to those produced by the body) progesterone reduces this anxiety and stress through its action on GABA receptors, the relaxing neurotransmitter—your body's natural Valium.[30]

Testosterone is also a wonderful brain-boosting hormone that improves mood, memory, motivation, and overall cognitive function. It drops significantly in women and men with age and has an enormous impact on quality of life.[31] But it drops mostly because of weight gain, lack of exercise, stress, and high-sugar diets—not because we are genetically designed to have less testosterone as we age.

The biggest reason I see low testosterone in men is insulin resistance. High belly fat drives insulin up and testosterone down. That's why men start looking like women and lose hair on their bodies, grow breasts, and have round, soft skin. It is because they are actually producing less testosterone and more estrogen. At the point that their estrogen levels exceed their testosterone levels, they sort of become women!

Correcting insulin problems by eating whole foods, cutting out sugar and white flour, and doing some exercise to build muscle may naturally raise testosterone levels. And if you are a man, be sure you root for the winning sports team, because research shows that when your team loses, your testosterone levels drop![32]

I find, especially in older men, that giving them a little topical bioidentical testosterone helps them build muscle and bone and lose weight; it re-lieves depression, stabilizes mood swings,[33] improves memory and concen-tration,[34] and improves sexual function.[35] Even women benefit from the use of bioidentical testosterone in some cases.

Hormone replacement therapy must be carefully administered under a doctor's supervision after adequate testing. I strongly advocate the use of "nature-made" molecules to support normal function, rather than "new to nature" or man-made substances, which often have many unwanted and dangerous effects.

That means supplementing your system with chemicals it already uses, like vitamins or minerals, is usually a better treatment than using medications.

This applies to hormones as well, which is why I recommend only *bioidentical hormones*. Used intelligently, at the right time, for the right pa-tient, in the right dose, for the right amount of time, they can be lifesaving.

But 80 percent of the time, simply changing your diet and lifestyle, detoxifying, addressing stress, and rebalancing all the other seven keys to UltraWellness can often help you regain balance without taking hormones.

To do this, you need to know what is sending your hormones out of bal-ance to begin with.

Why Are Our Sex Hormones Out of Balance?

Sex hormones can become unbalanced in both men and women. But *why* does this happen?

PMS and perimenopausal symptoms most women experience are be-cause their hormones are out of balance. Estrogen levels actually increase, especially from the age of about thirty to fifty, and progesterone levels de-crease either relatively or absolutely. Testosterone levels drop off in men and women, leading to a loss of energy, depression, and low sex drive.[36]

Many things promote these imbalances in hormones, such as a high-sugar, refined carbohydrate diet, caffeine, stress, dairy (if you are sensitive to it), hormones in the food supply in dairy products and meat, and estrogen-like toxins from pesticides, plastics, and pollution.

Exercise also helps keep hormones in balance. If you don't get enough of it, they will get out of balance.

Alcohol damages the liver and prevents it from excreting excess estro-gen, yet another factor that influences hormonal imbalance. Men who drink too much literally grow breasts along with their beer bellies!

In addition, constipation and imbalances in the gut bacteria can lead to the reabsorption of estrogen from the gut back into your blood, even after your liver has tried to get rid of it.

Before I close this chapter, there is one more issue I want to discuss that has a major impact on all the hormones and many other biological processes as well—sleep. You need it if you are going to stay in balance.

Lights Out: Why We Need More Sleep

Most people don't know that sleep deprivation leads to depression, chronic pain, heart disease, diabetes, and makes you fat!

In fact, beside eating whole foods and moving your body, getting enough sleep is the most important thing you can do for your health.

Yet it is estimated that 70 percent of Americans are sleep-deprived.

The era of Starbucks has been surpassed by prescription stimulants to keep people awake and functioning, like dexadrine and Ritalin, otherwise known as "speed" or amphetamines.

Surprisingly, I see an increasing number of patients prescribed these uppers by their psychiatrist because coffee is not enough. If we can't do ten things at once, then something must be wrong with us, right?

Wrong!

Our bodies and biological rhythms, which keep us healthy, produce cyclic pulses of healing and repair hormones, including melatonin[37] and growth hormone.[38; 39] When those rhythms are disturbed by inadequate or insufficient sleep, disease and breakdown get the upper hand. Sleep also helps us maintain low levels of cortisol—the stress hormone that makes us depressed and fat (see chapter 12).

Most of us need at least seven to eight hours of restful sleep a night.

Getting this is more and more difficult. Yet we evolved along with the rhythms of day and night. Our bodies use these rhythms to signal a whole cascade of hormonal and neurochemical reactions that keep us healthy by repairing our DNA, building tissues and muscle, and regulating weight and mood chemicals.

The lightbulb changed all that.

However, not following the normal rhythms of day and night can be deadly. In fact, when I learned that shift work (like I did in when I worked in the emergency room) leads to a shortened life expectancy, I quit.[40]

When we are sleep-deprived our cortisol rises with all its harmful effects, including brain damage and dementia, weight gain, diabetes, heart attacks, high blood pressure, depression, osteoporosis, reduced immune function, and more.

Sleep deprivation also leads to depression, decreased cognitive performance, and even decreased reaction times.[41]

Good sleep is not something that just happens (unless you are a baby or teenager). There are clearly defined things that interfere with or support healthy sleep. By following the six-week plan in Part III of *The UltraMind Solution,* you may restore your natural sleep rhythm.

It may take weeks or months, but using these tools in a coordinated way will eventually reset your biological rhythms.

But you have to prioritize sleep!

When I first started practicing, I thought M.D. stood for "medical deity" and meant I didn't have to follow the same sleep rules as every other human being. Was I wrong! Working one hundred hours a week, sometimes sixty hours straight, being up at night delivering babies, then working all day in the office, had a catastrophic effect on my health, and ultimately contributed to my chronic fatigue syndrome.

Our lives are infiltrated with stimuli and we stay stimulated until the moment we get into bed. This is not the way to get restful sleep.

Is it any wonder we can't sleep well when we eat a late dinner, answer e-mails, surf the Web or work, and then get right into bed and watch the evening news about all the disaster, pain, and suffering in the world?

We must take a little "holiday" in the two hours before bed. Creating a sleep ritual, a special set of little things you do before bed to help ready your system physically and psychologically for sleep, can guide your body into a deep healing sleep. In Part III, I will teach you how to achieve a sound and restful sleep every night.

So remember—*don't skimp on sleep.* It is one of the most powerful healing treatments for your body that is available to you every day. In Part III you will learn how to restore healthy sleep.

SPECIAL NOTE: SLEEP APNEA

Do you snore? Are you tired most of the day? Do you have trouble focusing, concentrating, and feel depressed? Do you nod off when you sit down to watch TV or read, or worse when you are driving? You could be one of the 18 million people (80 percent of whom are *not* diagnosed[42]) who have sleep apnea, a condition where your airway closes off periodically at night, interrupting your sleep as well as leading to high blood pressure, weight gain, and even heart failure. If you think you may have this problem, ask your doctor about testing and treatment. It could save your life.

Balance Your Hormones

Balance is the key to staying healthy. Nowhere is this truer than in the world of hormones.

Do not think of your hormones separately but as interconnected parts of the whole that affect one another.

Hormones are also influenced by imbalances in the seven keys. Our body is one whole system where everything is linked to everything else. So improving your nutrition, reducing inflammation, fixing your gut, and getting rid of toxins all support normalization of hormone function, which translates into better mood, more focus, and enhanced brain function.

Everyone has a different balance point and needs a little more tweaking here or there to get in balance, but following the basic six-week Ultra-Mind Solution in Part III will provide a strong foundation. Then you can customize your approach based on where you find you are most out of balance using the steps in Part IV.

Balancing your hormones is a process, and sometimes it has little twists and turns, but by sticking with it, you can figure out how to restore yourself to the vital, happy, alert, brilliant, and thriving being you are.

In the next chapter you will learn how brain inflammation has been linked to everything from autism to Alzheimer's, from depression to ADHD. Our brains are on fire. Find out why and what to do about it.

CHAPTER 8

KEY #3: COOL OFF INFLAMMATION

———

Can your brain become inflamed? Can you have a "swollen brain" like a swollen, arthritic knee? Can you have a "sore brain" like a sore throat? Until recently, except in cases of brain infections (such as meningitis or encephalitis), brain inflammation was considered rare.

However, new evidence links hidden brain inflammation to almost every known "brain disease," from depression to dementia, from autism to anxiety, from schizophrenia to sociopathic behavior.

The brain is on fire in the twenty-first century. If one in three Americans suffers from a mental illness, and 14 million Americans will soon have Alzheimer's, and nearly all mood disorders and age-related brain diseases are symptoms of an inflamed or "sore" brain, then this problem touches nearly everyone.

Of course, inflammation doesn't affect only the brain. We are seeing the flames in every disease, including autoimmunity (24 million), allergy (50 million), and asthma (30 million), as well as cardiovascular disease (60 million), cancer (10 million), and diabetes (14 million). These, it has been recently discovered, are primarily inflammatory conditions.

You might say we are all on fire.

The problem is that it's sometimes hard to locate the source of this fire. Because systemic inflammation, which contributes to all of these conditions, *is* systemic, it can be difficult to figure out what is fueling this unseen, internal inflammation in the first place. Why do our bodies become inflamed?

Finding an answer to this question is the key to healing all chronic illness, especially mental and brain disorders.

Then, once we find the fire, we have to learn how to cool it *way* down.

But the fire often comes from many unexpected places—foods we eat, toxins in the environment, hidden infections, unknown allergens, and stress. If you want to address your swollen, inflamed brain, you have to find the source of the fire and stomp it out.

Let's start by understanding what systemic inflammation is, what problems are caused by brain inflammation, and, finally, the causes of this unseen fire in the body.

But first, find out if your brain is on fire.

Take the following quiz to find out how inflamed you are and how this affects your brain.

In the box on the right, place a check for each positive answer. Then find out how severe your problem is using the scoring key below.

INFLAMMATION QUIZ*

I have seasonal or environmental allergies. ☐
I have food allergies or sensitivities or I don't feel well after eating (sluggishness, headaches, confusion, etc.). ☐ ☐
I work in an environment with poor lighting, chemicals, and/or poor ventilation. ☐
I am exposed to pesticides, toxic chemicals, loud noise, heavy metals, and/or toxic bosses and coworkers. ☐
I get frequent colds and infections. ☐
I have a history of chronic infections such as hepatitis, skin infections, canker sores, cold sores. ☐
I have sinusitis and allergies. ☐
I have bronchitis or asthma. ☐
I have dermatitis (eczema, acne, rashes). ☐
I suffer from arthritis (osteoarthritis/degenerative—wear and tear). ☐
I have an autoimmune disease (rheumatoid arthritis, lupus, hypothyroidism, etc.). ☐
I have colitis or inflammatory bowel disease. ☐
I have irritable bowel syndrome (spastic colon). ☐
I have neuritis (problems like ADHD, autism, mood and behavior problems). ☐
I have heart disease or have had a heart attack. ☐
I have diabetes or am overweight (BMI greater than 25—a BMI chart has been printed in *The UltraMind Solution Companion Guide* for your convenience.) ☐
I have or my family has a history of Parkinson's or Alzheimer's. ☐
I have a stressful life. ☐
I drink more than three glasses of alcohol a week. ☐
I don't exercise more than thirty minutes three times a week. ☐

---

* For your convenience, this quiz has been reprinted in *The UltraMind Solution Companion Guide.* Simply go to www.ultramind.com/guide, download the guide, and print out the quiz.

Scoring Key—Inflammation

Score one point for each box you checked.

Score	Severity	Care Plan	Action to Take
0–6	You may have a low level of inflammation.	*The UltraMind Solution*	Complete the six-week program in Part III.
7–9	You may have a moderate level of inflammation.	Self-Care	Complete the six-week program in Part III and reduce your inflammation using the self-care options in chapter 24.
10 and above	You may have a severe level of inflammation.	Medical Care	Do both of the steps above and see a physician for additional assistance. I have outlined some of the options you should discuss with your doctor in chapter 24.

What Is Systemic (Whole-Body) Inflammation? The Smoldering Fire Within

Most of us are familiar with inflammation. Classic signs are pain, swelling, redness, and heat. Think about a bad sore throat, a swollen knee, or an infected fingernail. In each case, the part of your body that's affected is inflamed.

Inflammation is part of the body's natural defense system against infection, irritation, toxins, and foreign molecules. When your body detects problems like these, a cascade of events occurs in which white blood cells and chemicals called cytokines (*see the text box on page 175 to learn more about these important chemicals*) mobilize to protect you from foreign invaders.

In this capacity, inflammation is a good thing. It fights foreign invaders of all types.

However, when the natural balance of your immune system (which produces just enough inflammation to keep infections, allergens, toxins, or other stressors under control) is disrupted, the immune system shifts into a chronic state of alarm, spreading a smoldering fire of inflammation throughout the body.

In essence, the part of your immune system that is designed to protect you from foreign invaders starts attacking the cells and tissues of your own body. When this happens it can create *major* problems.

This fire in the heart causes heart disease, in our fat cells causes obesity, in the whole body causes cancer, in the eyes causes blindness, and, when this fire spreads to your brain, it can cause depression, dementia, autism, ADHD, Alzheimer's, forgetfulness, and a host of other problems.

This inflammatory process may go awry, not only in individuals with inflammatory diseases but in otherwise healthy people whose lifestyles and/or environments expose them to substances the body perceives as irritants, such as low-grade infections from gum disease, food allergens, toxins, and even inflammatory foods such as sugar and animal fat. (You will learn more about each of these specific causes of inflammation later in the chapter.)

While inflammation is sometimes obvious, such as when an injured area becomes swollen, red, and warm to the touch, science is teaching us that inflammation can occur silently and insidiously, without any symptoms.

To understand how profound inflammation can be to brain health, I want to look at three conditions that may be caused by inflammation: autism, depression, and Alzheimer's. If we understand how inflammation plays a role in these conditions, we will have an opportunity to treat all problems of brain function in a radically different way.

Most psychiatric and neurological problems, in some way, are just the brain on fire.

CYTOKINES:
THE MESSENGER MOLECULES OF YOUR IMMUNE SYSTEM

Cytokines are a class of proteins that are the "language" of your immune system, much in the way neurotransmitters are the "language" of your nervous system, and hormones are the "language" of your endocrine system or hormone-secreting glands.

These chemicals can either promote or reduce inflammation. They are the main communication system that controls inflammation and directs your immune system to heal.

When triggered by toxins, infections, allergens, stress, a bad diet, or a sedentary lifestyle, cytokines run out of control starting fires all over the body and brain. There are 400,000 scientific studies on the role of these immune

(continued)

messengers in almost every disease. Inflammation does not respect the artificial boundaries of medical specialties.

In fact, when it comes to chronic illnesses—whether physical or mental—everywhere we look, there they are. Dementia, depression, ADHD, autism, chronic fatigue, obesity, heart disease, cancer, and, of course, allergic and autoimmune diseases are *all* related to elevated levels of cytokines and systemic inflammation. They can cause problems in every organ, in every part of the body.[1]

"Brain Disease" and Inflammation

Often we think of bad moods, unusual behavior, hyperactivity, or trouble concentrating as evidence of some psychological problem, much like we once thought autism and schizophrenia were the result of poor mothering. But new scientific findings are shaking up our thinking.

The Role of Inflammation and the Example of Autism

The most startling and convincing story comes from the world of autism. As I have said before, autism is just an extreme example of what can go wrong with our brain. The same things happen in depression, Alzheimer's, or almost any psychiatric or neurological problem.

As the nature of disease gets uncovered, the common underlying roots of all illnesses become apparent. Autism and Alzheimer's are almost the same disease showing up at the opposite end of the age spectrum—the metabolism, biochemistry, and causes all map over one another.

Martha Herbert, M.D., Ph.D., an assistant professor of neurology at Harvard Medical School, has put together a remarkable story of autism, which is like a hologram through which we can see the systemic nature of most illness. Her landmark paper, "Autism: A brain disorder, or a disorder that affects the brain?"[2] will change forever our thinking about mental and brain illness.

Dr. Herbert looked very carefully at autistic children's brains on MRI scans. She noticed their brains were bigger than children who did not have autism.[3] The question that remained was why.

That's where Dr. Diana Vargas and her group from Johns Hopkins came in. They examined the brains on autopsy of eleven autistic children who had died.[4] They also looked at the spinal fluid of living autistic children. By examining and comparing these factors, they proved that these children's brains were swollen and inflamed, like a swollen ankle!

This brought up another question: why were their brains inflamed to begin with?

The short answer is allergens, toxins, infections, and nutritional deficiencies.

But where do problems like these come from and how do they affect the brain? Are they in the brain to begin with? Well, many times they may not be.

It has long been known that children with autism not only have misfiring and wiring of their brain, but that 95 percent of autistic children have gastrointestinal problems and swollen bellies. It has also been noted that autistic children have frequent infections and allergies, and have often had multiple courses of antibiotics. And according to the MIND Institute at the University of California at Davis, more than 70 percent of children on the autistic spectrum have altered immune function.[5]

Most doctors assume these are annoying but secondary problems, meaning they have nothing to do with why autistic children's brains are not working properly or why their brains are swollen and inflamed.

But according to Dr. Herbert, the opposite seems to be true. These gut, immune, and toxicity problems are integrally related to and often the cause of what happens in the brain. In fact, she suggests that autism is really a systemic metabolic disorder that changes brain function. The brain and body function as a whole system. And multiple chronic, insidious triggers can throw the brain into chaos.

As you will learn in chapter 9 when I discuss the gut, more than 60 percent of the immune system is in the digestive tract. When that key system in the body is thrown out of balance, your immune system is triggered and widespread systemic inflammation can often result.

We insult our digestive tract every day. We do everything to harm it and hardly anything to help it work as it was designed. We eat food low in fiber, high in sugar, and full of antibiotics, pesticides, and hormones; we drink alcohol and caffeine; we take antibiotics, acid-blocking medication, anti-inflammatory drugs, hormones, and steroids; we are under constant stress; and we are exposed to thousands of environmental toxins, all of which damage the gut.

These factors create widespread inflammation because our gut immune system reacts to all the foreign proteins in food and all the myriad of bugs and gets "angry" and inflamed.

So if inflammation starts in the belly (and so many autistic children have swollen bellies), then spreads to the brain, it can literally lead to a swollen brain. And the effects can be disastrous.

Imagine the extraordinary beauty and dance of the brain where everything is exquisitely regulated. The timing and coordination of nerve-cell firing and the amplitude (or volume) of the message has to be just right. Filters that modulate our sensory inputs must let in only the information we need. The activity of the brain must be exquisitely synchronized for us to be awake, alert, receptive, interactive, communicative, flexible, and happy.

But what if the signals start misfiring and the coordination and synchronization break down because of multiple metabolic disturbances such as ineffective enzymes or cell function due to insults from toxins, infections, allergens, or nutritional deficiencies?

This is the net effect of inflammation, whatever the original cause. It triggers a runaway cascade of damaging effects. All mental processing slows, neurotransmitters can't do their job, cell membranes don't function the way they were designed, cellular enzymes get hijacked or derailed, cells get sent into a death spiral called apoptosis and the delicate network of cellular connections and communications is interrupted and altered.

How does that show up? As autism or Alzheimer's or depression. It depends on the unique genetic makeup and environment of each individual person. In the children discussed above, the result of this inflammation is autism. In you, it may be anything from a bad mood to dementia to hyperactivity and difficulty focusing.

Whatever the case, at the end of the day we are all suffering from swollen brains.

These problems may not show up on the radar of conventional testing, but they wreak havoc in your body and your brain. We see this havoc as altered behavior, mood, and memory. It is precisely in these metabolic disturbances that we need to look for answers.

Inflammation has enormous implications for treating autism and most "brain disorders." Our broken brains may be due to *fixable* metabolic problems created by digestive imbalances, toxins, foods, allergens, and hidden infections, and worsened by nutritional deficiencies.

Scientists are now asking the question why? Why do we find more mercury in autistic children? What is the effect of mercury on the brain? Why do these children have altered immune function? Why do they have more viral infections? Why do we find measles virus in the intestinal lining of these children and in their spinal fluid? What is the effect of giving babies nine immunizations at one doctor's visit, or twenty-seven by the time they are two years old? How do these all trigger inflammation and how does this cause autism?

Questions like these force us to ask how biology, brain, and behavior connect.

There Is No Gene for Autism: Looking at All the Causes

Researchers have been searching for the one autism gene, or the one location in the brain that is damaged, that leads to autism. Looking for these kinds of answers implies that the changes that cause autism (or other "brain disorders") are genetically hard-wired and therefore treatment is hopeless.

But these researchers are looking in the wrong place for the source of the problem.

These same metabolic and environmental problems hold true for the 1 in 6 children with some type of developmental problem, the 1 in 10 with ADHD, and the 1 in 150 with autism. Each of these may be problems related to underlying metabolic disorders, and *not* the result of genetically hard-wired diseases or damaged brains. It is all the same problem just showing up slightly differently in different kids.

Dr. Herbert suggests that many *different causes* can lead to the *same symptoms*, namely the lack of language and social connection and the rigidity and inflexibility of behavior seen in children with autism, as well as many "behavioral" problems in children such as those with ADHD. A few common pathways result in the same symptoms from a host of different insults. There may be many "autisms," each caused by slightly different factors.

Rather than studying drugs that affect the brain to treat autism, the better path may be studying treatments that target inflammation, toxins, allergens, infections, or fixing biochemical train wrecks (like problems with methylation and sulfation), and gut problems.

Treating the gut, or giving B_{12}, B_6, and folate, omega-3 fats, vitamins A or D, or magnesium and zinc, or eliminating gluten and casein (the protein in dairy that so many are sensitive to) from the diet, or detoxifying mercury and lead from their little bodies may be the best way to get autistic children's brain connections working again.

Quite a notion! **Treat the body, and heal the brain.**

The experience of thousands of children, parents, scientists, and doctors who are part of a unique collaborative effort called DAN!, or Defeat Autism Now! (www.autism.com), confirms that this approach helps children recover—some slightly, some miraculously—from a disorder that was thought incurable.

In the treatment of psychiatric and neurological disorders, we must look at the body. We need to look for the connections, patterns, and final common pathways that have enormous implications for so many "fixed" diseases. If recovery and improvement are documented in autism, what does that mean for Alzheimer's, chronic depression, bipolar disease, psychosis, eating disorders, or violent sociopathic behavior?

These problems, it seems, are not hard-wired into the brain, as we believed, but the result of a few common systemic problems that completely mess up the fine dance and coordination of the brain—problems that can be fixed metabolically and systemically.

Dr. Herbert's TRANSCEND (Treatment, Research, and Neuroscience Evaluation of Neurodevelopmental Disorders) research program at Harvard is breaking radical new ground in looking at the brain as part of the whole body system. Stay tuned, because I believe their work will change not only our perception of autism but of *all* disease and the nature of research itself by changing what questions we ask, how we ask them, and how we search for answers.

Now is the moment in medical science that parallels the shift in thinking that occurred when Christopher Columbus said the world was round or Galileo proposed that the earth was not the center of the universe but revolved around the sun.

The implications across the entire spectrum of suffering and illness are profound.

Is Depression a Systemic Inflammatory Disease?

How can exercise and fish oil often be a more effective treatment for depression than antidepressants? Could it be because they are both potent anti-inflammatories? Could it be that depression is a low-grade inflammatory disease of the brain?[6] Let's look at the evidence.[7]

1. Proinflammatory cytokines IL-1, IL-6, and TNF α (molecular messengers that set off the inflammatory response) and bacterial toxins (produced in our gut for reasons we will explore in chapter 9) produce symptoms of depression and anxiety.
2. Cytokines overactivate the HPA (hypothalamic-pituitary-adrenal) axis (the stress response), just as we find in depressed patients.
3. Cytokines increase the function of an enzyme (IDO) that breaks down tryptophan, leading to less serotonin in the brain.[8]

4. The immune system is overactive in severe depression, producing brain inflammation.
5. Using immune therapy like interferon (a cytokine) for diseases like hepatitis C or multiple sclerosis triggers depression.
6. Depression is more common in inflammatory diseases like autoimmune disease and heart disease.

As compelling as these pieces of information are, they are not the only indications that depression is caused by an inflamed brain.

Researchers from the Free University of Berlin discovered a new virus called Bornavirus found in the limbic system (or emotional center) of the brain in 30 percent of the population. One in six people who carry the virus have depression *and* can be cured by treatment with short-term antiviral medication. Think about it: a virus can cause depression and treating the virus can *cure,* not just reduce the symptoms of, depression. Even the best antidepressant drugs don't cure depression.[9]

And there is more evidence that inflammation can cause depression. A new technique called vagal nerve stimulation is very helpful in depression.[10] The vagus nerve is your calming, relaxation nerve. When you take a deep breath, meditate, or do yoga, the nerve is activated and it releases acetylcholine, which reduces the production of inflammatory cytokines.

There may be many reasons deep breathing and relaxation work, but certainly one of them is the fact that inflammation is reduced.

We also know that omega-3 fats help depression and produce remission.[11] They work through lowering inflammation, and also through their effects on cell membranes and communication.

Similarly, we know that exercise is an anti-inflammatory and works better than Prozac in treating depression.[12]

Another example comes out of Harvard. A group of researchers there discovered an increased number of "white matter lesions" or little white spots in the brain that are seen in autoimmune diseases like multiple sclerosis in depressed patients. This correlated with low levels of folate, which caused high levels of homocysteine, a molecule that causes inflammation in the brain.[13] So being vitamin-deficient produces toxic molecules that inflame the brain and cause depression.

Of course, we must ask, "What came first, the chicken or the egg? Does depression cause inflammation or inflammation cause depression?"

The answer is yes. It is a vicious cycle. Inflammation leads to depression, which leads to more inflammation.

The message is that to adequately treat depression we must look for, find, and eliminate the causes of inflammation and then help the body create balance in the immune system, turning off this vicious cycle.

All of the things that create inflammation not only cause depression but also anxiety, obsessive-compulsive disorder (OCD), and bipolar disease. Of course, we must remember that these are just names of collections of symptoms we give people. The causes may be very different from person to person. But within the seven keys we can find the causes, and we must treat all of them for people to heal.

Looked at as a whole, the pieces of the scientific puzzle make sense. In a separate but connected example, there is a form of OCD that is well documented in children called PANDAS (Pediatric Autoimmune Neuropsychiatric Disorders Associated with Streptococcal Infections). This condition causes children to suffer from the strange obsessions and compulsions "called" OCD—anything from repeatedly washing hands, or opening and closing doors, to counting objects, to involuntary movements. It is triggered by an infection with streptococcus.[14] The streptococcal bacteria release toxins that produce inflammation in the brain. Treat the bacteria with antibiotics, inflammation in the brain is reduced, and the OCD goes away.

Why aren't we looking at models like this one as a way to treat other "brain disorders"? Why do we insist on viewing them as "psychiatric problems" instead of systemic imbalances?

Surprising discoveries like the ones above break open new territory for treating mood disorders, particularly depression. Treating infections, eliminating allergies, learning to deeply relax, exercising, and taking vitamins and fish oil all can reduce inflammation and fix depression.

But we must remember that it is not either/or, it is *and*. Illness (whether it is mental or physical) is not usually one thing. It is often everything—just to different degrees in different people. Hundreds of my patients with mood disorders improve simply by addressing the inflammation. It is an "accidental" side effect of treating their other problems.

The lesson? Treat the fire, not the smoke.

Just like I did for Elizabeth.

*E*lizabeth *was a twenty-one-year-old woman who suffered, as many of my patients do, from a long list of problems.*

At the top of the list were mood problems that had plagued her since childhood. She had been diagnosed with anxiety, depression, and even borderline personality disorder because of her wild mood swings.

At work, people avoided her, never knowing what to expect, and she was always fighting with her parents.

She was high strung, irritable, and also had trouble concentrating. Sugar cravings drove her to the fridge every day after work—pudding, pizza, and junk food were staples and late-night snacking was hard to control.

She had been on Zoloft since she was thirteen. Now, an adult and five-foot-one-inch tall, her weight ballooned up to 170 pounds. Not only was she tired (though she was sleeping ten hours a night) but she also had allergies, postnasal drip, sinus congestion, fluid in her ears, and snored.

Her delayed or IgG food-allergy tests showed she was highly sensitive to eggs, wheat, rye, dairy, and yeast. She also had low levels of omega-3 fats.

I put Elizabeth on an elimination diet—giving her a break from foods that triggered her immune system. I added a few vitamins, including vitamin D and B_6, and omega-3 fats.

Two months later she came back. She had lost twenty-three pounds and her cravings were gone. But it was the mood change she experienced that was truly astounding. Her mood changed for the first time in her life. She no longer had wild mood swings or irritability.

Her energy level dramatically improved as well. She needed only seven to eight hours of sleep to feel fully and vitally awake.

After five months she had lost thirty-three pounds without trying, felt deeply happy for the first time in her life, and was thriving at work and in her family. All her other symptoms—sinus problems, postnasal drip, and premenstrual syndrome—were gone as well.

Alzheimer's: The Brain on Fire

When we look at an autopsy of an Alzheimer's brain we see a brain on fire. Considering that the fastest-growing segment of the population is people eighty and older (and more than half of them will get Alzheimer's), we must focus on finding the cause. The good news is that we are closer than ever to understanding what goes wrong.

The inflammation story is repeated over and over in all disease, and dramatically so in aging and the brain. This is why sugar, trans fats, saturated fat, stress, infections, lack of exercise, autoimmune disease, obesity, diabetes, vitamin deficiencies, celiac disease (from eating wheat and gluten), and colitis, which are inflammatory digestive diseases, all increase the risk of dementia and neurodegenerative diseases like Alzheimer's.[15] They all promote inflammation. It is also why anti–inflammatory drugs like Advil may reduce the risk of dementia. But don't take them to reduce your risk. Over 100,000 people per year end up in the hospital and 16,000 people die every year from intestinal bleeding caused by these medications.

Everyone is searching for the one thing that causes diseases like Alzheimer's. But there is no one thing. Complex interactions between multiple factors from your lifestyle and environment interacting with your genes create problems. We have to address all the factors to succeed in helping the brain become healthy and recover.

Like in autism and depression, many cases of dementia and Alzheimer's can be slowed and even reversed if all the causes are dealt with. The brain has extraordinary powers of healing and recovery if we provide the right conditions. But the answer is not taking aspirin or Advil! We must deal with the underlying causes of disease—causes like inflammation.

That is what I did for Christine, and her recovery from early-stage dementia was remarkable.

*U*ntil her seventies, Christine was mentally sharp, and while still highly intelligent, she noticed increasing trouble with her memory. By the time I saw her at eighty-one her memory was failing. Her ability to live on her own was being questioned by her children, who took her to see a neurologist and psychologist. After extensive neuropsychiatric and memory testing she was told she had early dementia. No treatment was recommended.

Her daughter brought her to see me and we found a high level of inflammation (C-reactive protein), along with a number of other factors that all contributed to this inflammation—low vitamin D; undiagnosed autoimmune thyroid disease; low levels of B_6, folate, and B_{12}; and a high level of mercury and lead.

Any one of these factors may not have been enough to cause problems, but added together in the body of an eighty-one-year-old woman, they caused her brain and body to start shutting down.

Over a period of six months we aggressively treated her with a fresh, whole foods, anti-inflammatory diet, gave her omega-3 fat supplements, and replaced all the vitamins she was missing—vitamins D, B_6, folate, and B_{12}.

We treated her thyroid and helped her gently reduce the level of mercury and lead in her body.

After this treatment Christine had her three-hour battery of neuropsychiatric and memory tests repeated, and they all improved.

Normally dementia is progressive and—according to conventional wisdom—cannot be reversed. But after cooling inflammation, improving nutrition, and helping her detoxify, Christine regained a lost part of herself.

In cases like these, the inflammation itself is caused by something. So let's have a look at what the major causes of inflammation are.

C-REACTIVE PROTEIN

If you are concerned about your level of inflammation, I would strongly recommend that you talk to your doctor about testing your levels of *C-reactive protein,* or *CRP.* CRP is a protein found in the blood and it's the major marker for inflammation. Its presence is the best indicator we have of a heightened state of inflammation in the brain and body. I give a more extensive list of tests to identify the causes of inflammation in *The UltraMind Solution Companion Guide.* Go to www.ultramind.com/guide to download this important information. The more information you have about how inflamed you are, the better position you are in to respond to this condition.

The Causes of Inflammation

Everything in the body is connected and there are only a few things that cause inflammation.

The list is short.

1. Our *inflammatory diet,* which consists of enormous amounts of sugar (158 pounds per person per year), refined flours, as well as trans fats and saturated fats.
2. *Food allergens*—mostly delayed reactions to food or hidden allergens that lead to "brain allergies" (allergic reactions in the body that cause inflammation in the brain).
3. Imbalances in *digestive function* and the gut immune system that produce widespread systemic effects.
4. *Toxins* such as mercury and pesticides (and the 85,000 mostly untested toxins in our environment), which have been linked to immune dysfunction and autoimmune diseases.
5. Low-grade, hidden, or *chronic infections* such as HIV-associated dementia, syphilis, and Lyme disease, which can cause many neurological and psychiatric "diseases," or PANDAS that leads to OCD.
6. *Stress*—emotional or physical, such as trauma.
7. *Sedentary lifestyle.*
8. *Inadequate sleep*—fewer than seven hours a night.
9. *Nutritional deficiencies* such as vitamin C, B vitamins, vitamin D, zinc, and omega-3 fats.

The inflammatory markers or cytokines that we see in almost all disease are now being discovered in autism, Alzheimer's, depression, and so many other neurological and psychiatric diseases. But cytokines are just the smoke signals. The real question is what causes the cytokines to send messages of inflammation and spread the fire.

The few basic causes noted above explain nearly all the complex phenomena of disease we see. They are all connected in one way or another to all the seven keys of UltraWellness.

The problem in medicine is that most researchers and doctors are like a group of blind men examining an elephant. One feels the leg, another the ears, another the tusks, another the trunk, and another the tail. All have a different story to tell about the nature of the elephant, but they see only one piece. They are all right, and they are also all wrong because they miss the whole picture.

Remember even within the paradigm of Functional Medicine, inflammation is just one (albeit very important) factor. The other six keys outlined in Part II of this book are equally critical.

But all of them connect back to the list of problems above.

Let's take a moment to look at some of the specific ways in which two of these factors (excess sugar in your diet and food allergies) lead to inflammation in the brain. Keep in mind these are only two of the more important factors that lead to brain inflammation and the problems that can result. There are others, but to cover them all in this book would be impossible. Similar problems result from each of the other issues mentioned above as well.

A Sweet Brain Is an Unhappy and Forgetful Brain

By far the most important factor in brain aging and inflammation in America is sugar. The sheer flood of sweet things and processed refined foods into our bodies is a tidal wave that leaves destruction everywhere we look.

As we saw in chapter 7, the insulin triggered by this flood of sugar sets into motion an entire inflammatory parade.

As I have already mentioned, Alzheimer's (which we now know is, at least in part, caused by inflammation) is now being called type 3 diabetes. We know that type 2 diabetics have four times the risk of getting Alzheimer's. Excess sugar in your diet is linked to brain diseases.

The inflammation triggered by sugar leaves in its wake a sea of disease beyond the brain—heart disease, obesity, cancer, diabetes, and rapid aging. The evidence is overwhelming and irrefutable.

Sugar (or anything that quickly turns to sugar, the "white foods" such as potatoes and pasta) is an enormous stress on the body, triggering a surge in stress hormones like cortisol and adrenaline. If you notice your kids bounce off the walls after a big sugar load, it is because the sugar produced a jolt of adrenaline.

The surge of insulin in the body also turns on cellular switches that increase the inflammatory cytokines, just as happens when you have the flu. Except it doesn't go away, but persists for decades, doing its damage slowly.

There is no scientific controversy here. The evidence is in. Sugar causes inflammation. The insulin-resistant fat cells you pack on when you eat too much sugar produce nasty inflammatory messengers (cytokines) like TNF α and IL-6, spreading their damage to the brain.

In fact, researchers have suggested calling depression "metabolic syndrome Type II" because instead of just having a fat swollen belly, you also get a fat swollen (and depressed) brain.[16] And psychiatrists are starting to treat depression and psychiatric disorders with anti*diabetic* drugs like Actos![17] These drugs lower blood sugar, lower insulin, *and* reduce inflammation.

But sugar is not the only thing that creates inflammation. I want to highlight one more important factor in brain malfunction. Hidden food allergies. This is a much more controversial area.

Do You Have Brain Allergies?

What is food for some may be poison for others.

TITUS LUCRETIUS CARUS, *A.D. first century*
De Rerum Natura (On the Nature of Things)

Do you have brain fog, trouble focusing, feel brain fatigue, or feel sad or angry after eating? Does fasting or skipping meals make you feel alert, focused, and clear? If so, something you are eating is eating at you. You may be allergic to your food. But what are food allergies, and how do they affect your brain?

Allergies are an inflammatory response. When you ingest molecules you are allergic to, your body believes a foreign intruder has entered its midst. Never mind that the molecule may not be truly harmful—it may simply be a food you have eaten—allergies make your body "think" this intruder is out to do you harm.

As a result your body sets in motion a host of inflammatory reactions to stop this intruder from harming you. What reactions are set off depend on your individual genetic makeup and can range from mild skin irritation to brain fog to aggressive behavior, anxiety, depression, and more.

What Are Food Allergies Anyway?

There are two main types of food allergies: acute (or immediate) and delayed.

Everyone knows about the *acute form (or IgE allergies)*, because they happen immediately and in a big way. If you eat a peanut and your throat closes, you get hives, and you can't breathe, you will never eat a peanut again. You know you are allergic to peanuts.

But *delayed allergies (or IgG allergies)* are sneaky. You may eat a piece of bread on Monday and be depressed on Wednesday, or have a piece of cheese today and get a migraine tomorrow. You never make the connection, because you don't even realize food can have this kind of impact on you.

This type of allergy is mostly ignored by conventional medicine. Yet addressing this in my practice is one of the most powerful things I do to help people recover from nearly any problem.

Allergic diseases of both types (IgE and IgG) are on the rise for many reasons.

We are becoming hypersensitive to our environments, perhaps because we live in an oversterilized environment and our immune systems don't mature properly. Or because we are eating hybridized and genetically modified (GMO) foods full of antibiotics, hormones, pesticides, and additives that were unknown to our immune systems just a generation or two ago.

The result?

Our immune system becomes unable to recognize friend or foe—to distinguish between foreign molecular invaders we truly need to protect against and the foods we eat or, in some cases, our own cells. In Third World countries where hygiene is poor and infections are common, allergy and autoimmunity are rare.

But delayed allergies, more specifically, occur because many of our twenty-first-century habits lead to a breakdown of the normal barrier that protects our immune system from the outside world of foods, bugs, and toxins.

That barrier is our gut. Right under that barrier is 60 percent of your immune system. When the lining of your gut breaks down, your immune system is activated by food particles that it misinterprets as foreign invaders. This sets off a chain reaction leading to inflammation throughout your body, including your brain.

In chapter 9, where I discuss the gut, you will learn more about why the barrier breaks down and how this is linked to so many mood, behavioral, and neurological problems.

For now, recognize that if that barrier is weakened by a nutrient-poor diet high in sugar and low in fiber, by nutritional deficiencies of zinc and omega-3 fats, by overuse of antibiotics and hormones, by exposure to environmental toxins, and by unprecedented levels of mental and emotional stressors, then the outside environment "leaks" into your body (and your brain) and you develop allergies and systemic immune problems. This is called a leaky gut.

In fact, much of what we see go wrong in the epidemic of mood and brain disorders is because of a "leaky brain."

This happens when outside influences from our diet and our environment somehow directly or indirectly cause changes in our brain function that we "diagnose" as neurological or psychiatric problems. There is a breakdown in the normal barrier protecting our brain and it then reacts, leading to brain inflammation. Toxins, small peptides from gluten and dairy, antibodies we make to the foods we eat, or infections and bugs and the cytokines they trigger, all get into our brain.

This is manifested as "brain allergies"—specific responses to the foods you eat that occur inside your brain. These allergies are a little bit like "nasal allergies." It's like you have a runny nose inside your brain. But the symptoms show up as fatigue, memory loss, brain fog, or, in more extreme cases, depression, anxiety, OCD, autism, Alzheimer's, dementia, and other "brain disorders."

Most of us accept that small amounts of food, pollen, mold, chemicals, dust, or dander can cause inflammatory reactions in our skin, lungs, and digestive system that give us hives, make us cough or wheeze, and give us diarrhea. But we somehow think our brain is insulated from the inflammation triggered by these allergens.

We now know differently. Food allergies create a metabolic disorder that can lead to a whole host of "mental" symptoms, including fatigue, brain fog, slowed thought processes, irritability, agitation, aggressive behavior, anxiety, depression, schizophrenia, hyperactivity, autism, learning disabilities, and even dementia.[18]

One study of thirty patients suffering from anxiety, depression, confusion, and trouble concentrating were tested using a placebo-controlled trial to see if food allergies contributed to their problems.[19] Indeed, food allergies lead to severe depression, nervousness, and lack of motivation, brain fog, and anger without cause.

Other studies have linked eating gluten (the protein found in wheat, barley, rye, spelt, kamut, and oats) to everything from depression[20] to anxiety, from schizophrenia[21] to autism,[22] and even dementia.[23]

And a recent groundbreaking study showed that children who were overweight and had the beginnings of cholesterol plaques in their arteries all had higher levels of IgG antibodies, which indicate more delayed food allergies and inflammation than normal-weight children.[24]

This remarkable study clearly shows that food allergies can make you fat and trigger inflammation and metabolic syndrome, which we know cause brain injury. Inflammation can be triggered in many other ways, but food allergies are clearly an important one.

Like gluten, casein, a protein found in dairy, also has negative effects that can lead to mood disorders and altered brain function.[25]

In fact, partially digested dairy and wheat particles (called *caseomorphins* and *gliadomorphins*) are found in the urine of severely depressed patients (as well as children with autism and ADHD). These odd proteins change brain function and can lead not only to depression but also psychosis and autism.

I have treated autistic children who begin to speak simply after going on a gluten and casein-free diet.

So if you think allergies to food don't affect your brain like your body, you are sadly mistaken.

How Food Allergies Affect Your Brain

Every part of your body and every cell in your body communicates with every other part of your body and every other cell. Everybody's talking at the same time. Making sense of all that conversation is called health. Good communication is good health.

There is *a lot* of talking going on between your brain, immune system, gut, and hormones.

We call this the PNEI, or "psycho-neuro-endocrine-immune system." In fact, the gut is called the second brain because it has its own nervous system and many neurotransmitters like the brain. It is through this system that your gut and immune systems talk to your brain. And it governs how food triggers a cascade of events through the body and the brain.

The immune system and the brain have much in common. They are both responsible for perceiving or "seeing" our world, and for remembering those perceptions. They sense things and remember things.

The nervous system "sees" the big world through our five senses and remembers things in the memory cells (neurons) of the brain. The immune system "sees" the microscopic world of little particles from food, and microbes, pollens, and dust mites, and remembers their unique identity in the immune cells (or lymphocytes). So, you see, they have a very similar job.

Problems arise when the immune system (or the nervous system) over-reacts to normally innocuous substances like food proteins or microbes that normally live in harmony with us.

Three basic abnormal reactions to foods can trigger brain injury. First, they can trigger inflammation, which in turn inflames the brain. Second, small partially digested food proteins, called peptides, from gluten and casein can act to disturb the normal neurotransmitter function in the brain, and third, they can act as "excitotoxins," increasing glutamate (an excitatory neurotransmitter) and creating a chain reaction that overexcites, injures, inflames and ultimately kills brain cells.

Hence we develop the brain allergies I discussed above. Our immune system overreacts to the foods we eat and our brains are damaged as a result.

Hidden food allergies are a major unrecognized epidemic in the twenty-first century. Despite the fact that the immune system and the brain are intimately linked and food has a *major* impact on your brain and body, most of us (including physicians) don't make the connection between what we eat and what we feel. In fact, most physicians practicing today don't acknowledge the critically important role food allergies play in health.

The result is that we have an undiagnosed epidemic of people whose lives are affected by low-grade, delayed food sensitivities or allergies. What they eat causes allergic reactions that make them feel badly, but no one is making the connections.

There are blood tests that can help you identify problems with food allergies. These can be helpful, but they aren't always 100 percent accurate and you will have to find a practitioner of Functional Medicine to run them for you—most traditional physicians will, unfortunately, tell you they are a waste of time and money.

Or you can take some simple measures on your own to heal from brain allergies. You just have to take away the substances that most often cause allergic reactions for a few weeks and let your immune system cool down.

Then you can systematically reintroduce these foods to test which ones you are allergic to. This is called an elimination/reintroduction diet. It is a simple, very effective solution for identifying the foods that cause your brain allergies, and it is one of the core components of the UltraMind Solution.

What Are the Most Common Food Allergies?

So what have I found after years of testing people for IgG allergies and teaching people how to use elimination diets to help them recover from their chronic symptoms and illnesses?

While everyone is different and you can become sensitive to many different kinds of foods, there are some foods that irritate the immune system more than others. You may have to eliminate all these foods for a few weeks and then reintroduce them one by one to see which affect you adversely. They are:

- Gluten (wheat, barley, rye, oats, spelt, triticale, kamut)
- Dairy (milk, cheese, butter, yogurt)
- Corn
- Eggs
- Soy
- Nuts
- Nightshades (tomatoes, bell peppers, potatoes, eggplant)
- Citrus
- Yeast (baker's yeast, brewer's yeast, and fermented products like vinegar).

A SPECIAL NOTE ON GLUTEN

Problems with gluten are widely underdiagnosed. The most serious form of allergy to gluten, celiac disease, affects 1 in 100 people or 3 million Americans, most of whom are not diagnosed.

Milder forms of gluten sensitivity are even more common, affecting up to one-third of the American population.

While there are tests to help you identify this condition, the only way you will know if this is really a problem for you is to eliminate all gluten (wheat, rye, barley, oats, spelt, kamut, triticale) for a short period of time and see how you feel.

Then eat it again and see what happens. This teaches you better than any test.

See www.celiac.com for more information and help identifying hidden sources of gluten.

Despite the fact that this epidemic of food allergies is still largely unrecognized by the medical community at large, new research in the prestigious journal *Science*[26] and in the journal *Gut*[27] confirms the connection between what you eat and how you feel that is being ignored by the rest of medicine.

Dealing with food allergies is essential to creating wellness of mind, body, and brain!

In Part III I will outline an elimination/reintroduction diet that will help you identify the foods you are allergic to and heal your brain allergies. Because this plan is specifically designed to help you overcome brain disorders, I will focus on the major allergens that lead to brain problems—dairy, gluten, and a few other substances.

If you are suffering from a brain disorder of any kind, it is likely these substances are a problem for you. Using the elimination program in this book may help you overcome your brain allergies.

However, they may not be the *only* foods you are allergic to. Though in most cases the elimination diet that the UltraMind Solution is based on helps heal brain disorders, there are a small percentage of cases where you may have other allergies.

So if you get through this program and don't see all of the results you expect, it may be time for a more radical approach to eliminating food allergens. In that case I would recommend you try *The UltraSimple Diet*, which offers a more detailed explanation of food sensitivities, how and why we overreact, and a more extended program that tells you how to fix *all* of your food allergies.

Cool Off Inflammation

The bottom line is that an unhappy, chaotic, disorganized, disengaged, forgetful brain is an inflamed brain. The trail of scientific clues leads us to a few final common pathways for all illnesses, and inflammation is a key pathway.

Doctors of the future will become experts not only in identifying inflammation (which we are already becoming increasingly good at), but in navigating to the ultimate causes of that inflammation and putting out the fire instead of just dealing with the smoke.

To treat depression, autism, Alzheimer's, or any disease that affects mood, behavior, or the brain, we must learn how to get rid of the causes of inflammation and restore the normal immune balance through the food we eat, nutrients, exercise, sleep, and stress management.

I will teach you specifically how to do this in Part III, where I outline my basic program for optimal brain health. If you have additional problems in this area, you can optimize this key using the strategies outlined in Part IV.

In the next chapter you will learn how your gut and brain are connected in surprising ways, and that often the first thing to do to fix your brain is to fix your gut!

CHAPTER 9

KEY #4: FIX YOUR DIGESTION

We all have had gut feelings. And we know what it is to feel something in our gut. In Japan, the gut is viewed as the seat of the mind and soul. A Japanese business mogul was once asked how he knew whether to do a deal, and he replied, "I swallow it, and if it feels good in my belly, I do it."

Your gut has a mind of its own . . .

The "mind" of the gut talks to your brain every day. We are familiar with signals for hunger, or elimination. But a new conversation is being discovered between the gut and the brain, a bidirectional conversation in which the brain speaks to the gut and the gut speaks to the brain.

We will explore how this conversation has dramatic implications for new ways to cure mental illness and neurodegenerative disease. The gut is the literal and figurative center of our health. If you start by fixing your gut, many things fall into place.

Here is what we will explore:

❖ The Second Brain
  ❖ The "second" nervous system in the gut
❖ Bad Bugs Below
  ❖ How errant bugs in the gut bug your brain
❖ Odd Neuropeptides
  ❖ Mischievous molecules from the gut—signals gone awry
❖ The Gut as the Center of the Immune System
  ❖ A source of inflammation in the brain
❖ You Are What You Absorb
  ❖ Nutritional deficiencies and the gut (vitamin B_{12}, vitamin D, zinc, omega-3 fats)

But before we do, take the quiz below to find out if your inner tube of life is broken.

In the box on the right place a check for each positive answer. Then find out how severe your problem is using the scoring key below.

GUT QUIZ*

I have a bloated or full feeling, and/or belching, burning, or flatulence right after meals. ☐

I have chronic yeast or fungal infections (jock itch, vaginal yeast infection, athlete's foot, toenail fungus). ☐

I feel nauseous after taking supplements. ☐

I feel fatigued after eating. ☐

I have heartburn. ☐

I regularly use antacids (Tums, Maalox, acid-blocking drugs, etc.). ☐

I have chronic abdominal pains. ☐

I have diarrhea. ☐

I have constipation (going less than once or twice a day). ☐

I have greasy, large, poorly formed, or foul-smelling stools. ☐

I find food that is not fully digested in my stool. ☐

I have food allergies, intolerance, or reactions. ☐

I have an intolerance to carbohydrates (eating bread or other sugars causes bloating). ☐

I have thrush (whitish tongue). ☐

I have anal itching. ☐

I have bleeding gums or gingivitis. ☐

I have geographic tongue (maplike rash on tongue indicating food allergy). ☐

I have sores on the tongue. ☐

I have canker sores. ☐

I crave sweets and bread. ☐

I drink more than three alcoholic beverages a week. ☐

I have excessive stress. ☐

I frequently use or have frequently used antibiotics in the past (more than one to two times in three years). ☐

I have a history of NSAID (ibuprofen, naproxen, etc.) or other anti-inflammatory use. ☐

I have taken birth-control pills or hormone replacement. ☐

I have taken prednisone or cortisone. ☐

I have any of the following diseases or conditions:

- ❖ Autism ☐
- ❖ ADHD (attention deficit hyperactivity disorder) ☐
- ❖ Rosacea (dilated blood vessels in the nose and cheeks giving a red appearance) ☐

(continued)

- ❖ Acne after adolescence ☐
- ❖ Eczema ☐
- ❖ Psoriasis ☐
- ❖ Celiac disease (gluten allergy) ☐
- ❖ Chronic autoimmune diseases ☐
- ❖ Chronic hives or urticaria ☐
- ❖ Inflammatory bowel disease ☐
- ❖ Irritable bowel syndrome ☐
- ❖ Chronic fatigue syndrome ☐
- ❖ Fibromyalgia ☐

* For your convenience, this quiz has been reprinted in *The UltraMind Solution Companion Guide*. Simply go to www.ultramind.com/guide, download the guide, and print out the quiz.

Scoring Key—Gut

Score one point for each box you checked

Score	Severity	Care Plan	Action to Take
0–8	You may have a mild problem with your gut.	*The UltraMind Solution*	Complete the six-week program in Part III.
9–12	You may have a moderate problem with your gut.	Self-Care	Complete the six-week program in Part III and optimize your gut using the self-care options in chapter 25.
13 and above	You may have a severe problem with your gut.	Medical Care	Do both of the steps above and see a physician for additional assistance. I have outlined some of the options you should discuss with your doctor in chapter 25.

The gut is a snakelike, disgusting, and smelly thing that we hope will silently do its job of digesting, absorbing, and assimilating our food. We trust it will prevent toxins and bacteria from intruding into our systems, while eliminating our wastes in a timely and efficient manner without the least awareness on our part. Just do your job, please.

Unfortunately, while the gut is a source of great intelligence, is it is also the source of great mischief for millions.

Nearly 70 million people suffer from some form of digestive disorder. More than 6 million diagnostic procedures are done for digestive problems and 45 million people visit the doctor for gut problems every year. Forty percent of all visits to internists are for "functional bowel" disorders such as reflux and irritable bowel syndrome. And the cost for treating digestive disorders is $107 billion a year.[1]

You would think by now we would have a clear understanding of the causes of irritable bowel syndrome, constipation, diarrhea, reflux, and inflammatory bowel disease, just a few of the common problems experienced by millions. You would also think we would have developed effective treatments to fix these problems.

Unfortunately, our understanding and treatments of this highly sophisticated and integral part of our body are still quite primitive despite the explosion of scientific research on what *Science* magazine called "the inner tube of life."

Over the last fifteen years of practice and research, I have found the gut to be the source of inestimable suffering. And I have found remarkable discoveries and cures that hold the promise of getting relief not only from common "functional" gastrointestinal symptoms (and most allergic and autoimmune diseases that originate in the gut) but from everything from depression to autism, to OCD, to ADHD, to dementia and Parkinson's disease.

Let's start our exploration of the inner tube of life by discussing what it does. Then we will review what the research has to say about how gut function is connected to brain function, how the gut is put out of balance, and how you can restore balance to achieve an UltraMind and UltraWellness.

Your Gut's Job: A Day at Work

The gut plays a number of remarkable roles in our overall health. Here are just a few of the main jobs:

- ❖ Breaks Down Your Food
    - ❖ Breaking down and digesting our food with the help of adequate stomach acid, digestive enzymes, and bile.
- ❖ Lets in the Good Stuff
    - ❖ Absorbing only the molecules we need, such as amino acids, fats, sugars, and vitamins and minerals through a one-cell-thick layer barrier to keep us properly nourished.

- ✢ Keeps Out the Bad Stuff
    - ✢ While letting in the nutrients essential for life, it must prevent, block, or neutralize nasty toxins, bugs, and chemicals that flow through our inner tube of life.
- ✢ Makes Stuff
    - ✢ Bacteria that live in your gut (about three pounds' worth containing five hundred different species) produce vitamins and health-giving molecules that are all part of your gut ecosystem.
- ✢ Protects You
    - ✢ Your gut immune system makes up 60 percent of your total immune system and is called the GALT (or gut-associated lymphoid tissue). It lies under that one-cell layer I mentioned above through which nutrients are absorbed. Its job is to protect you from illness. When it is in balance, you are well. When it is out of balance, a host of problems can occur, including those discussed in the last chapter as well as others I will outline in this chapter.

That's a lot of work. And it all has to function seamlessly for you to be properly nourished, to have a balanced immune system, and to adequately detoxify.

The gut has to be completely in balance for your brain to be in balance. The brain experiences everything that happens in your gut directly through nervous system feedback, immune activity, cytokines, and other assorted mischievous molecules made in your gut.

Despite its critical importance, few people look to the gut as the seat of health and happiness. Nowhere is this truer than when it comes to our broken brains. Who would ever think that problems in your brain originate in your gut?

When it comes to the gut, most physicians and scientists miss what is right in front of us, because we are looking for solutions in the wrong place. How could the cure for autism start in the gut? How could depression be rooted in bacterial imbalances in the gut? How could dementia occur from eating wheat?

We have no model for seeing this. So we don't.

Luckily, a few revolutionary doctors and scientists are looking at how the gut is connected to the brain. And what they are finding is astonishing.

The Brain-Gut Connection:
Your Gut Is Your Second Brain

Dr. Michael Gershon, of Columbia University, has called the gut the "second brain." In fact, your gut has a mind of its own, literally. While it is connected to the brain through an extensive network of wiring and communication systems, it is also the only "organ" besides the brain that has its own nervous system.

We call it the ENS, or enteric (or gut) nervous system, as opposed to the CNS, or central nervous system. The small intestine alone has as many neurons as the spinal cord. Ninety-five percent of the body's serotonin (remember, that's the happy mood chemical) is produced by the gut nerve cells, and every class of neurotransmitters found in the brain is also found in the gut.

The question is how does this nervous system below interact with the one above?

The gut brain actually comes from the same embryonic tissue as the "brain" brain. And it is still connected via the autonomic nervous system—the sympathetic and parasympathetic nerves.

Acting completely independently, it has a number of important jobs: it keeps everything moving in the right direction from the top down by coordinating the contraction of muscle cells; it triggers the gut hormones and enzymes to be released from cells to promote digestion; it helps keep the blood flowing so that when you absorb your food it can get to where it needs to go, and it controls the immune and inflammatory cells in the gut.[2]

All that happens in the background and is communicated back up to your brain via the autonomic nervous system. Think of it as two independent, but interdependent, businesses that must coordinate and communicate but can act independently.

But how does this interaction affect us?

Nearly everyone has experienced "butterflies" in the stomach, or had diarrhea under acute stress, or, worse, became incontinent in life-threatening situations. Clearly, we can have a "nervous" stomach because of our thoughts and feelings and external events. But can we have a "nervous" brain (or a depressed or hyperactive or autistic or demented brain) because of mischief originating in the gut—specifically due to problems with digesting food, the gut immune system, or signals that go haywire on the way from our gut-brain, or ENS, to our "brain" brain?

In medical training, most doctors think pejoratively of people with "functional bowel" disorders. Doctors see nothing with the tools they use—scopes, X-rays, and scans. No tumors, ulcers, or blockages. Nothing "real." So these patients are just neurotic people with emotionally triggered symptoms. Right?

The evidence is directing us otherwise.

The suffering for millions is real. So the question becomes, are these tens of millions of Americans "crazy," with "psychosomatic symptoms" that lead them to be irritable, anxious, depressed, and obsessed with their digestive system? Or are we missing something?

Thankfully, new science is shedding light on this topic.

Over the years I have seen emotional, psychiatric, and behavioral symptoms triggered by problems in the gut. One of my patients was a thirty-year-old executive who would experience anxiety and insomnia whenever his irritable bowel would act up. Another was a little boy who would have explosive bouts of anger whenever his stomach was a little "swollen" with gas. Yet another was a woman who found herself free of lifelong depression after a course of antibiotics (metronidazole) we used to clear out bad bacteria from her gut.

When psychiatric symptoms are "coincidentally" cleared up with antibiotics, that gets my attention.[3] How could this happen? An autistic boy I treated actually began to speak after changing his diet and eliminating gluten and dairy, which altered the "information" that went into his gut.

These remarkable stories are all evidence of the intimate connection between your gut and your brain.

Doctors often blame a patient's psychiatric problems for their gut symptoms. They are "psychosomatic" illnesses created in the brain of people whose anxieties get the best of them.

But perhaps, very often, it just may be the other way around. Mischief in the gut causes disturbance in the brain. Fix the gut, and mood, behavior, and cognition all improve.

Many different factors affect gut—and brain—health:

- Unfriendly bacteria in the gut and other bugs like yeast that produce brain toxins.
- Fermentation of starches from your diet, which produce gas and toxic levels of ammonia.
- Odd, partially digested food proteins that interfere with normal brain operations.
- Activation of the immune system because of digestive imbalances

that damage the protective barrier, which normally keeps the outside world from entering through the gut.

Why are millions of us having all these gut problems?

The answer is that we are not very kind to our gut. We eat a SAD diet (Standard American Diet), which is low in fiber and nutrients and rich in sugar, additives, and chemicals, which changes the ecosystem of our gut.

We are under chronic stress, which damages the normal intestinal barrier and affects the ENS.

Our drug culture pushes antibiotics, anti-inflammatories, aspirin, steroids, and acid-blocking medications that all disrupt our gut's ability to stay in balance and do its job.

And we are exposed to toxins such as mercury, which damage our normal gut function.

All in all, we live in dangerous digestive times.

An article in the *Journal of the American Medical Association* by Dr. Henry Lin[4] mapped out a new way of thinking about irritable bowel and the psychological symptoms seen in irritable bowel patients.

He turns the current view on its head by saying that bacterial mischief in the small intestine (from bacteria that migrate up from the large intestine into a normally sterile territory) triggers an immune and nervous system response that sends messages back to the brain, which lead to insomnia,[5] "sickness behavior," anxiety, depression,[6] and impaired cognitive function.[7] The gut immune system "speaks" to the brain, sending messages of inflammation, which increases levels of CRF (corticotropin releasing factor) in the hypothalamus (which, in turn, increases stress hormones like cortisol),[8] and changes neurotransmitter levels.[9]

Your gut is talking to your brain. And when these bacteria are involved, the communication isn't good.

So, bottom line—little bacteria in our gut start a cascade of immune and neurological events that stop our brain from doing what it was designed to do and this creates poor connections and communication all around.

This is one of the major ways your gut sends signals of ill health to your brain that can manifest themselves as any type of broken brain and many other illnesses.

I want to discuss how this happens. Let me start by telling you the story of one of my patients, who suffered from this problem.

Bugged Out: How Bugs in Your Brain Make You Crazy

*T*he most remarkable story of how bugs in the gut can affect your brain is from a woman who came to see me with the typical "whole list" of problems (which is why I call myself a "whole-listic" doctor).

Most of her problems started in her gut—she had the usual diagnoses of irritable bowel syndrome with terrible bloating after meals as well as acid reflux, and she also had an autoimmune disease with joint pains and lots of inflammatory symptoms such as allergies and rashes.

She also had metabolic syndrome, or prediabetes, thyroid problems, and chronic stress.

In addition to all these problems, she also suffered from debilitating obsessive-compulsive disorder. She was an educated, otherwise well-balanced human being, and there was nothing odd about her on the surface. But she could not pick up anything off her floor or clean or move anything in her house because of this weird obsession—for years!

In the ten years before she came to see me, she had become increasingly withdrawn because of her severe fatigue and her frustration and exhaustion from these quirky behaviors.

Actually she had been given many "diagnoses" over the years by many different doctors, including depression, anxiety, OCD, and sleep disorder. She also had severe fatigue for many years.

As a result, she took many drug cocktails over the years, including Ritalin and Dexedrine—or speed. When I first saw her she was on Provigil (a new drug to wake up the brain), and Depakote, a seizure drug given to OCD and bipolar patients, as well as two antidepressants, Celexa and Wellbutrin. She was also on a highly controlled new drug for sleep called Xyrem (which was the knockout date rape drug, or GHB). This was quite a collection of mood stabilizers, uppers, and downers—this woman was a walking pharmacy.

We found she was allergic to gluten and dairy and she was making very odd peptides (little proteins) because of poor digestion. These are morphinelike proteins that result from incomplete digestion of casein (from dairy) and gluten (from wheat), which have been linked to many psychiatric disorders, especially autism and ADHD.[10]

She also had vitamin D and magnesium deficiency, which can contribute, as you learned in chapter 6, to depression and anxiety.

When we looked at her gut environment with a stool analysis, we found there weren't any of the normal healthy bacteria growing, her gut lining was inflamed, and some strangers had taken up residence in her gut, including yeasts and odd bacteria.

A gut is a veritable ecosystem—like a rain forest. There are over five hundred *species of bacteria living there weighing in at a whopping three pounds. There is more bacterial DNA in your body than human DNA. All of them need to be in balance and in the right place (mostly in your large intestine) for your gut to function properly.*

There are good bugs and bad bugs. The good bugs help digest your food, produce vitamins, control inflammation, boost immune function, and more. The bad bugs produce toxins, ferment starches leading to bloating and gas, and sometimes move into areas of the bowel like the stomach and small intestines where they create terrible mischief. We generally want to get rid of the bad bugs and add more good bugs or probiotics to keep the gut healthy.

As part of this woman's gut cleanup, I gave her a new treatment pioneered by Dr. Mark Pimentel, of the University of California at the Los Angeles School of Medicine.[11] *A nonabsorbed antibiotic called Xifaxin clears out abnormal bacteria in the small bowel. I expected her bloating and even some of her inflammatory symptoms to clear up by fixing her gut. But I was surprised by what she told me after she took the antibiotic.*

Overnight her OCD disappeared; after years of unsuccessful treatment with psychotherapy and psychiatric medications, she was suddenly able to clean her entire house and pick up everything off the floor. The lights in her brain had come on for the first time in ten years.

A high level of ammonia in her blood caused her OCD. Ammonia is a neurotoxin that excites and damages brain cells and the mitochondria (the site of energy production in all cells—see chapter 11 for more information). Bacteria in the gut produces ammonia, and when the liver can't detoxify it, or there is just too much, it causes brain damage.

Every physician knows this because since the 1960s doctors have been treating a condition known as "hepatic encephalopathy,"[12] *a form of temporary insanity common in patients with liver failure. The brain dysfunction results from too much ammonia and is cured by clearing out the ammonia-producing bacteria in the gut with antibiotics. So this idea shouldn't seem strange to most doctors.*

But it occurs in many patients—not just those with liver failure.

When we rechecked her ammonia level after treatment, it had returned to normal. After a few months, the bacteria came back, and so did her OCD symptoms, and once again treating the bacteria cured her OCD. The link was clear.

And this is just one of many ways abnormal gut bacteria can affect your thoughts and cognitive function.

In fact, Pimentel talks about seeing common symptoms like brain fog and fatigue in patients with irritable bowel syndrome that clear up when the toxic bacteria are cleaned up using the treatment he created. A bloated belly leads to a bloated brain. The symptoms can vary from OCD to depression to anxiety to autism or even psychosis.

So what else do we know about how bugs down below affect command central up on top?

Bad Bugs Below and Above: Intestinal Bugs and Your Brain

Beside ammonia, there are also many odd, toxic molecules that are produced by the five hundred species of bugs that make their home in your intestinal tract, populating the surface of your gut, which is a hundred square meters in surface area, but only one cell thick.

These good bugs are very busy living in a symbiotic manner with you. You give them a place to live in your gut, and they reciprocate by helping you digest your food, make necessary vitamins (like vitamin K and biotin), detoxify poisons, produce energy for your intestinal cells (butyrate), regulate cholesterol metabolism, and keep normal pH balance.

They also compete for real estate with bad bugs—parasites, yeast, and toxin-producing bacteria. These bad bugs take over because you took too many antibiotics or don't eat enough plant foods with lots of fiber (which the good bugs love to eat) and eat too much sugar (which the bad bugs love even more). Then the whole ecosystem is disrupted, leading to a bigger set of disruptions that alter your mood and brain function.

Let me tell you another story.

*O*ne spring afternoon, a beautiful little six-year-old girl walked into my office with her mother and sister. On the surface she seemed quite normal, but then the story of her tragic life unfolded.

This first-grade student was extraordinarily aggressive with her sister and her peers—kicking, pinching, and hitting them. She threatened to kill herself regularly.

She cut her mother and sister out of family pictures. She was anxious, negative, and hopeless. Temper tantrums, mood swings, and attention seeking were regular patterns of behavior.

She was also diagnosed with OCD and "perfectionism."

She didn't make friends at school, and her mother was called daily about her disruptive behavior in class.

Genetics might have set her up for problems. One cousin was bipolar and another cousin had Asperger's, a mild form of autism.

She had all the regular childhood immunizations, including diphtheria, pertussis, tetanus, measles, mumps, rubella, hemophilous, varicella, and hepatitis B. She was a very colicky baby, had frequent diaper and vaginal yeast infections as a child, with vaginal and rectal itching (which gives you a pretty strong idea that yeast is hanging around), and had very sensitive skin.

And she loved sugar and refined pastries and carbs.

While I see children all across the spectrum of mood and behavior problems, hers were particularly extreme. So I began my medical detective work.

She had no digestive complaints, but I have learned that even if a child or adult doesn't complain about their gut, mischief can still be brewing. The bacteria and yeast literally ferment the sugary, starchy foods in the diet, producing "auto-intoxication" with alcohol—a by-product of this process.[13] *Violent, aggressive behavior so commonly seen in drunks can occur from alcohol produced by yeasts in the gut. I wondered if this little girl had a little auto-brewery in her belly.*

On my detective hunt I found she was low in magnesium, which can make you pretty irritable, and was deficient in zinc, so important to helping your digestive enzymes break down your food. That may have contributed to why she had those little toxic opiumlike peptides from gluten running around her brain (we will talk more about these in a moment).

She also had delayed food allergies (IgG) to wheat, rye, oats, and barley (all gluten-containing grains).

And, of course, she had low levels of DHA—the brain-balancing omega-3 fat.

She also had the typical problems with her methylation train—evidence of severe B_6, B_{12}, and folate deficiency—and major problems with the sulfation train, with low levels of glutathione, the body's main detoxifier. (We will talk more about the sulfation train and glutathione in chapter 10.)

And she had a lot of trouble making enough energy in her cells (see chapter 11 on energy).

These problems occur in patterns, because they are all connected. It is not usually one thing. It is almost always everything. But the gut is often at the center of the problem—even if there are no digestive symptoms.

The most incredible finding in this young girl's case was the sky-high indicators of overgrowth of bacteria and yeast in her gut. I had never seen levels this high in anyone.

Just getting her on a gluten- and dairy-free, whole foods, organic diet; some cod liver oil; magnesium; methylation helpers like B_6, B_{12}, and folate; a multivitamin; and some probiotics improved her condition.[14]

But when I gave her an antibiotic to clear out the bad bugs in her gut,[15] *followed by an antifungal, she transformed into a well-behaved little girl.*

Her aggressiveness, negativity, and hopelessness were gone. Her mother said she used to be punished ten times a day and got into trouble at school every day. All that stopped when we cleared up the bad bugs in her gut and helped her get her flora and gut ecosystem back in balance.

She was suffering from "autointoxication," which leads to crazy behavior. This process of a bug producing toxins that actually modulate brain chemistry is just one way the gut can affect the brain. There are many more.

Many studies have shown abnormal, toxin-producing flora in children with developmental problems like these.[16] Normal kids have normal flora.

While I have been using children with ADHD, behavioral problems, and autism as examples throughout this book, these principles apply to everyone with mood, behavioral, or memory problems.

Of course, behavioral and psychotherapeutic approaches are also necessary to help manage emotions, beliefs, attitudes, thinking patterns, and poor behavior, but it is much easier to work on yourself if your brain is not in chaos, if signals and communication systems in your brain are not incoherent and unsynchronized by toxins, allergens, infections, nutritional deficiencies, and stress.

An integrated, comprehensive approach to regain balance is always necessary and often remarkably effective.[17] Treating the gut is almost always one piece of that puzzle.

Changing diet and tuning up biochemistry with nutrients have profound effects on brain and behavior. In one study[18] 207 patients with severe, violent behavior disorders were treated with a comprehensive metabolic and biochemical systems approach. They were tested, and their problems with metals, methylation, blood sugar, nutrient deficiencies, and gut problems were all corrected.

Seventy-six percent of the group actually followed the program. More than 90 percent of the participants significantly reduced violent behavior, and 54 percent had total elimination of their severe behavior problems.

This study should be headline news. But you don't hear about it, because it is not a new drug or procedure but a simple diet and nutrient-based approach.[19]

These simple treatments help restore normal metabolism and biochemistry. Things can go quite awry in the brain when digestion doesn't work. One possibility is toxic chemicals that are sometimes created when bad bugs get into your gut, as discussed above.

Besides diet, new research about peptides—little toxic proteins from partially digested food—give us another clue as to what can go wrong with the communication between your gut and your brain.

Peptides and Your Brain

*T*wo sisters, nine and seven years old, came into my practice struggling with behavior problems in school, short attention spans, outbursts, tantrums, and mul-
*tiple medical diagnoses, including bipolar disease and attention deficit hyperactivity
disorder. Their doctors prescribed the usual cocktail of stimulants and antidepressants.*

*Both had many digestive problems, including food allergies, yeast, and odd
bacteria.*

*But what was most striking in their case were the high levels of peptides (little pro-
teins) that were produced by lack of adequate digestion of gluten (from wheat) and casein (from dairy).*[20] *The proteins are called gluteomorphins and caseomorphins,
because they affect the morphine or opium receptors in the brain.*

Gluteomorphins and caseomorphins are absorbed from the gut and find
their way to the brain, causing much mischief, manifesting as mood and behavior problems. In the case above, I found out about this problem through
a urine analysis. Peptides can be measured in the urine, because after they
are absorbed into the body they must be excreted. These funny molecules
cause their mischief in one of two ways.

First, they look "foreign," so the body's immune system reacts, leading to
overall inflammation, which can show up as autoimmunity, autism, ADHD,
depression, or psychosis as you learned in chapter 8.

Second, peptides leak into the body and brain. Because they are
"opium-" or "morphine-like" in nature, these peptides mess up brain function just as heroin or a psychedelic drug would.

One of the reasons these peptides are created has to do with digestive
enzymes.

Many people with weak digestion have low levels of or poorly functioning digestive enzymes. Some of these cases are genetically determined. Toxins such as mercury, which can come from silver dental amalgams or large
predatory fish like tuna, inactivate these digestive enzymes. In other in-
stances, the digestive enzymes are not activated because of low stomach
acid, poor pancreatic function, or zinc deficiency (zinc is often needed to
turn on these enzymes).

One important link between digestive enzymes and peptides is the failure of a particular enzyme called DPP-IV.[21; 22] This enzyme is important in
breaking down foods, particularly gluten and casein. When it malfunctions,
these noxious peptides are often created in the gut and end up in the brain.

That is why using special digestive enzymes as part of treatment is so important in helping recovery from autoimmune and inflammatory disorders, including inflammation of the brain!

F or the two little girls above, I connected the dots. When I cleaned up their guts by improving their diet, got rid of food allergens like gluten and casein, and gave them digestive enzymes, not only did their mood and behavior normalize, but those odd little peptides also disappeared from their urine.[23; 24] Clearing up the gut imbalances, and removing casein and gluten, stopped the production of these mood- and brain-altering peptides. This returned their mood and behavior to normal. Remember, everything is connected to everything else in the body.

And it isn't just little kids who have autism and behavioral problems who suffer from these peptides. They have also been linked to depression[25] and schizophrenia.

The critical point to understand is that the total load of insults to your system disrupts normal things from happening in the body—things like digesting the food you eat, distinguishing friendly molecules from foreign ones at the interface between you and the outside world (like the one in the gut), and the activation of the gut immune and gut nervous systems.

This has broad implications for every type of chronic illness, as well as the mood, attention, behavior, and neurodegenerative diseases like Alzheimer's and Parkinson's disease we see exploding in our culture.

Next, I want to tell you about the remarkable discoveries of Dr. Andrew Wakefield in autistic children, because they have implications for all of us who have inflamed guts and inflamed brains.

The Gut Immune System and the Brain

Many medical discoveries are made by accident. Some smart doctor observes something and asks why.

For the most part, doctors and scientists have ignored the fact that up to 95 percent of autistic children have intestinal problems, especially big swollen bellies. How can their belly problems destroy their brains, interrupt their language, and lock them in their own private world?

Dr. Wakefield asked why. He happened to notice inflammation (or lymphoid nodular hyperplasia) in the bowels of some children with autism. Could this observation be brushed off as coincidence? Dr. Wakefield dug deeper and discovered this is common in autistic children.

In a study of 148 children with autism compared to thirty normal controls (children without autism), 90 percent of autistic children showed inflamed bowels on biopsy compared to only 30 percent of controls. This makes me wonder if many nonautistic children have bowel inflammation from poor diet and allergies as well.[26]

He also realized that the inflammation was much more severe in autistic children. Food allergens, bacteria, viruses, and toxins (such as mercury) could all be the cause. These same things are the common causes of all disease and create imbalance in every key system of the body—toxins, infections, allergens, poor diet, and stress.

Making Sense of Measles Vaccine Controversy

Other studies have linked the live measles virus from vaccinations to an inflamed gut. Living measles viruses have been identified in people with inflamed guts. How does this happen? And how does it relate to autism?

Normally, when you get a vaccine, even with an "inactivated" live virus, it just stimulates the body's own immune system to create antibodies, which will defend you in the event of a real infection. But sometimes, as in the case of autistic children, their weakened immune systems can't handle this "inactivated" live virus, and can't fight it off. So the live virus hangs around in the body creating inflammation on a low-grade level—both in the gut and the brain.

In fact, a study of children with developmental delay found that seventy-five of ninety-one patients with autism and inflamed bowels had live measles virus detected in samples of their intestinal tissues. Only seven of the seventy normal patients (or controls) were found to have the measles virus in their gut.[27]

In another study, DNA analysis was performed on the measles strains found in autistic children and compared to nonautistic children with inflamed bowels. The shocking finding was that the DNA of the measles virus in autistic children came from *vaccine strains* of measles (the ones made specially for vaccines), not wild types (the type of measles virus that comes from a community-acquired infection).[28]

This doesn't mean that *all* children who get vaccinated have problems, but for some reason autistic children are unable to handle the live measles virus used in immunizations, and it triggers an inflammatory response in the gut as well as the brain. These children can't handle the vaccine (maybe because mercury suppresses their immune system) and then the normally benign live measles virus in the vaccine takes root in the body and sends these kids into an even deeper spiral of brain dysfunction.

What is even more alarming is that vaccine strains of measles virus seem to migrate into the brains of children with autism. That means it may not be only gut-related inflammation that is causing the problems, but the measles virus may take root in the brain itself. How this all happens is not clear, but the trail from vaccine to the gut to the brain is smoking hot. Vaccine measles strains have been isolated from the spinal fluid of autistic children.[29]

Large-scale population studies show no connection between MMR or measles vaccine and autism.[30] That's because in such large populations the effect on children susceptible to MMR is "washed out." If you study large groups of people, you won't pick up small effects on genetically or biochemically unique individuals. Looking at the problem using this kind of statistical analysis is unhelpful for treating individual patients.

Oddly, in the major study "disproving" this connection, the authors noted an *increase* in the diagnosis in the six months after the MMR vaccine but dismissed it as unimportant because "this appeared to be an artifact related to the difficulty of defining precisely the onset of symptoms in this disorder." If your child had autism or autistic behaviors you would know it and you would know when it started! This is yet another example of conventional science seeing what it believes instead of believing what it sees.

The vaccine probably affects only a few genetically susceptible children who are biochemical and immunological train wrecks because of toxic overload. The methods of these larger population studies are not designed to ferret out the uniqueness of individuals. If they examine all the genetic subgroups in the population, then there can be meaningful data. If they do intestinal biopsies and spinal fluid examinations on affected and unaffected kids as Dr. Wakefield did, then we may get some meaningful information.

But in the absence of that we are duped into a false sense of security by studies that are destined to fail because of how they were designed. You only get the answers to the questions you ask. Don't ask the right questions and you won't get clear answers.

Roger Williams, the author of *Biochemical Individuality*, said that, "Nutrition [and medicine] is for real people. Statistical humans are of little interest. People are unique. We must treat people with respect to their biochemical uniqueness."

Functional Medicine and the model of treatment used in this book offer a method to do that.

In addition to all the potential digestive problems that autistic children face, it also seems they are more susceptible to allergies and gut inflammation triggered by certain foods such as gluten and casein.[31]

The extreme inflammation in the guts of autistic children contributes to their inflamed brains. (For more specifics on how inflammation in the body leads to inflammation in the brain, see chapter 8.)

The bottom line is that the guts of these genetically susceptible autistic children are damaged for many reasons—live measles vaccinations, toxic metals, overuse of antibiotics, abnormal gut flora, and food allergies.

The net result is that their digestion breaks down. Digestive enzymes don't work properly. Food particles (especially from gluten and dairy) are partially digested and become brain-fogging toxic compounds (like the peptides mentioned above). The immune system in the gut is switched on and activated by toxins, viruses, bacteria, and food allergens, leading to brain inflammation. Toxic bacteria and yeasts take over, releasing compounds that change normal brain operations. All this overwhelms the system and creates chaos between the brain and the gut immune system.

While this whole discussion on digestive problems in autistic children is interesting, you might wonder how this relates to depression or Alzheimer's or just feeling a little brain fog.

Through the extreme example of autism we can see one end of a spectrum of disorders that affects millions in small and large ways, from full-on psychosis and dementia to mild anxiety and a little depression. Dealing with gut inflammation is a back door into healing the brain.

People who have celiac disease[32] or inflammatory bowel disease are more likely to get dementia. And even schizophrenia has been linked to bowel inflammation and autoimmune response to gluten.[33]

Learning what causes brain inflammation and how to heal the gut are central to the UltraMind Solution.

One of the key causes of this inflammation is food allergy. We covered food allergies in chapter 8, where I discussed inflammation, but they are so connected to gut inflammation specifically and are so important in healing the brain that we need to revisit how damage to the gut leads us to become so allergic—and how to fix it.

Food Allergies Revisited: More Mischievous Molecules

Why do we become sensitive or allergic to foods?

In the last chapter we learned that food allergies cause inflammation and that this occurs because of imbalances in the gut. So what sends our gut out of balance? Why do we become allergic to the foods we normally should be able to digest easily?

All the factors that cause imbalances in the other keys—a poor diet, inflammation, overuse of medications, environmental toxins, and the rest—damage the surface of our intestinal lining in the small intestine.

You will remember that this surface, if laid out flat, would be the size of a tennis court, but it is only one cell layer thick. When this delicate surface is damaged, inflammation spreads throughout the brain and body.

Damage to this delicate barrier creates a *leaky gut* (known in medical terms as increased intestinal permeability).

Our digestive enzymes reside on this delicate one cell layer of intestinal cells. When it is damaged we cannot digest our food properly. Suddenly we have partially digested food particles from normally innocuous foods "leaking" into our bloodstream through the leaky gut.

Since 60 percent of our immune system is located right under that one-cell layer of intestinal cells lining our digestive tract, our bodies react by increasing our immune response and generating inflammation. Our immune system, normally used to seeing fully digested foods (like proteins broken down to amino acids, fats broken down to fatty acids, and carbohydrates broken down to simple sugars), suddenly "sees" foreign (meaning partially digested) proteins.

So the immune response does what it is designed to do—attack and defend—and this is how we create antibodies and develop IgG allergies to common foods. This is what makes us sick and fat, toxic and inflamed, depressed and anxious, forgetful and foggy.

It is sometimes helpful to get blood tests for IgG allergens and work with a doctor or nutritionist trained in dealing with these delayed and often hidden food sensitivities.[34] But following the basic six-week plan in *The UltraMind Solution* may help you find out if your mood, behavior, attention, or memory problems or other brain fog are related to food allergies.

Eliminating food allergens from your diet for six weeks, and taking digestive enzymes, zinc, and probiotics can all help repair the damaged intestinal lining and bring your digestive system, and your brain, back into balance.

THE DANGERS OF ACID-BLOCKING DRUGS

Are millions of us born with a genetic defect that makes us produce too much stomach acid? And do we need powerful, acid-blocking drugs to prevent heartburn (a condition that has recently been renamed GERD, or gastroesophageal reflux)? Do we have a major evolutionary design flaw?

Or is something out of balance?

At least 10 percent of Americans have episodes of heartburn every day, and 44 percent have symptoms at least once a month. Overall reflux, or GERD, affects 25 to 35 percent of the United States population.[35]

After Lipitor and Plavix (drugs for cholesterol and heart disease), an acid-blocking drug is the third top-selling drug in America's $252 billion drug market.[36] In fact, three of the drugs to treat reflux—Nexium, Protonix, and Prevacid—are in the top twenty bestselling drugs and account for $12.1 billion in sales annually!

The problem is that these medications have long-term side effects with significant implications for your brain (as well as your gut, immune system, bones, and more).

When I was a medical student and these drugs first came on the market, the pharmaceutical representatives warned us how powerful they were. We were told not to use them any longer than six weeks and only for patients with documented ulcers.

Now they are given like candy to anyone who ate too many hot dogs at a ball game. One drug, Prilosec, whose patent ran out, is currently available without prescription.

The funny thing is, when I was a medical student, GERD was not even on the radar as a significant disease. People had heartburn, and then there were people with ulcers. That was it for the most part.

Drug companies invent diseases to create markets for their drugs. They attempt to make us think that humans can't feel good and live with normally functioning digestive tracts without help from powerful drugs with dangerous side effects. This is absurd.

The pharmaceutical companies have great commercials showing a family rushing to stop their father from eating a big sausage with fried onions and peppers—and he tells them not to worry because he took his acid-blocking pill!

I know someone who used to work for the makers of Pepcid (an acid blocker). When the drug first became available over the counter, teams of drug company representatives would stand at the gates of county fairs and Southern barbecues and hand out free samples!

Let's look at some of the recent research on the dangers of these drugs, and why they cause problems.

What do these drugs do that are so bad? Well, their "good" effects—shutting down stomach acid—also have a "bad" effect.

Stomach acid is necessary to digest protein and food, to activate digestive enzymes in your small intestine, to keep bacteria from growing in your small

(continued)

intestine, and to help you absorb important minerals like calcium and magnesium. And it helps you absorb vitamin B_{12}. We now know how all these things are also essential for optimal brain function.

Does the research prove that these things do occur? Absolutely.

Taking acid-blocking drugs can prevent you from properly digesting your food, cause vitamin and mineral deficiencies, and lead to irritable bowel syndrome, depression, hip fractures because you cannot absorb calcium, and more.

First, studies show that people who take long-term acid-blocking medications can become vitamin B_{12}-deficient, which can lead to depression, anemia, fatigue, nerve damage, and even dementia, especially in the elderly.[37]

Second, research has revealed that taking these drugs can cause dangerous overgrowth of bacteria in the intestine called Clostridia, leading to life-threatening infections.[38] For many more people, low-grade overgrowth of bacteria in the small intestine leads to bloating, gas, abdominal pain, and diarrhea. (By the way, these are many of the common "side effects" noted in the drug warnings for these drugs.) These side effects can cause irritable bowel syndrome and many other toxic effects, including bad effects on the brain, as we have seen.

Acid blockers can occasionally be necessary for short-term use, but if we deal with the causes of digestive imbalance, most of the time, reflux and GERD can be managed without medication.

Nutritional Deficiencies: Fallout from a Damaged Gut

As you learned in chapter 6, nutrients such as the omega-3 fats, magnesium, zinc, and vitamins D and B_{12} are critical for normal operations in the brain and a robust mood and mental functioning. These nutrients also have the most trouble being absorbed when things go wrong in the gut.

When the gut is damaged, inflamed, and filled with nasty bugs that don't normally belong there; when enzymes are damaged by mercury and other toxins; when you take acid-blocking drugs that lower the essential acid necessary to absorb minerals and vitamin B_{12}, it is hard to absorb these essential ingredients for life and be well nourished.

Keeping your digestive system healthy is critical for proper brain function, because ultimately you are not only what you eat; you are truly only what you absorb.

Fix Your Digestion

I imagine this has been an eye-opening chapter, and I recognize that the discoveries I have told you about are mostly off the radar of conventional medicine. But not for long. The emerging story from the research is clear. The evidence I have seen in my patients is irrefutable.

In a healthy body, our bacterial tenants and our brains are locked in a fine dance. Your "brain" brain is in constant and synchronous communication with your gut brain.

Our gut must tangle with potentially mischievous neuropeptides from omnipresent gluten and dairy in our diet. It must contend with an onslaught of toxins, allergens, and bugs that interact with our gut immune system with widespread effects on our health and brains.

And it must try to stay nourished all the while to provide the "neuro" nutrients necessary for optimal brain function.

This is not an easy task, but it is very much within our reach if we understand how our bodies work, what goes wrong, and how to fix it. The road map for this new territory is *The UltraMind Solution*.

In Part III and Part IV I will give you the detailed tools and instructions for achieving energy, vitality, happiness, and a sharp, focused, alert mind and brain for life. This is a major part of UltraWellness. One of the keys to unlocking it is learning how to give your gut what it needs to stay in balance and avoid the things that send it into chaos.

If you want to eliminate morphine-like molecules that poison your brain, if you want to eliminate the possibility of "autointoxication," if you want to reduce the inflammation in your gut that is setting your brain on fire, the solution is simple: eliminate the dietary and environmental factors that are traumatizing your gut and feed it what it needs so you can live in harmony with it. Later in the book I will show you how.

For now let's turn our attention to toxins, how they affect our brain, and how they lead to systemic breakdown that contributes to almost every brain- and mood-related problem we face.

CHAPTER 10

KEY #5: ENHANCE DETOXIFICATION

There are two things most physicians never learn in medical school:

1. The role of nutrition and food in health and disease.
2. The role of toxins and the importance of detoxification in health and disease.

And they are probably the two most important things we need to know to cure disease and create health.

In today's world, food and toxins are more important than ever. The nutritional value of our food has been compromised by factors that range from corporate agribusiness, overfarming, and depleting the nutrient levels of the soil to food conglomerates like Kraft, Nestlé, and Nabisco putting highly processed, high-glycemic-load foods on the market that contribute to every health problem we see today, from heart disease to dementia.

The poor nutritional value of our food is further complicated by the extraordinary amounts of toxic chemicals that have entered our food supply and our bodies. Since the 1800s, more than eighty thousand new, largely untested chemicals have been introduced into the environment. Today, many are used as pesticides to "protect" our food supply.

And our exposure to poisonous substances doesn't end there. Toxins are everywhere—from household cleaning products to plastics in our kitchenware, phthalates and bisphenol A in our plastic water bottles, and even in our tap water and air supply.

We live in a sea of toxins, and a large body of growing evidence shows that these toxins are, in part, responsible for the epidemic of disease we see in the twenty-first century. Toxic exposures affect the health of all brains, young and old.

We must also deal with all the by-products and toxic metabolic wastes created by our own bodies. These self-produced toxins make us sick if our kidneys or livers fail or work at less than optimal levels.

In this chapter we will review the scientific evidence of the dramatic impact toxins have on the health of your brain. I will explain how I came to understand the importance of toxins in health and disease, and I will tell you how you can avoid the toxins that may be making you lose your mind.

But first, take the quiz below to find out if you are toxic.

In the box on the right, place a check for each positive answer. Then find out how severe your problem is using the scoring key below.

TOXINS QUIZ*

I have hard, difficult-to-pass bowel movements every day or every other day. ☐

I am constipated and go only every other day or less often. ☐

I urinate small amounts of dark, strong-smelling urine only a few times a day. ☐

I almost never break a real sweat. ☐

I have one or more of the following symptoms: ☐

- ⁙ Fatigue
- ⁙ Muscle aches
- ⁙ Headaches
- ⁙ Concentration and memory problems

I have fibromyalgia or chronic fatigue syndrome. ☐

I drink unfiltered tap or well water or water from plastic bottles. ☐

I dry clean my clothes. ☐

I work or live in a "tight" building with poor ventilation or windows that don't open. ☐

I live in a large urban or industrial area. ☐

I use household or lawn and garden chemicals or get my house or apartment treated for bugs by an exterminator. ☐

I have mercury amalgams (silver fillings) in my teeth. ☐

I eat large fish (swordfish, tuna, shark, tilefish) more than once a week. ☐

I am bothered by one or more of the following: ☐

- ⁙ Gasoline or diesel fumes
- ⁙ Perfumes
- ⁙ New car smells

(continued)

- Fabric stores
- Dry cleaning
- Hair spray
- Other strong odors
- Soaps
- Detergents
- Tobacco smoke
- Chlorinated water

I have a negative reaction when I consume foods containing MSG, sulfites (found in wine, salad bars, dried fruit), sodium benzoate (preservative), red wine, cheese, bananas, chocolate, even a small amount of alcohol, garlic, or onions. ☐

When I drink caffeine I feel wired up, and also experience an increase in joint and muscle aches or have hypoglycemic symptoms (anxiety, palpitations, sweating, dizziness). ☐

I regularly consume any of the following substances or medications: ☐

- Acetaminophen (Tylenol)
- Acid-blocking drugs (Tagamet, Zantac, Pepcid, Prilosec, Prevacid)
- Hormone-modulating medications in pills, patches, or creams (birth-control pills, estrogen, progesterone, prostate medication)
- Ibuprofen or naproxen
- Medications for colitis, Crohn's disease, recurrent headaches, allergy symptoms, nausea, diarrhea, or indigestion

I have had jaundice (turning yellow) for any reason or I have been told I have Gilbert's syndrome (an elevation of a liver test called bilirubin). ☐

I have a history of any of the following conditions: ☐

- Breast cancer
- Smoking-induced lung cancer
- Other type of cancer
- Prostate problems
- Food allergies, sensitivities, or intolerances

I have a family history of Parkinson's, Alzheimer's, ALS (amyotrophic lateral sclerosis) or other motor neuron diseases, or multiple sclerosis. ☐

* For your convenience, this quiz has been reprinted in The UltraMind Solution Companion Guide. Simply go to www.ultramind.com/guide download the guide, and print out the quiz.

Scoring Key—Toxins

Score one point for each box you checked.

Score	Severity	Care Plan	Action to Take
0–6	You may have a low level of toxicity.	*The UltraMind Solution*	Complete the six-week program in Part III.
7–9	You may have a moderate level of toxicity.	Self-Care	Complete the six-week program in Part III and detox using the self-care options in chapter 26.
10 and above	You may have a severe level of toxicity.	Medical Care	Do both of the steps above and see a physician for additional assistance. I have outlined some of the options you should discuss with your doctor in chapter 26.

A Poisoned Doctor: My Own Brain Failure

As you know from Part I, I learned about the importance of toxins and detoxification the hard way . . . in my own life . . . as a patient.

I had a fascination and love for China and the Orient, which probably started because of our regular Sunday dinner trips to Chinese restaurants during my childhood. Little did I know going to China would damage my brain and derail my life.

At Cornell, I majored in Asian Studies and studied Mandarin Chinese. I then went on a three-month sojourn through the remotest areas of China in 1984, after my first year of medical school, with the woman who would become my wife.

I loved the culture, the people, and the way food is treated as medicine. In China, people "eat" their medicine. The words for "take your medicine" are *"chi yao,"* which means eat your medicine. Food and healing are intimately connected. In China, food is pharmacology.

I returned to China ten years later to live and work in Beijing and develop a medical center. In one decade the landscape had changed from a city of 10 million people wearing Mao suits and riding bicycles to a frenzied, money-chasing city filled with Audi limos, cell phones, high heels, and business suits.

But the homes of the 10 million were still heated by raw coal, sending a dark cloud over the city on the brightest winter days. People walked the streets with surgical masks to filter out the black air. At the time, I was unaware that coal burning is the most significant source of mercury emissions. I breathed that air every day.

At the time I knew nothing of mercury, nor had I heard about genetic polymorphisms. But it turns out that I am missing a key gene necessary for the detoxification of mercury and many other twenty-first-century poisons, the GSTM1 gene.

About half our population is missing this gene. It turns out that it is the sick half!

Shortly after I returned home to the beautiful Berkshire mountains of western Massachusetts, I became ill with chronic fatigue syndrome (CFS).

How could this happen? Why was I sick? Certainly the stress of sleepless nights working in the emergency room weren't good for me and getting a severe intestinal infection from a lake in Maine didn't help either, but suddenly I was sick.

After I spent a few years searching for the cause of my illness, a colleague mentioned that many people with CFS are toxic.

So I checked my hair for mercury. It was high. Perhaps growing up on daily tuna fish sandwiches, receiving multiple immunizations, using contact lens fluid with thimerosal, and my love of sushi all became too much to handle once I inhaled a toxic load of mercury from the cold, dark winter air in Beijing.

I took a urine test to see the total mercury load in my body. I used a chelating substance, which binds up metals in the body and carries them out in the urine and stool. "Normal" levels of mercury are less than 3 mcg/g of creatinine. My level was almost 200 mcg/g of creatinine. Anything over 50 mcg/g of creatinine is considered "poisoning."

Through a long learning process, experimentation on myself, and conversations with dozens of experts, I was able to rid my body of mercury using a careful, deliberate detoxification process that included detoxifying foods, supplements, intravenous glutathione and vitamin C, metal chelators, and saunas.

I also worked on healing my gut by eliminating food allergens and using probiotics and enzymes, but it didn't get completely better until I got the mercury out of my system.

The brain fog, depression, insomnia, severe memory deficits, and slowed thinking that are the symptoms of CFS lifted, and I got my brain and my health back.

Unfortunately, this is a story repeated over and over in our society. We live in a sea of toxins—6 million pounds of mercury emissions a year, and 2.5 billion pounds of 80,000 other toxic chemicals.

These industrial emissions threaten our health and the health of our planet. Global warming and chronic health problems are triggered by the same emissions. How can these known neurotoxins not affect our brains? How exactly do they harm our brains? What can we do to protect and detoxify ourselves?

These are questions that medicine must face and answer. Each person responds differently to toxins. Some are great detoxifiers; others, like me and those with autism, ADHD, Alzheimer's, Parkinson's, and depression, are often not.

Let's look at what the research has to say about which toxins affect your health most dramatically. Remember, these are only examples. Every chemical currently in use that has not been tested for toxicity by public health agencies is a potential health threat. Keep in mind that only about 0.6 percent of all chemicals now in use have been tested.

As a doctor, one of the things that concerns me most is the impact these untested chemicals may have on our health as we age.

Mercury and Illness: Demented or Toxic?

Few topics are so politically and scientifically charged and have such enormous implications for our health and our economy that we avoid them as the impact of heavy metals (and mercury in particular) on our health.

But, like nutrition, poisoning with heavy metals such as mercury and other toxins and the importance of detoxification is not something we learn about in medical school.

So we have few tools to address this toxic exposure, which is contributing to many of the health epidemics we see in today's world. Once we start looking a little deeper, the effects of toxins are not hard to document.

Thankfully, though, the human organism has an extraordinary capacity for resiliency, regeneration, recovery, and renewal. I have seen this over and over, not only in relation to my own mercury-toxic brain and its recovery, but also in the recovery of so many patients with depression, behavior problems, ADHD, autism, dementia, and Parkinson's disease.

So, even if you haven't been treated for toxins you have certainly been exposed to, there is still hope—even in extreme cases. We need to look under the "hood" and see what dirt and poisons we may find, then clean up the metabolic, immunological, and biochemical mess.

So how do toxins connect to dementia?

Dementia is a "brain disease" that may affect cognitive function, language, attention, memory, personality, and abstract reasoning. In severe forms people's memories disappear, they forget their history, they stop talking, and their personality evaporates. A terrifying, progressive, irreversible process, dementia does not have a good medical treatment except for toxic medications with many side effects that, at best, may delay entry into a nursing home by a few months.

Dementia is a big problem and growing every day. Ten percent of sixty-five-year-olds, 25 percent of seventy-five-year-olds, and 50 percent of eighty-five-year-olds will get Alzheimer's (which is a form of dementia) at a cost of $60 billion a year to society. Scientists predict that the number of people with Alzheimer's will triple in the next few decades. It is now the seventh leading cause of death.[1]

And basically the medical community has no solution for it.

I was recently speaking on a panel for PBS-TV at the American Association of Retired Persons convention in Boston. The topic was dementia. A woman with mild cognitive impairment (MCI) was on the panel—MCI is sort of like pre-Alzheimer's or predementia—and everyone on the panel (including the Harvard neurologist) agreed that memory loss is *not* a normal part of aging. But now 22 percent, or 5.4 million people over seventy have "predementia."[2]

The sad part was that the doctors on the panel didn't have much to offer in the way of prevention—just a very bad and pretty ineffective selection of drugs with many nasty side effects.

But there is a way to prevent, treat, and sometimes even reverse the memory loss in dementia. That is where my patient, George, comes in.

George had a diagnosis of dementia and came with his wife to see me. He could no longer manage his business affairs, had become increasingly unable to function at home, and had to withdraw from family and social relationships.

He was desperate as he felt himself slipping away.

As I said above, there is no effective known treatment for dementia. But we do know a lot about what affects brain function and brain aging: our nutrition, vitamin deficiencies, omega-3 fat deficiencies, inflammation from food, infections and the gut, environmental toxins, stress, exercise, hormonal imbalances, and trouble producing energy in our cells.

These factors and how they related to George's genetic background gave me the hints I needed to help him heal.

How the Environment Affects Your Genes: George's Mercury Poisoning

Your specific genetic variations set the stage for health or disease, including heart problems or depression, diabetes or dementia.

When it comes to dementia specifically (and keep in mind this is just an example of how *all* disease works), many genes have been found to contribute to the condition. Chronic diseases like these are usually multigene disorders. No one gene is responsible, but the interaction between many genes, their variations (or single nucleotide polymorphisms), and the way these genetic variations interact with the environment, can put someone at risk for a chronic disease such as dementia.

That is why we will *never* find *the* gene for Alzheimer's, or heart disease, or cancer, or autism, or depression. There isn't one. There are many genes that influence our predisposition to certain systemic imbalances and many others that determine how these systemic imbalances show up in each of us as a "disease."

This is the loaded gun each of us lives with. But we don't have to pull the trigger. It is our environmental influences (our diet, stress levels, toxic exposure, the amount we exercise, etc.) that do that for us. Even if we are predisposed to certain illnesses, that doesn't mean we are *destined* to have them.

Remember:

Genes + Environment = Disease

We know that many things affect how our genes function—our diet, vitamins and minerals, toxins, allergens, infections, stress, lack of sleep, exercise, and more.

Even though no long-term studies have been done that look at treating dementia based on genes and environmental influences, there are many scientific threads creating a picture of how and why our brains age and what genes are involved.

CAN YOU CHANGE YOUR GENES?

I want to take a minute to clarify something very important. Many people know you can change your environment to reduce toxins by eating organic food; filtering your water; avoiding mercury-containing fish, vaccines, dental fillings; and more. But most people don't think you can change your genes.

(continued)

Well, you can.

You can't trade your genes in for new ones (well, at least not yet), but you *can* change how those genes *function*. You can change how they work, which ones are turned on or off, and how they control your biochemistry and physiology.

In fact, you influence your genes with every bite of food you eat and every thought you think.

So if you are born with genes that predispose you to certain problems, you can work around them, help them do a better job, and prevent disease or health problems. You can boost your ability to detoxify by turning on the right genes and turning off the wrong ones. You can help by giving them everything they need to do a good job, such as the right vitamins and minerals and phytonutrients. For example, eating two cups of kale or cabbage will supercharge your detox system and the genes that control it.

Know this: though you may have been dealt a certain genetic hand, it is what you do with that hand that determines the course of your life and your health.

For George, whose mind and life were evaporating, I looked deeply into his genes and the biochemistry his genes controlled and found places where we could improve things.

He had a gene called apo E4, which is a high-risk gene for Alzheimer's disease,[3] one that also made it hard for him to lower his cholesterol or detoxify mercury from his brain.

This gene predisposes people to dementia for many reasons. One of them may be that people with this gene cannot easily remove mercury from their brains.[4] This certainly seemed to be the case for George, who had some of the highest levels of mercury poisoning I have ever seen.

When your brain can't detoxify mercury, the mercury accumulates there over a lifetime. This mercury may come from many sources, including vaporization of dental fillings, environmental exposures, tuna fish, or air pollution.[5] Wherever it comes from, the effect can be severe.

In one study of 465 patients with chronic mercury toxicity, 32 percent had severe fatigue, 88 percent had memory loss, and almost 30 percent had depression. These symptoms and mercury poisoning were much more common in people with the apo E4 gene. Today about 20 percent of the population has this gene.

The good news that came out of this study is that removal of amalgam fillings combined with a mercury detoxification program resulted in significant symptom reduction.[6]

However, apo E4 was only the beginning of George's genetic problems.

Some genes are critical for optimal detoxification of metals and other toxins. One of the most important is the GST gene. George had a version of this gene (glutathione-S-transferase, or GST)[7] that was very inefficient. This gene helps increase the levels of glutathione, the body's main detoxifier and antioxidant. George's inefficient GST gene made George accumulate even more toxins over his lifetime.

Having the combination of a problem with GST and apo E4 puts people at even more risk for dementia.[8; 9]

In another study, people with an absent GST gene were likely to have much higher levels of mercury in their system.[10] So the interaction between genes and the environment is the problem. People like George aren't genetically programmed to have dementia, but they are living with a loaded gun, and their toxic environment pulls the trigger.

Luckily, we know how to work around these genes that are better adapted to a pollution-free world. We do it with diet, supplements, and other detoxification methods.

George also had another gene we found through his blood tests called MTHFR,[11] which made him require very high doses of a special kind of folate (MTHF) to lower homocysteine in his blood, which is a substance that is very toxic to the brain.

Again we see problems with methylation show up (I discussed these problems in detail in chapter 6).

The very *core* of nearly all chronic illness is the breakdown in the process of moving around methyl groups (CH3) in the body (the methylation train), and creating the most important detoxifier and antioxidant in our bodies—*glutathione* (the sulfation train, which I will discuss in detail later in this chapter).

Amazingly, these two biochemical cycles are completely tied together. All the biochemical steps along the way have to work in order for you to methylate and to sulfate, which is the process by which your body produces glutathione, the mother of all detoxifiers and antioxidants.

For the glutathione in the body to be produced, you must have enough folate, B_6, and B_{12} and the methylation train must run efficiently. As I have said many times, everything is tied together.

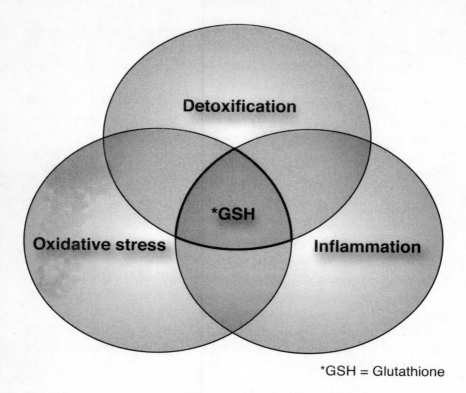

*GSH = Glutathione

Figure 12: Connections between detoxification, oxidative stress, and inflammation

Often problems with these same metabolic pathways show up in very different diseases—such as autism or Alzheimer's—but the underlying mechanisms are the same: jammed-up biochemistry leads to oxidative stress and inflammation common to all psychiatric and neurological illness (and to all other diseases), because these are the final common mechanisms of destruction in the body. And they are all connected at the core by a deficiency of glutathione.

*T*he last gene George had a problem with is called CETP. This gene is involved in cholesterol transport and we know that high cholesterol promotes Alzheimer's. People who have a problem with this gene don't make enough of the HDL, or good cholesterol, to shuttle out the bad cholesterol. We know high cholesterol leads to dementia and Alzheimer's disease. Combine this gene with the apo E4 gene and your risk of dementia goes way up.[12]

So George seemed to be a genetic train wreck. Every gene made him in one way or another susceptible to environmental insults from mercury overload, folate, or B_{12} deficiency, and elevated cholesterol.

GENES THAT INFLUENCE BRAIN HEALTH

The following are the most important genes for brain function. They not only have an impact on your ability to detoxify, but can affect all seven keys to Ultra-Wellness.

Gene	What It Does	How to Improve Its Function
MTHFR (methylenetetra-hydrofolate reductase)	Controls methylation.	High doses of folic acid or activated folate called methyl-folate.
Apolipoprotein E4	Carries cholesterol and heavy metals.	Whole foods, low-glycemic-load diet; exercise.
GSTM (glutathione-s-transferase, M, isoform) GSTP (glutathione-s-transferase, P, isoform)	Helps your body detoxify and produce glutathione.	Adequate intake of B_{12}, B_6, folate, and sulfur-containing amino acids such as NAC; eat two cups of cruciferous vegetables a day.
CETP (cholesterol ester transfer protein)	Transports cholesterol away from arteries.	Whole foods, low-glycemic-load diet; exercise.
COMT (catechol-O-methyltransferase)	Metabolizes neurotransmitters and hormones through methylation.	Adequate intake of B_6, B_{12}, and folate.
SOD-2 (superoxide dismutase-2)	Powerful intracellular antioxidant.	Take zinc, manganese, and copper in your multi-vitamin; eat plenty of phy-tonutrient antioxidants.

The good news is that these genes are not static, but are highly influenced by the way we live, the food we eat, our nutritional status, and our level of toxicity. We can address all these environmental factors and reduce the risk significantly. We can even stop or reverse the effects of toxicity.

That is what I did for George. But to understand how, you need to know a little more about what George, specifically, was facing.

George grew up and lived his life in steel country, so he had long-term exposure to coal-burning steel plants. He and I were very much alike in this regard. Coal-burning industrial plants or heating homes with coal is the major source of mercury in the environment—it is the same environmental factor I was exposed to in China that caused me to get chronic fatigue syndrome. George, it turned out, was suffering from severe, chronic mercury poisoning.[13]

We found that he had high levels of mercury. After we gave him a test for mercury using DMPS (a heavy-metal binding or chelating agent),* we found he had a level of 350 mcg/g of creatinine. Normal is less than 3. This was one of the highest levels of mercury I had ever seen.

Taking a blood sample tells you only what is floating around in your blood if you have been breathing polluted air, or eating too much sushi, but a challenge test (sort of like a cardiac-stress test or glucose-tolerance test for diabetes) picks up buried problems—in this case mercury. Studies have found that using DMPS increases mercury excretion from 3 to 107-fold.[14] The chelating agents or drugs, DMPS and DMSA, are both used to test for and to treat heavy metal toxicity.

Just doing one thing wouldn't help George. So we worked hard to get everything in balance. The most important thing we did was to have his dental fillings[15] removed safely† and slowly chelate out the mercury. Mercury toxicity was the core of his problem, and solving it would be the core of his solution.

We helped him detoxify from this mercury poisoning with foods such as kale, watercress, and cilantro; herbs such as milk thistle; nutrients such as selenium and zinc; and chelating medications that helped him overcome his genetic difficulties getting rid of toxins.

We lowered his cholesterol with diet, herbs, and exercise.

We lowered his homocysteine with high doses of folate, B_{12}, and B_6 to overcome his weak MTHFR gene. And we added an extra, special form of folate called methyl-folate, the active form that bypasses the ineffective gene. After a year of aggressive therapy that was matched to his genes and his own quirky biochemical train wrecks—not his diagnosis—he had a remarkable and dramatic recovery.

Before I saw him, he could not manage his business, nor did his grandchildren want to be around him. After matching his treatment to his genes, he was again able to function, and his grandchildren loved being with him. His memory improved, he could read and remember what he read, and run his business affairs. He no

---

* Testing for heavy metals is performed by taking a chelating agent, then collecting your urine to measure the amount your body excretes. This test is usually done only by Functional Medicine doctors or doctors specially trained in detoxification.

† Removal of dental mercury or silver fillings should be performed only by a biological dentist. See www.iaomt.org to find a biological dentist.

longer isolated himself at home, but became an engaged member of his family and community.

While this area of genetic testing and nutrigenomics (see chapter 2, page 37) is new, and more research is needed to help us refine our understanding, new doors are opening onto an entirely new era of medicine—one that no longer focuses on the disease, but on the person and that individual's uniqueness.

The ways that toxins such as mercury affect your health and the methods we now have to heal from toxicity are some of the most exciting possibilities this new science offers. We are swimming in toxins today. It's astounding that the human body can detoxify from these chemical agents that it was never designed to encounter.

But it can, and learning how to do that is one of the keys to Ultra-Wellness.

Chemicals and Neurodegenerative Illness: Can We Protect Ourselves?

The one disease that even conventional doctors now know is irrefutably linked to toxic chemicals is Parkinson's disease. This first came to light in 1979, when young drug addicts consumed heroin tainted with the toxin MPTP and developed Parkinson's. Recently Michael J. Fox, Janet Reno, and Muhammad Ali have increased awareness of Parkinson's disease.

But Parkinson's is a bigger problem than most people think. It affects over a million Americans, costs society $23 billion a year, and is second only to Alzheimer's as the most frequent neurodegenerative disease.[16]

Though genes influence the risk of getting Parkinson's, one study of 193 identical twin pairs found that genetic factors do not play a major role in causing typical Parkinson's disease.[17]

Then what causes it?

Over the years, even in my relatively small patient population (a few thousand people), the link between my Parkinson's patients and toxins stares me in the face. My patients with Parkinson's all had clear, documented, and serious toxic exposures.

The owner of a vineyard loved to care for his grapes himself, showering them with the pesticides that he carried in a barrel on his back. He developed rapidly progressive Parkinson's and died.

Or the woman who grew up in a rat-infested apartment in the Bronx and had a phobia about pests. She had her house sprayed with pesticides monthly inside and out for years. And she kept tubs of the toxic and banned pesticide chlordane in her garage. Her Parkinson's started early, at age fifty-three.

And there was the woman who at fifty-one started to have a tremor. Her mouth was full of fillings, and her mercury level was over 300 mcg/g of creatinine.

Another man was an endurance athlete who swam around Manhattan Island in the polluted Hudson River every year and developed Parkinson's disease in his early fifties.

Reams of research confirm this link—exposure to toxins from any source puts you at risk: pesticide exposure; living in a rural farm environment; consumption of well water that contains runoff from all the nearby farms; exposure to herbicides; or living close to industrial plants, printing plants, or quarries.[18] In fact, farmers now wear gas masks, and farming is considered one of the most dangerous occupations.

But Parkinson's is not just a disease of slow-moving feet, or a tremor in the hand, or the lack of ability to show facial expression. Parkinson's also comes with depression, dementia, hallucinations, and even psychosis, all of which are linked to toxic exposures as well.[19; 20]

Toxins must be excreted through the body's liver detoxification system. Detoxification happens in two phases, both dependent on different sets of enzymes to do the job. As we know, the effectiveness of the enzymes you produce depends on the genes that have the code for that type of enzyme.

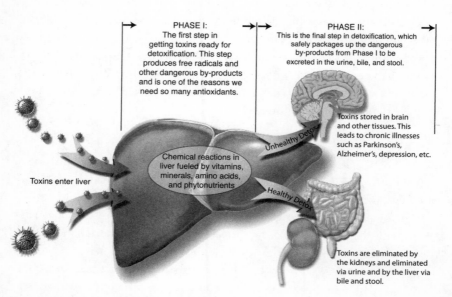

PHASE I:
The first step in getting toxins ready for detoxification. This step produces free radicals and other dangerous by-products and is one of the reasons we need so many antioxidants.

PHASE II:
This is the final step in detoxification, which safely packages up the dangerous by-products from Phase I to be excreted in the urine, bile, and stool.

Toxins stored in brain and other tissues. This leads to chronic illnesses such as Parkinson's, Alzheimer's, depression, etc.

Chemical reactions in liver fueled by vitamins, minerals, amino acids, and phytonutrients

Unhealthy Detox

Toxins enter liver

Healthy Detox

Toxins are eliminated by the kidneys and eliminated via urine and by the liver via bile and stool.

Figure 13: Two phases of liver detoxification

It might be hard to imagine, but nature has given us the remarkable ability to detoxify compounds that were not around at the time humans evolved, such as medications and environmental toxins. Drugs are metabolized or "detoxified" by enzymes, which are produced by ancient genes. Some of us are better detoxifiers than others and have an easier time getting rid of drugs and toxins.

Certain of those genes have been linked to Parkinson's. One particularly worrisome problem is the gene called 2D6, which controls one of the main enzymes for detoxifying drugs such as SSRIs (Prozac and Zoloft) and many other common drugs and most pesticides.

This gene is slow in 5 to 10 percent of Caucasians. The gene that produces the slow form of 2D6 is the gene more common in patients with Parkinson's disease.[21] So take someone with this gene, expose them to pesticides and antidepressants, and imagine what might happen.

While it is easy to despair about all the toxins we are exposed to from pesticides in our food and water, to plastics everywhere we turn, to mercury and lead from coal-burning power plants, there is a new strategy we can use to protect ourselves from these poisonous substances. It is the foundation of the UltraMind Solution.

Some have called this strategy "neuroprotection."[22] I am all for protecting our neurons, a proactive, optimistic strategy, and have used it successfully in patients all along the spectrum of mood, behavior, and neurodegenerative diseases, including Parkinson's disease.

Dr. Jeffrey Cummings from the department of neurology and psychiatry at UCLA emphasized how important it is for us to focus on prevention and detoxification as a deliberate and careful strategy to deal with our current epidemics of brain problems. He explains:

> *Advances in medical and surgical therapies have provided substantial improvement in the quality of life of patients with Parkinson's disease. Nevertheless, these approaches are largely directed toward symptom management and eventually must give way to identification of environmental hazards that can be eliminated and raising the level of public health, or to chemo preventive strategies that can be administered to exposed, at-risk, or minimally symptomatic individuals. The therapeutic nihilism traditionally implied in the term "degenerative" is giving way to the dissection of the sequence of the molecular events that lead from the initial trigger to cellular extinction.*[23]

Wow. So here in the most conservative medical journal, the *Journal of the American Medical Association,* we have a call to action to eliminate toxins and protect our brains through understanding the underlying causes of cellular breakdown.

Another key paper in the *Journal of the American Medical Association,* called "Neuroprotection in Parkinson Disease,"[24] lays out the exact model we must address to protect ourselves not only from Parkinson's but all types of brain damage.

The basic concept goes like this—

Environmental factors interact with susceptible genes to trigger this injury in the brain, and at each point of injury there are things we can do to stop or reverse the process.

Free radicals from toxins lead to oxidative stress, which damages our mitochondria, the cells' energy factory (see more on this topic in chapter 11). This leads to overexcitation of cells and inflammation. Ultimately, all this results in cell death and the symptoms we see as mood disorders and behavior problems, as well as Parkinson's and Alzheimer's.

The authors of the study suggest that if we can use antioxidants, energy boosters, and anti-inflammatory treatments along with compounds that reduce the overexcitation (excitotoxicity) of brain cells, which lead to cell death, then we can protect the brain and prevent, stop, or reverse this process.

These are exactly the same underlying factors that are the basis of the seven keys of UltraWellness, on which this program is founded.

The astounding fact is that changes in brain function can be seen on PET scans decades before the "disease" of Parkinson's occurs.[25] "Premotor" symptoms such as depression, poor cognitive function, and poor sleep often occur years before doctors can make the diagnosis of Parkinson's.

By the time the clinical diagnosis is made, more than 60 percent of the neurons related to movement (in the substantia nigra, the part of the brain that controls movement and is damaged in Parkinson's) are degenerated! So waiting till then is very late. The good news is that we can protect the brain. But we must start before all the brains cells are dead.

I have applied these concepts over and over in patients with every type of mood, behavior, or degenerative disorder and am often witness to miracles. Not everyone can be helped completely, though many can. Using these tools recovery is often possible.

It doesn't matter if it is mercury or lead or pesticides or any of the other eighty thousand—mostly untested—chemicals that we are exposed to. The end result, one of the final common pathways that leads to illness, is our overloaded detoxification system. This occurs in many chronic illnesses such as Parkinson's, depression, autism, dementia, chronic fatigue, cancer, heart disease, diabetes, and obesity.[26]

This process of oxidative stress, inflammation, toxicity, and cell death through injury to the energy system of the body or mitochondria is central to nearly all chronic illness. At the end of the day, our cells die when they lose energy or the ability to make more energy. You will learn more about this in the next chapter.

Let me tell you two stories of patients with whom I used this method and the remarkable results that occurred. They are wonderful examples of how balancing the seven keys, and enhancing detoxification, can mean the difference between a life of suffering and UltraWellness.

Is Depression a Form of Poisoning?

*J*oanne *was a thirty-six-year-old professional woman who came to see me after struggling for years with severe depression, fatigue, weight gain, severe PMS, and fibrocystic breast disease.*

Often, she said, she wanted to "hurt" herself.

Her story has many pieces but they all fall into the seven keys. Often when one thing goes wrong, such as detoxification, everything spins out of control. In all the clues she gave me, I found the answer.

She was toxic. She was unable to detoxify her hormones, which led to severe pre-menstrual syndrome, painful breasts, and heavy bleeding—a sign of too much estro-gen that couldn't be properly detoxified and eliminated from the body.

Prozac was prescribed for her for years without much benefit, as was a birth-control pill to "control" her cycles.

Joanne complained of being a sugar addict (which fuels the growth of yeast). She also took many antibiotics over the years for chronic sinus congestion (which kills the good bacteria and promotes yeast overgrowth), and had many vaginal yeast infections. (Think yeast in the gut.) No surprise.

She was always sick. Her skin was dry, her nails soft, and her hair thinning. (Think thyroid problems.)

Her blood work and other tests turned up many other clues.

A C-reactive protein blood test that picks up hidden inflammation was very high, with a level of 4.3 mg/L (normal is less than 1 mg/L). (See The UltraMind So-lution Companion Guide *online for testing details. Go to www.ultramind.com/ guide.) Her white blood cell count was low, with a high level of lymphocytes and a low level of neutrophils characteristic of a yeast infection. Her B$_6$ and folate levels were* *very low; they are needed to support mood and hormone metabolism. She also had antibodies working against her thyroid gland and a "borderline" thyroid level.*

But most alarming was her extraordinarily high mercury level of 260 mcg/g of creatinine (normal is less than 3 mcg/g of creatinine), accompanied by a mouthful of fillings.

Although the cause of her depression and many of her problems (including her weight gain) was mercury, we had to clean up all the collateral damage. We have to clean up the whole mess to restore optimum health. Treat the cause, yes, but also help people get relief from all the effects—in Joanne's case this included chronic sinus infections, yeast problems, PMS, hormonal imbalances, painful cystic breasts, thyroid problems, nutritional deficiencies, and inflammation.

So we went to work. We cleaned up the yeast with antifungals (medications used to kill yeast and other fungus in the gut); boosted estrogen detoxification with vitamin B_6, folate, and magnesium; supported her liver detoxification with herbs and essential fats like evening primrose oil, an anti-inflammatory omega-6 fat; cleaned up her sinuses with salt water irrigation; and gave her a small dose of bioidentical★ thyroid hormone called Armour thyroid (see chapter 7).

Then came the job of safely removing her mercury fillings[27] and using detoxifying foods such as broccoli sprouts, watercress, and kale, as well as metal chelators (medications that bind to heavy metals and help you excrete them more easily) to help her detoxify the mercury she had been exposed to. I also gave her herbs, and nutrients to support both methylation and sulfation—the keys to detoxification. (I will explain this connection in more detail in a moment.) And she began doing hot yoga and taking infrared saunas, which helped her promote the elimination of toxins through the sweat.

Slowly her mercury level started falling—from 260 to 150 to 27 (after her fillings were removed) to 10 mcg/g of creatinine. And, with each reduction, her depression, fatigue, and all her other symptoms got better and better until she was feeling alive again. She also lost forty-two pounds without trying.

I wish Joanne were a rare case of the havoc imbalances and toxicity cause. Unfortunately she's not.

The same pattern repeats over and over with a few variations. I see thousands of patients with nutritional deficiencies, hormonal imbalances, inflammation, gut problems, toxicity, and energy problems, the roots of all illness. All of these problems are a result of environmental factors over which we have a lot of control.

★ Bioidentical hormones are hormones identical to those made by your body, rather then synthetic hormone molecules, which have more side effects and increased risks.

More studies on the neurodevelopmental and neurobehavioral effects of mercury are being documented every day.

One study[28] found that workers exposed to mercury vapor while making fluorescent lightbulbs experienced higher levels of anxiety and depression, as well as many impairments in memory and motor function.

The workers at ground zero on 9/11 were exposed to high levels of toxic metals. In another study,[29] 160 of those workers had eight or more chronic symptoms, including depression, anxiety, insomnia, weight gain, high blood pressure, and fatigue.

After a chelation challenge test with DMSA (an FDA-approved metal chelator), they were found to have high levels of mercury and lead in their urine. After three to four months of detoxification treatment the workers experienced an average of 60 percent reduction in symptoms.

Mercury is often at the root of so many problems. But when was the last time your psychiatrist or neurologist checked for heavy metal poisoning before prescribing Prozac?

Addressing metal and chemical toxins and all their downstream effects on our biology is essential if we are to address our chronic disease epidemic and the burden of mood, memory, attention, and behavior disorders.

A Heavy Boy

Though the effects of toxins on adults are serious and lead to fatigue, depression, sleep disorders, cognitive loss, and dementia, the toll on our children is staggering.

I believe that an overload of heavy metals in children who are genetically susceptible to their effects is one of the root causes of our epidemic of ADHD, learning disorders, and autism, not to mention depression, anxiety, and bipolar disease. Today, a doctor who takes care of kids at summer camp has to be a psychopharmacologist trained in the dispensing and monitoring of psychoactive cocktails. What is wrong with this picture?

One little boy's story reflects the "heaviness" of the problem.

He was a wild child—uncontrollable, violent, unpredictable—in fact, mercurial. At the young age of three his "diagnoses" ranged from severe ADHD, to bipolar disease, to Asperger's (a mild form of autism), to oppositional defiant disorder (defiance of authority).

His pupils were always dilated like someone in constant pain or danger, and like many children on the autism spectrum, he couldn't look directly into your eyes.[30] Autistic children look at you sideways, not because they don't want to look into your eyes, but because they can see better out of the corners of their eyes. This may have to do with the effects of vitamin A and omega-3 fat deficiencies on the retina and the way the proteins (rods and cones) that do the "seeing" are out of alignment in "sick" cell membranes.[31] *(Cod liver oil, which contains vitamin A and omega-3 fats, often corrects this "sideways" seeing.)*

His mother had to use her fingers to remove his feces every day from his rectum, and every night he wet his bed, problems all too common in these children.

At social outings to the pool or park, the other parents would chastise his mother. "Can't you control your kid?" He was asked to leave every type of activity he joined. At school he had to have one-to-one supervision every day, and still couldn't be controlled. He was kicked out of a special behavioral therapy group for children who couldn't be in groups, and was not allowed into a special camp for kids who couldn't be in a regular camp.

Aside from starkly autistic children, I had never encountered a more difficult child.

It turned out he was weighed down by an extraordinary amount of metals. I have performed over ten thousand tests for heavy metals in my patients. This boy had the highest level of lead I had ever seen and a load of mercury on top of that.

His mother had plenty of mercury fillings; he was born at the time of peak immunization schedules, before the thimerosal was removed from vaccines, and he grew up in an urban, industrialized area, where the mercury and lead from emissions ends up in the soil and on the floors of homes. (Perhaps we should be like the Japanese and remove our shoes before entering our homes so we don't track in the pollution from the soil and streets.)

Because his genes made him susceptible, he accumulated these poisons instead of naturally detoxifying them.

How did he get better?

Parents, doctors, and scientists track the benefits of every type of treatment given to autistic children whose parents or doctors are connected to the Autism Research Institute (www.autism.com) and the DAN! group, which work closely together (see the box on page 237 to read about the exciting new discoveries DAN! is making).

By far the most beneficial treatment is the detoxification of heavy metals, which unblocks the metabolic and biochemical traffic jams that create problems. Then immune, gut, and brain function can resynchronize and rebalance.

Our little boy was "heavy" with metal poisoning. So we slowly chelated out his mercury and lead; fixed his gut; improved his diet; removed the sugar and dairy from his diet; boosted weak metabolic pathways with B_{12}, folate, and B_6; calmed his nervous system with magnesium; and used zinc[32] *to help him digest his food and activate enzymes (called metallothionein) that naturally eliminate mercury and lead.*

Now he is twelve years old and thriving. He has no aide in school, and he can look you straight in the eye and have a normal conversation. He doesn't wet his bed and goes to the bathroom normally. When I asked him how he felt after all this treatment with pills and dietary changes, he said, "I feel like my brain is not short-circuiting all the time."

DEFEAT AUTISM NOW!

A few dedicated parents, scientists, and doctors led by Sidney Baker, M.D., John Pangborn, Ph.D., and the late Bernard Rimland have created a new map for this terrifying territory where we now find ourselves (see www.autism.com). Through their group, the DAN! (Defeat Autism Now!) think tank, their work makes it clear that many children on the autism spectrum, and those with ADHD and even learning difficulties, have become poisoned.[33]

Autistic children have low levels of glutathione, the major detoxification compound in the body, so they cannot excrete metals. (I will talk more about glutathione in the next section.) Their hair shows *low* levels of mercury because genetically they can't excrete it,[34] but *higher* levels in their baby teeth.[35] But when given a chelation challenge test with DMSA or DMPS, autistic kids have more mercury and other metals than normal children.

METALS JAM UP OUR CHEMISTRY

Mercury and other heavy metals block many metabolic pathways, including those related to building new hemoglobin molecules (oxygen-carrying molecules inside your red blood cells). The biochemical pathway that is damaged by mercury involves something called porphyrins. Studies show that markers of abnormal porphyrins can be found in the urine of patients whose biochemistry is jammed up by toxic metals.[36] Genetic quirkiness in porphyrin metabolism or processing by the body seems to be linked to the development of neurotoxic and neurobehavioral effects from mercury exposure.[37]

In addition, having a quirky or "polymorphic" gene for BDNF (brain-derived neurotrophic factor), which we learned is so important in helping the brain repair and heal—BDNF is needed to prevent depression and dementia—significantly increases the risk of mood, cognitive, and motor problems even at very low levels of mercury exposure.[38; 39]

This explains why some of us are more susceptible to heavy metal poisoning than others, and why studies of large populations often show no harmful ef-

(continued)

fects from toxins. If 95 out of 100 children can detoxify metals and are not affected, they are 100 percent fine. But for the 5 percent of children who cannot
detoxify well, the problem is huge and the effect severe.

But remember, it is not just the porphyrin gene, or BDNF gene, or GST gene,
or MTFHR gene, or any one of the genes that is a problem. The unique combination of all your genes combined with the toxic environment in which you live
makes you sick. Our environmental influences pull the trigger and cause sickness. If you had those genes but lived in a more pristine time without toxins, you
would likely not get sick.

Each one of us is susceptible. Some of us break down at very low levels of
toxicity—like those with autism or Parkinson's, they are the yellow canaries
warning the rest of us that something is wrong with the "air."

But how many of us are just a little more depressed or mentally slow or forgetful or distracted or anxious because we are toxic?

We may never know and that is why it is important for all of us to reduce our
total exposure to toxins and maximize our body's own detoxification system,
which I will show you how to do in Part III of the program.

Getting Thoughts and Feelings to Stick: The Secret of Sulfur

In chapter 6 I described how the methylation train gets off the tracks and all
the collateral damage that occurs. I also briefly explained how the methylation and sulfation trains always run together, intersecting and interacting.
Breaks in the tracks anywhere along the line to optimal methylation and
sulfation often lead to dramatic and serious consequences, not only for our
brains, but for our entire well-being.

Let's dig a little deeper so you can understand, appreciate, and hopefully
act on the information I am about to give you.

What is the most important molecule you need to stay healthy and prevent disease? Why have most of you never heard of it? Why is it the secret to
prevent aging, cancer, heart disease, dementia, and more? Why is it necessary
to treat everything from autism to Alzheimer's? Why are there more than
seventy-six thousand medical articles about it yet your doctor doesn't
know how to address the epidemic deficiency of this critical life-giving
molecule?

What is it?

The mother of all antioxidants, the master detoxifier, and the maestro of the immune system is *glutathione* (pronounced "gloota-thigh-own"), a sticky, smelly sulfur (like a rotten egg, or a sulfur hot springs) molecule that is the ultimate product or destination of the sulfation train. Think of it as a sponge that your body uses to soak up and get rid of toxic molecules. It is the body's workhorse of detoxification.

Glutathione needs to be continually rebuilt and replenished from our diet with the help of specific vitamins (B_6, B_{12}, and folate), and can only be produced if *both* the methylation and sulfation cycles, or "trains," are running on time and at full speed. Any break in that process leads to toxic build-up and more free radicals and oxidative stress and more inflammation.

Your body produces its own glutathione.

The bad news is that our poor diet, pollution, toxins, medications, stress, trauma, aging, infections, and radiation all deplete your glutathione. Thus depleted, you are susceptible to unrestrained cell disintegration from oxidative stress and free radicals, and to infections and cancer.

Your liver also gets overloaded and can't keep up with the need to make more glutathione, making it unable to do its job of detoxification.

In treating chronically ill patients using Functional Medicine for more than ten years, I have found that glutathione deficiency is found in nearly all very ill patients—those with depression, mood disorders, chronic fatigue, heart disease, cancer, chronic infections, autoimmune disease, diabetes, autism, Alzheimer's, Parkinson's, arthritis, asthma, kidney problems, liver disease, and more.[40]

At first I thought that this was just a coincidental finding, but over the years I have come to realize that our ability to produce and maintain a high level of glutathione is critical to recovery from nearly all chronic illness, to preventing disease, and for maintaining optimal health and performance. And so have the authors of the seventy-six thousand medical articles on glutathione!

So what is glutathione?

What does it do for us?

How can we get more of it?

How is it connected to the methylation and sulfation trains?

Glutathione is a very simple molecule that is produced constantly in your body. Glutathione is composed of a combination of three simple building blocks of protein or amino acids—cysteine, glycine, and glutamine.

But the secret of its power is the sulfur (SH) chemical groups it contains. This sulfur acts like flypaper and all the bad things in the body stick to it—

from free radicals to toxins like mercury and other heavy metals. Think of it as the UPS or FedEx system in your body that packs everything and ships it out in the urine and stool.

We make it from foods that contain sulfur—garlic and onions, cruciferous vegetables, egg yolks, and most forms of protein. All these contain an amino acid called cysteine, the basic building block of glutathione. Add a few more amino acids like glycine and glutamine and a few vitamins (B_6, B_{12}, folate), and voilà, the magic of the methylation and sulfation trains pops out a little glutathione molecule.

Normally glutathione is recycled in the body—except when the toxic load becomes too great (which explains why we are in such trouble now in our hyperpolluted world).

In my practice I test the enzymes involved in glutathione production as well as the genes involved in producing enzymes that allow the body to manufacture and recycle glutathione. GSTM1 and GSTP1 are just two of the genes that can be tested for.[41]

We all evolved in a time before the eighty thousand toxic industrial chemicals were introduced into our world, before electromagnetic radiation was everywhere, and before we polluted our skies, lakes, rivers, oceans, and teeth (with dental amalgams) with mercury and lead.

We used to get by with just the basic version of the genetic detoxification software encoded in our DNA, which is mediocre at ridding the body of toxins. We didn't need more. But who knew we would be poisoning ourselves and eating a processed, nutrient-depleted diet?

So why is glutathione so important?

Glutathione recycles antioxidants. I will discuss antioxidants more in the next chapter. For now you simply need to know that antioxidants are critical for cleaning up free radicals that, when left unchecked, lead to massive cell destruction.

Dealing with these free radicals is like handing off a hot potato. They get passed around from vitamin C to vitamin E to lipoic acid (which are all antioxidants in their own right) and then finally to glutathione, which cools them off and recycles the other antioxidants. Then the body can "reduce" or regenerate another protective glutathione molecule. And we are back in business.

This antioxidant function is critical. When it doesn't work well, cells are damaged and cannot produce the energy we need to live (see chapter 11).

Problems occur when we are overwhelmed with too much oxidative stress, or too many toxins, or when the methylation or sulfation trains are derailed, or we are not getting enough sulfur in our diet, or enough methylation nutrients such as B_6, folate, and B_{12}.

Then the glutathione becomes depleted, leading us toward some terrible illness. We can no longer protect ourselves against free radicals, and we can't get rid of toxins that accumulate in our bodies and brains. Then we become sick.

Glutathione is also critical in helping your immune system[42] do its job of fighting infections and preventing cancer. Studies show it can even help in the treatment of AIDS.[43]

We need glutathione to reach peak mental and physical function. Research has shown that raised glutathione levels decrease muscle damage, reduce recovery time, increase strength and endurance, and shift metabolism from fat production to muscle development. Oxidative stress and glutathione deficiency have also been connected to dementia, depression, Parkinson's, autism, and ADHD.

If you are sick or old or just not in shape, you likely have glutathione deficiency. The top British medical journal, *Lancet,* found the highest glutathione levels in healthy young people, lower levels in healthy elderly, lower still in sick elderly, and the lowest of all in the hospitalized elderly.[44]

Keeping yourself healthy, optimizing brain function, treating mood and brain disorders, boosting your performance, preventing disease, and aging well all depend on keeping your glutathione levels high.

Glutathione is responsible for keeping many of the keys to UltraWellness (which are the basis of the UltraMind Solution) optimized. It is critical for immune function and controlling inflammation; it is the master detoxifier, and the main antioxidant, protecting our cells and making our energy metabolism run well.

Glutathione is the center of good health because it is the *key* to protecting us against oxidation, controlling inflammation, and getting rid of toxins. When those systems break down, disease results.

Thankfully, we can easily boost our own glutathione production.

First you must get the methylation train running properly, because if it stalls, so does the sulfation train. Sometimes you can take glutathione itself, or the compounds that help your body make more glutathione, such as NAC (n-acetylcysteine), alpha lipoic acid, or milk thistle.

But you can also eat your way out of trouble. Using phytonutrient "super foods" from a plant-based diet should be the foundation for everyone's diet and health.

Broccoli sprouts are the biggest inducers of glutathione production, but you can load up on all the members of the broccoli family daily. Take your pick: collards, kale, cabbage, kohlrabi, mustard greens, rutabaga, turnips, bok choy, Chinese cabbage, arugula, horseradish, radish, wasabi, and watercress.

In Part IV I will give you a specific program for boosting glutathione. I will also teach you how to detoxify and boost your own detoxification system. This promises to protect you from the deadly toxins that infiltrate our lives more and more every day and cause the epidemic of brain disorders.

Even if you suffer from little more than a bad mood, detoxification can help. If you are coping with a chronic illness (whether physical or mental), it is an absolutely critical step on the path to UltraWellness.

Enhance Detoxification

Clearly we must face the enormity of our addiction to "modern" life, which is dependent on energy, coal burning, and industrialization, and has dumped billions of pounds of metals and toxins into our environment.

This poison echoes across the brains of the very young with autism and ADHD, the very old with Alzheimer's and Parkinson's, and the rest of us with depression and anxiety.

Ferreting out the toxins, making different choices, cleaning up our lives, going "green," filtering our water, eating organically, and learning how to optimize the body's own detoxification system are essential if we are to regain our health and reduce our impact on the planet and all its inhabitants.

I remember an old saying from the 1970s: think globally, act locally. The time has never been riper for each of us to be actively engaged.

That starts with your own health and the environment you occupy. I will teach you some steps on how to detoxify your body, your diet, your home, and your life in Parts III and IV. I strongly encourage you to follow those steps and become actively engaged in detoxifying our world.

Next we will learn about why conserving and making energy is so important to your brain and what can go wrong. You will learn how all these toxins, bugs, poor nutrition, hormonal imbalance, and inflammation ultimately lead to cell destruction and death by a common mechanism, literally depleting us of our life energy.

Making energy from food and oxygen to run all our cells is essential to life. And the system that does that for us—the mitochondria—is very sensitive to injury. If you want more energy and you want to learn how to protect your brain, read on.

CHAPTER 11

KEY #6: BOOST ENERGY METABOLISM

Ultimately everything comes down to energy.

We need it, we want it, we lose it, and we try to get it back until finally we can't make energy anymore. That's called death!

Most of us don't think much about where our energy comes from, why sometimes we have more or less of it, how it might affect our brain, or even the whole process of aging.

But in fact, everything we have explored in the first five keys influences our health directly through energy.

Enough energy means a happy, healthy, focused, and sharp brain. Lack of energy means slowed mental function, autism, mood disorders like depression, and ultimately Parkinson's and dementia.[1]

The part of your body that uses the most energy is your brain, which has the most *mitochondria,* the little factories inside your cells that produce energy. Energy is necessary for memory, learning, and the whole information flow inside you that creates the synchronous, harmonious firing of neurons and brain cells.

No energy = abnormal cell function and cell death.

Abnormal cell function and cell death = chronic illness and brain disease.

Is this is why your brain is broken? Take the following quiz to see if your mitochondria are damaged and you are losing energy.

In the box on the right, place a check for each positive answer. Then find out how severe your problem is using the scoring key below.

LOSS OF ENERGY QUIZ*

I have chronic or prolonged fatigue. ☐
I have aching muscle pain or discomfort. ☐
I have sleep problems (trouble staying or falling asleep or
waking up early). ☐
My sleep is not refreshing. ☐
I have a poor tolerance for exercise, with severe fatigue after. ☐
I have muscle weakness. ☐
I have trouble concentrating or remembering things. ☐
I am irritable and moody. ☐
Fatigue prevents me from doing things I would like to do. ☐
Fatigue interferes with work, family, or social life. ☐
I have been under prolonged stress. ☐
My symptoms started after acute stress, an infection, or trauma. ☐
I have chronic fatigue syndrome or fibromyalgia. ☐
I have a history of chronic infections. ☐
I overeat. ☐
I have been exposed to environmental chemicals (pesticides,
unfiltered water, nonorganic food). ☐
I have Gulf War syndrome. ☐
I have a neurological disease, such as Alzheimer's, Parkinson's,
ALS, etc. ☐
I have autism or ADHD. ☐
I have depression, bipolar disease, or schizophrenia. ☐

---

*For your convenience, this quiz has been reprinted in *The UltraMind Solution Companion Guide*. Simply go to www.ultramind.com/guide, download the guide, and print out the quiz.

Scoring Key—Energy Loss

Score one point for each box you checked.

Score	Severity	Care Plan	Action to Take
0–6	You may have a mild loss of energy.	*The UltraMind Solution*	Complete the six-week program in Part III.
7–9	You may have a moderate loss of energy.	Self-Care	Complete the six-week program in Part III and optimize your energy metabolism using the self-care options in chapter 26.

10 and above	You may have a severe loss of energy.	Medical Care	Do both of the steps above and see a physician for additional assistance. I have outlined some of the options you should discuss with your doctor in chapter 26.

Want More Energy? Heal Your Mitochondria

To understand how energy is produced and how its production affects your mind, mood, and behavior (not to mention your health and your weight), we must start with the energy-producing factories inside your cells—your mitochondria.

Mitochondria are the parts of your cells that take the calories you consume, combine them with oxygen, and turn this mixture into energy used to run everything in your body. A single cell may have anywhere from two hundred to two thousand or more mitochondria.

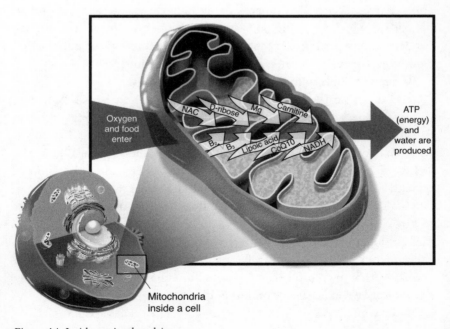

Figure 14: Inside a mitochondrion

Mitochondria are built to convert calories and oxygen into energy the body can use—ATP (adenosine triphosphate). Our cells contain a total of one hundred thousand trillion mitochondria, which consume 90 percent of our oxygen intake. This oxygen is necessary to burn the calories we eat in food. But free radicals are produced as a by-product of this combustion, much like exhaust that comes out of the tail pipe of your car.

These free radicals are dangerous because they damage or oxidize molecules and cells throughout the body. This damage is called oxidative stress. More damaged cells equals more oxidative stress or "rusting"—which is essentially what oxidative stress is. This, in turn, leads to damaged DNA, damaged cell membranes, rancid or oxidized cholesterol (which is what truly makes cholesterol harmful), stiff arteries that look like rusty pipes, wrinkles, and brain damage. Oxidative stress is a central feature in dementia[2] as well as autism.[3]

We have our own built-in antioxidant factories that produce molecules, whose job it is to seek out free radicals and clean them up before they rust our bodies. But these systems are easily overwhelmed by a toxic, low-nutrient, high-calorie diet like the ones most Americans eat.

We can get even more of these important antioxidant molecules if we eat the right foods. But we don't, so we aren't getting them that way either.

This problem is further complicated because the critical antioxidant enzymes we make (called superoxide dismutase, catalase, and glutathione peroxidase, which helps the body use glutathione to protect you) are dependent on essential dietary nutrients to help them work well. These include zinc, copper, manganese, vitamin C, and selenium.

We are in trouble with free radicals for two reasons.

First, the typical American diet is one that causes an escalation in free radicals because it has too many empty calories and not enough antioxidants.

Second, our reduced nutrient intake (vitamins and minerals) limits the ability of our antioxidant enzymes to function. For example, without enough zinc or selenium, these enzymes can't do their job.

That's why our self-manufactured antioxidants are not enough to protect us.

The single most important controllable factor regulating the oxidative stress in your body is your diet. Eating too many calories and not enough antioxidants from colorful plant foods results in the production of too many free radicals, wreaking havoc on our bodies and our minds.

Here's why.

Mitochondria are exquisitely sensitive to our nutrient-deficient, highly processed, sugar-laden, omega-3 fat–deficient, excitotoxin-rich (MSG, aspartame) diets. They bear the brunt of our nutritional deficiencies. Empty, high-calorie, refined, and processed diets that lack nature's colorful plant-based antioxidants set the stage for trouble.

Mitochondria are also extremely sensitive to inflammation and toxic damage. I have shown in previous chapters how critical diet is in regards to inflammation and toxicity.

The combinations of these insults lead to more oxidative stress (or rusting) than your body can handle. As a result, your mitochondria literally rust and stop, just like a rusty wheel.

Colorful plant pigments—the dark green, yellow, red, orange, blue, and purple colors in our diet—are our major source of antioxidants. For example, blueberries, red grapes, sweet potatoes, and collard greens—the "rainbow diet."

Your mitochondria depend on all your antioxidant defenses being optimized. If you don't eat this rainbow diet, your defenses are not at their best. The result is that your mitochondria are injured by the very free radicals they produce as a by-product of their energy production, and they stop making enough energy for your cells to operate optimally. Then you get sick and ultimately die.

The energy assembly line depends on many steps to produce the little packets of energy called ATP (adenosine triphosphate) that run every single cell in your body. And every step depends on vitamins and minerals and special nutrients such as carnitine, NADH, lipoic acid, and coenzyme Q10.

When you don't get enough of these vitamins and minerals, your mitochondria have a much more difficult time producing energy, compounding the problem they face from the onslaught of ever more free radicals.

The result is that they produce less energy and all of the processes in your body slow down. Your brain cells fire more slowly, your metabolism slows, and your ability to process toxins shuts down, to name just a few. Every function in your body would eventually cease if you stopped producing enough energy to keep it functioning.

This is what aging ultimately is—the slow destruction and damage to our mitochondria that result from nutritional deficiencies, low levels of antioxidants, exposure to toxins, allergens, infections, and stress. In short, imbalances in any of the keys to UltraWellness cause problems by damaging the mitochondria.

If you don't eat enough healthy fats, you can't build fluid, flexible, functional mitochondrial membranes, which keep your mitochondria healthy and prevent them from dying.[4]

If you are deficient in the B vitamins or magnesium or other key nutrients, energy production slows down.

If the methylation and sulfation trains slow down, free radicals and oxidative stress increase because you don't have enough glutathione to protect yourself, and homocysteine (which is a toxic molecule in high amounts) increases, which creates even more oxidative stress. The result? Energy production slows, or worse, your cells die.

If your hormones are out of balance,[5] including high cortisol from too much stress,[6] or your thyroid function is slow,[7] your mitochondria slow way down. If you have inflammation[8] from any source, including the gut, you damage mitochondria. Toxins[9] of any kind do their damage, ultimately, by poisoning the mitochondria.

At the end of the day, loss of function or death of mitochondria accounts for much of what we see in most diseases—including problems with mood, behavior, attention, and memory.

Taking a journey through the scientific literature makes it clear that all these factors lead to oxidative stress and mitochondrial injury as the final common pathways of illness and disease.

Evidence links autism,[10,11] Alzheimer's,[12] Parkinson's,[13,14] depression,[15] bipolar disease,[16] and brain aging[17] in general to mitochondrial injury from oxidative stress, which can be triggered by poor diet, toxins, infections, allergens, hormonal imbalances, altered gut function, and stress.

This may sound far-fetched. How can this all be connected?

I will answer this question over the course of this chapter. However, trust me when I say that the research on oxidative stress and mitochondrial injury bears this out.

While most researchers work quietly in their labs sorting out all the pieces of the puzzle of human suffering, a few take a step back and ask, "What are the patterns, themes, and principles that link everything together?"

What these men and women have begun to realize is that there are a few unifying themes of disease that most scientists and doctors have come to accept. They are:

+ Inflammation
+ Oxidative stress
+ Mitochondrial injury

There are only so many ways the body can say "ouch" when insulted. And the final common pathway for most conditions is oxidative stress, mitochondrial damage, and the resultant loss of energy.

That is why so many "neuroprotective" strategies are under investigation and have shown promise, including lipoic acid, acetyl-L-carnitine, coenzyme Q10, and NADH. All help repair the damage to your mitochondria—damage from any source—and protect your "neurons." The result is improved brain function.

Neuroprotective strategies like these can be important (and supplementation is often a critical part of healing), but even when these methods are used they are often used late in the game (when the damage is already done), and they don't address the real core of the problem. Sure, if you have a tack stuck in your foot you can take a lot of aspirin, but the real treatment is taking out the tack. You have to work at both ends: find the cause and fix the collateral damage. If you have been poisoned by mercury, you must get rid of the mercury and support and protect your mitochondria with nutrients and antioxidants.

Similarly, you can give supplements and medications that boost mitochondrial function, but the treatment is removing the substances that lead to damage in the first place.

Since your mitochondria are so sensitive and can be damaged so easily, oxidative stress can come from anywhere—mercury poisoning, nutritional deficiency, hormonal imbalance, or inflammation.

The key is finding the cause and eliminating it. If you are mercury toxic, neuroprotective strategies will take you only so far. The treatment is to get rid of the mercury. The same is true for the other imbalances that cause mitochondrial distress.

Let's look at some of the key factors that lead to oxidative stress and the brain problems it brings. This will give you the power to treat the problem, not the symptoms. You can remove the "tack" that is making you crazy, depressed, and forgetful.

Locating the Causes of Oxidative Stress: A Few Among Many Factors

Is oxidative stress leading to your loss of energy? Take the following quiz to find out.

In the box on the right, place a check for each positive answer. Then find out how severe your problem is using the scoring key below.

OXIDATIVE STRESS QUIZ*

I am fatigued on a regular basis. ☐
I get less than 7 or 8 hours sleep a night. ☐
I don't exercise regularly or I exercise more than 15 hours a week. ☐
I am sensitive to perfume, smoke, or other chemicals or fumes. ☐
I regularly experience deep muscle or joint pain. ☐
I am exposed to a significant level of environmental toxins
(pollutants, chemicals, etc.) at home or at work. ☐
I smoke cigarettes or cigars (or anything else). ☐
I am regularly exposed to secondhand smoke. ☐
I drink more than three alcoholic beverages a week. ☐
I don't use sunblock, or I like to bake in the sun or go to tanning booths. ☐
I take prescription, over-the-counter, and/or recreational drugs. ☐
I would rate my life as very stressful. ☐
I eat fried foods, margarine, or a lot of animal fat (meat, cheese, etc.). ☐
I eat white flour and sugar more than twice a week. ☐
I eat fewer than five servings of deeply colored vegetables and
fruits a day. ☐
I have chronic colds and infections (cold sores, canker sores, etc.). ☐
I don't take an antioxidant-containing multivitamin. ☐
I am overweight (BMI more than 25—a BMI chart has been printed ☐
in *The UltraMind Solution Companion Guide* for your convenience).
I have diabetes or heart disease. ☐
I have arthritis or allergies. ☐

*For your convenience, this quiz has been reprinted in *The UltraMind Solution Companion Guide*. Simply go to www.ultramind.com/guide download the guide, and print out the quiz.

Scoring Key—Oxidative Stress†

Score one point for each box you checked.

Score	Severity	Care Plan	Action to Take
0–9	You may have a low level of oxidative stress.	*The UltraMind Solution*	Complete the six-week program in Part III.

† Note that for this quiz there are only two scores. Low-level problems are treated on the six-week program. If you have severe problems, I strongly encourage you to seek the assistance of a physician trained in Functional Medicine.

10 and above	You may have severe level of oxidative stress.	Medical Care	Complete the six-week program in Part III and see a physician for additional assistance. I have outlined some of the options you should discuss with your doctor in chapter 26.

As I have already said, many imbalances can lead to oxidative stress. Everything from nutritional imbalance to environmental toxins can contribute to this problem.

However, there are a few primary biochemical factors that are linked to the mitochondrial destruction that lead to so many brain diseases.

I would like to review a few of these here. These are examples of some of the key elements that push this key system out of balance. There are others. But these examples give a powerful explanation of the relationship between oxidative stress, reduced energy production, and the brain problems that result.

Balancing the Brain: Don't Get Too Excited

Much of the metabolic mischief that damages our energy-producing system occurs by the overactivation of something called the NMDA receptor[18] (the site of action for a new Alzheimer's drug called Namenda).

Think of NMDA as the on and off switch for your cells. All systems in the body have a way of staying in perfect balance. Just like Goldilocks and her porridge—not too hot and not too cold, but just right. In the same way you want to excite your brain cells so they can learn, remember, and focus, but you don't want to overexcite them so that you become hyperactive and can't retain any information. Not too hot, not too cold, but just right.

The balance in the brain is tightly regulated. A little excitement is good. Too much sends the cells into a death spiral. When the NMDA receptor is "excited" it opens a "gate," flooding cells with too much calcium.[19] The overload of calcium triggers a cascade of signals that produce free radicals, damage the mitochondria, and ultimately lead to cell death.

Many things—toxic foods such as aspartame and MSG, environmental toxins, infections, allergens, and even psychological stress—can trigger this overexcitement and stimulate the NMDA receptors to open the floodgates, damaging and killing brain cells.

The trick is keeping the balance. Not too much stimulation of the NMDA receptors, not too little.

The wondrous thing about the body is that it has so many systems to maintain balance, like yin and yang. All of them are necessary, but balance is the key. Just think of pH balance, or blood-sugar balance, or sleeping and waking, breathing in and out, the stress response and the relaxation response. Illness occurs when things are out of balance in any of these systems.

When your brain cells are injured by overexcitation or die, every one of the problems we have been discussing in this book ensues—ADHD, autism, depression, anxiety, Alzheimer's, Parkinson's, and more.

The good news is that we understand how to modulate this system naturally to prevent overexcitation and brain injury.

Many of the things we have found helpful to stabilize mood and an irritable nervous system and to prevent cell death work through their calming action. All slow down the overstimulation of this receptor.

Magnesium is the natural guard against too much stimulation of the NMDA receptor by glutamate, the neurotransmitter that normally flips the "on" switch. Zinc is also a natural relaxant. GABA, taurine, vitamin B_6, vitamin D, n-acetylcysteine (the glutathione booster), and even green tea all act as a brake on the overstimulation of the NMDA receptor.

On the other hand, mercury, arachidonic acid (an inflammatory omega-6 fat from dietary sources like meat and dairy), cortisol (the stress hormone), and homocysteine (because of a lack of folate, B_6, or B_{12}) all overexcite the NMDA receptor, leading to cell death.

Understanding this helps us learn how to prevent overexcitation and calm things down. Doing this is part of the brain-protective and balancing plan in Parts III and IV of *The UltraMind Solution*.

Live to Be 120 Years Old by Drinking 1,500 Bottles of Red Wine a Day

Another one of the key balancing acts you need to keep in mind to protect your mitochondria is your insulin and sugar balance. I am going to explain why in a moment, but before I do . . .

Did you know you can live to be 120 years old by eating as much as you want and drinking lots of red wine?

The only catch is that you have to drink about 1,500 bottles of wine a day, which would kill you, before you could live forever!

David Sinclair and his group at Harvard found that the red pigment in grapes called resveratrol could extend life in rats by protecting their mito-chondria. He so believes in this compound he started a company (Sirtris Pharmaceuticals, which has been purchased by Glaxo Smith Kline for $720 million) to produce a pharmaceutical derivative of the active compound in red wine, resveratrol.

Though he has discovered something very important, those who view this as the "magic pill" that will allow you to eat whatever you want and live forever are misguided. The body is much more complex than that. But he is onto something drawing the link between resveratrol, aging, and mito-chondria, something that affects brain health and has an impact on all chronic diseases.

Let me explain why a magic pill won't work, and what may really help you live longer and prevent all the diseases of aging, including all brain dis-eases. He is on the right track, but "magic pills" without more usually don't work. The focus must be on systems.

News about this new "drug," resveratrol, says it extends life span, lets you eat whatever you want, and gives you the fitness of a trained athlete without any exercise.

But it is not a drug at all, and the excitement only serves to reinforce the idea that a single molecule (whether it is from a drug or a plant) can solve all our health problems.

Resveratrol comes from grapes (hence the benefit of red wine), peanuts, berries, and a Chinese herb called *hu zhang* (polygonum cuspidate, also known as giant knotweed, which is a common ingredient in many Chinese herbal formulas). A natural plant defense molecule, resveratrol is only one of many beneficial plant compounds called phytonutrients, included in the class called polyphenols, of which there are thousands.

These phytonutrients act in many ways, the most important of which is as a genetic control system, turning on and off genes that help us stay healthy. This is the science of nutrigenomics—or how food is information that tells our bodies what to do, not just a source of calories we need for energy.

If treating people with a simple dose of resveratrol sounds too good to be true, it is.

As much as I support the use of supplements and know about the impor-tance of phytonutrients, all of this excitement about resveratrol is mis-guided.

Why?

Because looking for a quick fix is misguided. To find the real secret to longevity, healthy aging, and fitness we need to look at how this compound works and learn from that the lessons we need on how to keep ourselves healthy.

What is the real secret, and how does resveratrol really work?

In one word, mitochondria.

Two recent studies (one of which was done by Sinclair himself) shed light on how resveratrol works, how it impacts oxidative stress, and how mitochondrial function holds the key to health, brain wellness, weight loss, and longevity.

In the first study, published in *Nature*,[20] David Sinclair and his colleagues gave one group of mice a high-fat (60 percent of calories) diet. In middle age these rats all became obese, got diabetes, fatty livers, and died early.

He fed the same diet to another group of mice, but gave them resveratrol at a dose of 24 mg/kg of body weight—which is equivalent to the amount of resveratrol found in about 750 to 1,500 bottles of wine a day.

That group still got fat, but lived longer and did not get diabetes or heart disease. They were also more agile and had more endurance than the rats that didn't get the resveratrol. Interestingly, their cholesterol profiles didn't improve *but* they didn't get heart disease, showing that cholesterol is not the big evil we think it is.

So how does resveratrol have these effects? And what does this study on rats have to do with brain disease in people?

Let me explain how this relates to your brain. Anything that helps your mitochondria helps your brain, and anything that improves your blood-sugar control, improves insulin resistance and also helps your brain.

How Resveratrol Works

In the study above, resveratrol produced changes associated with longer life span and produced the following biologic effects:

1. Increased insulin sensitivity leading to better blood-sugar control.
2. Reduced insulinlike growth factor-1 (IGF-I) levels—a molecule related to a growth hormone that promotes cancer growth.
3. Increased AMP-activated protein kinase (AMPK)—a signaling system in the body that controls insulin sensitivity and can prevent diabetes.
4. Increased peroxisome proliferator-activated receptor—coactivator 1 (PGC-1) activity—which is a critical signaling system that turns

on genes that improves blood-sugar control and improves mitochondrial function.

5. Increased the number of mitochondria produced by the cells—
boosting the capacity to turn food into energy and to burn
calories.

6. Improved motor function, making the old rats more agile.

7. And finally the resveratrol worked by opposing the effects of
aging by modifying 144 out of 153 metabolic pathways, controlled by genes, many of which control mitochondrial function.

But what does this study really tell us—that aging, including much of
brain aging and disease, is controlled in large part by *sugar* and insulin function in the body! Sound familiar?

Too much sugar in your diet causes your body to produce too much insulin. This triggers more inflammation and oxidative stress leading to mitochondrial injury.[21] Mitochondrial damage, in turn, leads to even more
insulin resistance. That means anything that protects the mitochondria, like
resveratrol, will prevent at least part of the damage that leads to insulin resistance and hence mitigate many possible problems.

People with genetically underperforming mitochondria, like the children of diabetics, are more susceptible to mitochondrial injury if they have
a poor diet, don't exercise, and don't get enough of the right nutrients to
protect their mitochondria.[22]

The next study published in *Cell* by Johan Auwerx,[23] from the Institute
of Genetics and Molecular and Cell Biology in Illkirch, France, tested much
higher doses of resveratrol in mice, eighteen times as much, or 400 mg/kg
of resveratrol—equal to about 360 capsules of resveratrol for a 130-pound
person.

Their findings were even more dramatic. Imagine achieving the fitness
of a trained athlete, staying thin, preventing diabetes and heart disease, and
living to 120 years of age while eating a high-calorie, high-fat diet (and taking 360 pills a day of resveratrol!).

The rats fed the high doses of the resveratrol along with their high-
calorie, high-fat diet had the following effects:

1. They did *not* gain weight and reduced the size of fat cells.

2. They didn't get prediabetes or metabolic syndrome.

3. They increased the number of energy-producing mitochondria
in muscle cells.

4. It turned up their metabolic thermostat (thermogenesis) and increased fat burning in the mitochondria.

5. They increased their endurance and aerobic capacity (without exercise).
6. They maintained their cells' sensitivity to insulin, hence better blood-sugar control.
7. They had enhanced muscle strength and reduced muscle fatigue.
8. They had improved coordination.
9. There were *no* side effects on any organs.
10. They increased the activity of PCG-1 alpha, which in turn controls genes that improve the function of mitochondria and blood-sugar control.

This seems incredible. But it is plausible if you understand these two root causes of obesity, brain injury, aging, and disease—blood-sugar control and the health, number, and function of your mitochondria.

That taking *only* resveratrol even at high doses will allow us to live a depraved life of sloth and gluttony and live disease-free forever, is unlikely. But what these studies do tell us is *very* important.

When taken from a systems perspective—understanding *all* the influences on blood-sugar control, insulin, and our mitochondrial function (nutritional balance, hormone balance, inflammation, toxins, energy production, oxidative stress, and psychological stress—or the seven keys to UltraWellness, which lead to an UltraMind)—we can create a lifestyle and program that works to keep us healthy, happy, alert, mentally sharp, thin, and more likely to live to 120.

Finding the Gene Control Switch for Mitochondria

At a conference on longevity and aging I had a chance to have a conversation with Dr. Leonard Guarente from the Massachusetts Institute of Technology, who in 1995 discovered a gene called SIR-2 in yeast that controlled longevity. David Sinclair, who authored one of the studies above, was his student.

The SIRT-1 gene (which is what it is called in humans) or sirtuin family of genes works by protecting and improving the health of your mitochondria.[24] I asked him how this master gene controlled longevity, the gene through which the effects of this grape compound, resveratrol, did its magic.

His answer was quite simple really. *Sugar!* This gene is the master-control switch for healthy aging because it improves blood-sugar balance and insulin sensitivity through its effects on mitochondria.

When your mitochondria are running in top shape, you can metabolize or process all your calories and produce energy. But when they are overloaded with too many empty calories, they are unable to keep up, and too many free radicals are generated, slowing down your cells and your metabolism.

By increasing the activity of this master gene, you improve the overall function of your mitochondria, improve blood-sugar control and insulin sensitivity, and boost your antioxidant defenses. You live longer, and your brain works better.

This is no surprise, since all of the signs of aging such as hardening of the arteries and organ damage (especially brain damage) are increased through worsening blood-sugar control—even before you get diabetes. Diabetics, in fact, have smaller and more poorly functioning mitochondria and get cancer, heart disease, depression, and dementia at far greater rates than the general population.[25]

Remarkable new research links mood disorders to problems with insulin and blood-sugar control. In fact, some researchers suggest calling depression "metabolic syndrome type II," meaning that the changes in the brain from oxidative stress, inflammation, and mitochondrial injury lead to altered mood.[26]

So if we could fix our blood-sugar control and boost our mitochondria, we could live longer and disease-free.

Taking a big-picture view, we don't just want to take a magic pill that will be unlikely to work given all the other real life insults affecting us, such as poor diet, stress, environmental toxins, and sedentary lifestyle.

This just takes us back to the basic principles of systems biology and Functional Medicine at the foundation of *The UltraMind Solution*.

One of the keys to this program is to rebalance your diet by eating real, whole foods instead of the highly processed, high-calorie, high-fat diets that cause imbalance in your blood sugar and produce catastrophic effects on your mitochondria.

Or you could drink 1,500 bottles of red wine a day.

But what else can you do to boost your mitochondrial function and prevent the destruction of your brain?

Neuronutrients: Boosting Your Brain Power and Your Mitochondria

Taking supplements to enhance your mitochondrial performance is actually a well-founded scientific approach to overcoming oxidative stress. It's simply that taking huge quantities of resveratrol *alone* (or as some magic pill) without changing your lifestyle or using all the other nutrients needed for optimal mitochondrial function is a misguided approach. This is especially true considering the fact that resveratrol really has an impact on your insulin/sugar balance, which is more effectively treated with diet, exercise, and lifestyle changes anyway.

Many vitamins and minerals and "conditionally essential" nutrients are known to control energy production and to protect and defend your mitochondria. These "antiaging" or neuroprotective supplements work because of the way they help protect and optimize mitochondrial function, both directly and indirectly.

A number of "basics" are essential, including omega-3 fats, which make up the membrane of the mitochondria, and the two B vitamins, niacin (B_3) and riboflavin (B_2), which are necessary to help the enzymes involved in turning food into energy in your mitochondria.

We get others from our diet or our bodies produce them. But as we age, or are exposed to any type of physical, toxic, or emotional stress, we need to replace these nutrients.

The top mitochondrial nutrients are acetyl-L-carnitine,[27] alpha lipoic acid, coenzyme Q10, NADH, D-ribose, magnesium, riboflavin (vitamin B_2), niacin (vitamin B_3), and n-acetylcysteine (NAC). These mitochondrial nutrients and antioxidants can protect your critical energy-producing factories.

Dr. Bruce Ames, of the University of California at Berkeley, has been investigating the use of these mitochondrial protective nutrients with much success. In fact, he suggests that we should not just think of nutrients as compounds to prevent disease, but rather as substances that can give us a metabolic tune-up.[28]

He has shown that providing compounds such as alpha lipoic acid and acetyl-L-carnitine can reduce mitochondrial injury and the effects of aging on the brain, including memory, learning, and speed of motor function.[29] The key, he says, is not to get focused on just one nutrient, but to use a whole team of natural compounds to help the body function the way it was designed.[30]

A Metabolic Tune-Up: A Systems Strategy

All our efforts to help prevent aging and mitochondrial injury have to be coordinated. Here is what Dr. Ames says:

1. Problems with mitochondrial enzymes lead to less energy production and more free radicals and oxidative stress.

2. Enzymes can be made to work better by providing helpers, namely vitamins and minerals and conditionally essential nutrients (nutrients required under certain conditions such as unique genetic needs, extremes of age, stress, and sickness) like B_3, B_2, magnesium, D-ribose, coenzyme Q10, NAC, acetyl-L-carnitine, lipoic acid, and NADH.

3. The right nutrients can help the body induce its own antioxidant defenses. For example, zinc, copper, and manganese are needed for the function of one of our own most powerful antioxidant enzymes called SOD, or superoxide dismutase, and selenium is needed for the function of glutathione peroxidase, which helps your glutathione do its job as an antioxidant and detoxifier.

4. Use combinations of antioxidants to soak up free radicals and prevent overproduction of oxidants in the mitochondria.

5. Use phospholipids and omega-3 fats such as DHA and EPA to repair and rebuild the mitochondrial membrane.

The reason studies don't show benefit for this or that nutrient is that the studies are designed wrong. What if you put Michael Jordan on a court by himself against the worst team in the NBA? Could he win? Of course not.

Antioxidants and nutrients work as a team,[31] and giving just one compound in isolation can actually backfire, producing more damage.

Studies have shown that high levels of the antioxidants vitamin E and C in the diet are very powerful, and can lower Alzheimer's risk by 70 percent.[32] But people who eat diets high in vitamin C and E are eating a plant-based, nutrient-dense diet full of other nutrients and antioxidants.[33] The combination is the key.

The plant world is full of powerful protective compounds such as curcumin (the yellow color in curry) and green-tea catechins that can reduce the risk of Parkinson's disease and Alzheimer's.[34] We must focus on a plant-based diet first, and then boost our efforts with supplemental mitochondrial nutrients.

Another energy booster is coenzyme Q10,[35] which has been shown to stop or slow the progression of Parkinson's disease in a sixteen-month study of eighty people.[36;37] The dose given was very high, at 1,200 mg a day, but there were no side effects.

In fact, some patients with Parkinson's may have a defect in the enzyme that needs coenzyme Q10 to operate properly.[38] Therefore, if they have any increased oxidative stress such as from exposure to toxins, their mitochondria are much more susceptible to damage and loss of energy and they need much higher doses of coenzyme Q10 to protect themselves.

What concerns me is new research on the statin drugs (drugs designed to lower cholesterol, like Lipitor and Zocor), which shows that they are mitochondrial poisons. Statins block the body's ability to produce its own coenzyme Q10.[39] We know that statins cause muscle damage,[40] but even in people without any symptoms[41] or abnormal blood tests,[42] muscle biopsy shows cell injury.

How does this affect a susceptible population? Or someone already burdened by a load of mitochondrial toxins, inflammation, and other factors that create excess free radicals, which are so common in the twenty-first century?

One hundred years ago, heart disease was almost unknown and there were no statins. Some cardiologists now suggest putting these drugs in our water supply.[43] Should we be wondering what those more natural conditions were and what we should be eating and doing so we don't develop preventable lifestyle diseases? Or should we dump medications in our water supply?

Other nutrients have also been shown to be beneficial in animal studies of Parkinson's disease and Alzheimer's. These include creatine, nicotinamide,[44] and n-acetylcysteine.[45]

But lest you think that all this protection is just important for old brains, it appears that loss of energy production and oxidative stress are critical components of little autistic brains as well.[46]

So all across the age spectrum and all across the spectrum of different diseases that affect the brain (and almost everything else), we must focus on keeping our free radicals and oxidative stress in check and our mitochondria healthy.

A BRAIN WITHOUT ENERGY

I want to share a very important story with you. This is the story of another little boy who made a miraculous recovery using the same techniques you are learning about in *The UltraMind Solution*.

A desperate mother came to see me because her 2½-year-old son had just been diagnosed with autism. He was born bright and happy, breast-fed, and had the best medical care available (including all the vaccinations he could possibly have). He talked, walked, loved, and played normally—that is until after his measles, mumps, and rubella vaccination at twenty-two months.

He was vaccinated for diphtheria, tetanus, whooping cough, measles, mumps, rubella, chicken pox, hepatitis A and B, influenza, pneumonia, hemophilous, and meningitis—all before he was two years old.

I do not believe vaccines *cause* autism and I support the safe use of vaccinations, but we need to revisit how and when to safely provide them to our children. For a comprehensive perspective on this topic see Dr. Stephanie Cave's book, *What Your Doctor May Not Tell You About Vaccinations.*

After this string of vaccinations he lost his language, became detached, withdrawn, less interactive, and was unable to relate in normal ways to his parents and other children—all signs of autism. How could a normal boy be transformed so quickly?

He was taken to the best doctors in New York and it was "pronounced" that he had autism (as if it were a thing you catch like a bug), and told that there was nothing to be done except arduous, painful, and barely effective behavioral and occupational therapy techniques. The doctor told his mother the progress would be slow and she should keep her expectations low.

Devastated, this woman began to seek other options and found her way to me.

There is much yet to undo and peel, like the layers of an onion, but by seeing autism as a body disorder that affects the brain (highlighting the importance of the *body-mind effect*), there is so much that can be done.

Children treated this way, often called the "biomedical model" (see www.autism.com for more information, resources, and conferences for doctors and parents), can often have dramatic and remarkable (if not miraculous) recoveries.

So what did I find in this little boy that gave me clues about how to treat him?

When I first saw Sam, he was deep in the wordless inner world of autism. Watching him was like seeing someone on a psychedelic drug trip.

We dug into his biochemistry and genetics and found many things to account for the problems he was having.

He had a very high level of antibodies to gluten. He was allergic not only to wheat, but to dairy, eggs, yeast, soy, and about twenty-eight

(continued)

other foods in total. He had a leaky gut, which was very inflamed, and he had three species of yeast but no healthy bacteria growing in his inner tube of life, his intestines. Urine tests showed very high levels of D-lactate—an indicator of overgrowth of bacteria in the small intestine.

He was deficient in zinc, magnesium, manganese, B_{12}, vitamin A, vitamin D, and omega-3 fats. He had trouble making energy in his mitochondria (common in autistic children). The loss of energy in his cells led to his brain losing energy, so it couldn't do its job.

He was depleted in amino acids, necessary for normal brain function and detoxification.

His blood showed high levels of aluminum and lead and his hair showed very high levels of antimony and arsenic—signs of a very toxic little boy. His levels of sulfur and glutathione were low, indicating he couldn't muster the power to detox all these metals.

In fact his genes showed a major weak spot in glutathione metabolism, which is the main detox highway for getting rid of metals and pesticides and the main antioxidant in the body.

He also had trouble with methylation, which is required to make normal neurotransmitters and brain chemicals and critical for helping the body get rid of toxins. This showed up as low levels of homocysteine (a sign of problems with folate metabolism) and high methylmalonic acid (a sign of problems with B_{12} metabolism).

He also had two genes that set him up for more problems with his system (COMT and MTHFR, which both control this process of methylation). He had very high levels of oxidative stress or free radical activity, including markers that told me his brain was under free radical fire and inflammation.

It seems complicated, doesn't it? Actually it's not. I simply worked through the seven keys of UltraWellness, saw how everything was connected, and created a plan to get to the causes of the problems. Then I helped Sam deal with all the biochemical and physiological rubble that those causes had left along the road.

So what did I do with Sam?

Having the new road map of Functional Medicine and UltraWellness makes it straightforward.

Take away what's bugging him.

Give his body what it is missing and needs to thrive (based on his own biochemical uniqueness).

And his body does the rest.

• • •

This is what we did with Sam:

- Fixed his gut and cooled the inflammation in there.
    - Took away the gluten and food allergies.
    - Got rid of the yeast with antifungals.
    - Killed off the toxic bacteria in his small intestine with special antibiotics.
    - Put back healthy bacteria with probiotics.
    - Helped him digest his food with enzymes.
- Replaced the missing nutrients and coenzymes to help his genes work better.
    - Added back zinc, magnesium, folate, B_{12}, B_6, vitamin A, and vitamin D.
    - Gave him brain-supporting omega-3 fats.
    - Gave him coenzyme Q10 to help his mitochondria return to normal.
- Helped him detoxify and reduce oxidative stress.
    - Added high-dose B_{12} shots (with a special form of B_{12}—methyl B_{12}) to turn on his brain chemistry and get his detox system unstuck.
    - Gave him a chelating medication (DMSA) and detoxifying nutrients to help him get rid of the metals.

Does this sound familiar? Improve nutrition, reduce inflammation, heal the gut, and detoxify. It is the basis of the UltraMind Solution.

No matter what the disease, biology has basic laws we have to follow and understand. All the details of Sam's story fit into these laws. We just have to dig deep, peel back the layers, and understand what is going on.

After three weeks on a gluten-free diet during which we treated his gut, he showed dramatic and remarkable improvements. Sam got back much of his language and showed much more connection and relatedness to other people in his interactions.

After four months, he was able to enter a more mainstream school, was more focused, and used more words.

At ten months we retested him and found that his gut inflammation was gone, his overgrowth of gut bacteria was gone, and his detox system was working much better. The tests that showed his mitochondria and energy system weren't functioning well were now back to normal. His mitochondria, which were unable to provide the energy necessary for his brain to function, now were running at nearly full speed.

But most important, he went from nonverbal to verbally fluent and no longer qualified for a special school or special services because he "lost" his diagnosis of autism.

(continued)

> *Sam now has a wonderful sense of humor (typically completely absent in autistic children), and engages in spontaneous play and hugs with friends and family.*
>
> Remember, every child with behavior problems—whether it is ADHD, autism, or something else—is unique. Each has to find his or her own path with a trained doctor. But the gates are open and the wide road of healing is in front of you. You simply have to take the first step.

Boost Energy Metabolism

Energy is something we lose with age. But it can also be lost because of anything that triggers more free radicals and oxidative stress or damage to our mitochondria.

Even as we are learning how mitochondrial injury is one of the final common pathways in so many neurological and psychiatric disorders, we are also learning how to protect and defend ourselves.

Getting a metabolic tune-up is not only possible, but also necessary for most of us. Thankfully by eating a colorful plant-based diet, reducing toxic exposures, and supplementing with mitochondrial protective and antioxidant compounds we can protect and restore our energy metabolism to optimal function.

In the last chapter of Part II (chapter 12) we will look at how the mind influences the body. You have learned all the ways so far in which the body affects the mind. But remember, the communication is bidirectional: top down and bottom up. The body affects the mind *and* the mind affects the body.

Thoughts, feelings, beliefs, attitudes, and life traumas can all trigger damage to the brain. This brain damage occurs because stress itself causes depletion of nutrients from the body, changes our hormones, creates inflammation, damages the gut, has direct toxic effects, and increases oxidative stress.

Wow! All that just from negative thoughts.

As you learned so far, if you change your body, you will change your mind. In the next chapter, you will learn that if you change your mind you will also change your body.

CHAPTER 12

KEY #7: CALM YOUR MIND

Stress is the perception of a real or imagined threat to your body or your ego.

One man's meat is another man's poison.

Thoughts are things. They can heal or harm. Beliefs mold your brain. Perceptions can please or paralyze your nervous system. Life traumas and experiences rewire and reorganize your brain's connections and communications systems.

Other than eating breakfast regularly, and eating more fruits and vegetables, the one characteristic that is present in all the healthy aged is resiliency. Resiliency is that hard-to-measure quality of adapting to change, shifting with changing tides rather than drowning, seeing the glass half full, or knowing how to turn lemons into lemonade.

Plasticity is another way to describe this quality—being adaptable, changeable, and malleable. Remarkably, the nature of the brain mirrors the nature of our thoughts, beliefs, and attitudes. A stiff, rigid, "hard" personality is reflected in stiff cells, hard, rigid plaques in the brain, and a general loss of resiliency and the ability to renew, remember, and repair.

This is not just a figurative metaphor for what happens. Your brain literally stiffens, slows, and loses function in direct relationship to your thoughts, beliefs, and attitudes about you and your place in the world. How each of us responds to our life—to our perceptions—has enormous implications for how we feel, how we age, and the health of our brain.

Why is it that some can emerge from enormous strife and conflict, such as war, violence, abuse, and rape, with a deeper sense of life and beauty and connection to meaning while others are debilitated from minimal life traumas such as a minor car accident?

Victor Frankel, the internationally renowned psychiatrist and author of *Man's Search for Meaning,* is an interesting example of a man with extraordinary resiliency. Not only did he survive the Holocaust, but he used the horror he experienced to create what was in his time a revolutionary approach to psychotherapy *and* he wrote about his experience to try to help heal the world.

Whether you are consumed by the traumatic experiences in your life or ripen and learn from them is largely a question of perception, thoughts, and your sense of control and place in the world. How each of us measures our life, and creates meaning and purpose in the small and large things, determines, perhaps more than anything, our capacity for resiliency and wholeness.

Your mind affects your body. Your mental health affects your physical health. This in turn affects your mental health again. These are not two separate systems. They are intertwined and interconnected in subtle and sophisticated ways you need to understand if you are going to achieve UltraWellness.

While not all of the ways in which the mind influences the body are fully understood, in this chapter I will give you an overview of what the research does tell us and explain some of the ways your mind affects your body.

But first, take this quiz to assess your stress response, and the level of stress in your life.

In the box on the right, place a check for each positive answer. Then find out how severe your problem is using the scoring key below.

ADRENAL DYSFUNCTION QUIZ*

I have low blood pressure. ☐
I feel dizzy when I stand up. ☐
I have hypoglycemia (low blood sugar). ☐
I crave salt. ☐
I crave sweets. ☐
I have dark circles under my eyes. ☐
I have sleep problems (either falling asleep or staying asleep). ☐
I have nonrestorative sleep (don't feel reenergized). ☐
I have mental fogginess or trouble concentrating. ☐
I have headaches. ☐
I have frequent infections (catching cold easily). ☐
I don't tolerate exercise well and feel completely exhausted after. ☐

I feel stressed most of the time.   ☐
I feel tired but wired.   ☐
I retain water.   ☐
I have panic attacks or am easily startled.   ☐
I have heart palpitations.   ☐
I need to start the day with caffeine.   ☐
I have poor tolerance to alcohol, caffeine, and other drugs. ☐
I feel weak and shaky.   ☐
I have sweaty palms and feet when nervous.   ☐
I feel fatigued.   ☐
My muscles are weak.   ☐

*For your convenience, this quiz has been reprinted in *The UltraMind Solution Companion Guide*. Simply go to www.ultramind.com/guide download the guide, and print out the quiz.

Scoring Key—Adrenal Dysfunction

Score one point for each box you checked.

Score	Severity	Care Plan	Action to Take
0–7	You may have mild adrenal dysfunction.	*The UltraMind Solution*	Complete the six-week program in Part III.
8–10	You may have moderate adrenal dysfunction.	Self-Care	Complete the six-week program in Part III and optimize your adrenal function using the self-care options in chapter 28.
11 and above	You may have severe adrenal dysfunction.	Medical Care	Do both of the steps above and see a physician for additional assistance. I have outlined some of the options you should discuss with your doctor in chapter 28.

Facing the Greatest Danger

A human being is part of a whole, called by us the "Universe," a part limited in time and space. He experiences himself, his thoughts and feelings as something separated from the rest—a kind of optical

*illusion of his consciousness. This delusion is a kind of prison for us,
restricting us to our personal desires and to affection for a few persons
nearest us. Our task must be to free ourselves from this prison by
widening our circle of compassion to embrace all living creatures and
the whole of nature in its beauty.*

—*Ideas and Opinions*, ALBERT EINSTEIN, 1954

In 1986, I traveled to Nepal as part of an expedition to study the public
health problems of a small village near the Tibetan border. Along the way I
encountered a remarkable man who had faced grave threats to his life and
his place in the world. He was a Tibetan doctor captured in 1959 during the
Chinese invasion and sent to a Chinese gulag for twenty-two years. Interested in Tibetan medicine, I had asked our guides to introduce me to this
Tibetan doctor. We waited outside his office.

An old monk with long white whiskers and enormous ears that fanned
like sails from his head informed us we could see the doctor.

He came out of his room, which adjoined the small clinic. He was
dressed in long maroon robes, his head shaved. Thick, black-rimmed glasses
were held around his head by a red lama string (a sacred red string used to
serve as a reminder of the Buddha) nowhere near his ears. His face radiated
a serene and happy interior. The doctor sat cross-legged on a platform in
front of his desk listening to my questions.

I looked around the small room. In one corner was his desk, and behind
it along the wall was an assortment of herbal preparations in the form of
small, mud-colored round pills, carefully labeled and stored in Horlick's
malt jars. In each corner, bags upon bags of these medicines were stacked, all
brought overland from Tibet.

There were a few chairs, one bed frame without a mattress, and a
large photograph of the Dalai Lama wearing a great crescent-shaped yellow hat.

Though spartan, the room, the medicines, and the monk/doctor, priest/
healer gave me the feeling of safety and protection.

Slowly and in pieces his story unfolded. He was sixty-eight years old and
was born in western Tibet. There he learned medicine as a young monk as
an apprentice to another doctor—learning the texts, the herbs and plants,
and the techniques for preparation most doctors learn in formal medical
schools. His remote village had no medical schools. He learned the subtle
skill of pulse diagnosis and stool and urine analysis from his teacher, and engaged simultaneously in the life of a novice monk.

He carried on with his work until 1959, when the Chinese invaded Tibet, jailed and murdered religious and political leaders, and oppressed the elite class. He remained for twenty-two years in China's jails, where he was made to serve as a laborer, carrying wood for the first eight years he was in prison.

He was moved several times, first into western Tibet, then Xiagatse, and then near Lhasa, the traditional capital of the country. He did not practice medicine for the first eight years of his imprisonment. However, once the Chinese realized his talents they thought he could serve them better as a clinic doctor in jail.

He worked there, still a prisoner, until they gave him his own clinic of Tibetan medicine, which he ran for a few years near Lhasa. In 1981, he was given the choice to stay in Lhasa or return to his native village in western Tibet. He chose the latter. After a few months in his village, at the age of sixty-three, he escaped across the Himalayas into Dharmsala, India, to visit the Dalai Lama, who told him to go to Katmandu to practice.

I found it difficult to reconcile the serene, calm, happy man who dispassionately told me of his twenty-two-year imprisonment in a Chinese gulag, where he was stripped of his community, his place in the world, prevented from practicing Buddhism, tortured, and abused.

I asked him about the greatest danger he faced during his twenty-two years of imprisonment. I expected him to say the physical and psychological torture and relentless, sophisticated brain-washing techniques designed to force him to renounce his spiritual beliefs and monkhood and embrace Communist ideology.

"The greatest danger I faced during my imprisonment was the few moments I thought I might lose my compassion for my Chinese captors," he said.

Meaning, Purpose, and Health

The lack of meaning in life is a soul sickness whose full extent and full import our age has not as yet begun to comprehend.

—C. G. JUNG

Meaning makes a great many things endurable—perhaps everything. Through the creation of meaning . . . a new cosmos arises.

—C. G. JUNG

The same event or experience can have a different impact on different people. Most of us cannot imagine worrying about having compassion for those who kept us locked away from everything we value and believe in for twenty-two years.

Yet somehow, in small and large ways, our sense of control, our sense of meaning, purpose, and connection in life is one of the most powerful factors that determines our health and well-being.

What do you feel connected to? What gives you meaning and purpose in life? Answers to questions like these define who we are, not only mentally, but also physically.

Many of our beliefs, attitudes, and perceptions are learned behaviors that can be unlearned. Sudden shifts happen. But more often a slow, gradual examination of our lives and our place in the world are necessary to emerge from the chronic stress of "half-empty" perceptions and ANTS (automatic negative thoughts) in our brain.

We all know those people in life who see everything negatively. For them, nothing can be right or good. The glass is always half empty. I would hate to see their brains on an MRI.

Disconcertingly, studies show that it is not lifestyle or even socioeconomic status, but the perception of our place in the world that determines health. One would think disease risk factors commonly associated with poverty or low socioeconomic status such as smoking, consumption of alcohol, junk food, obesity, and lack of exercise should explain the higher rates of disease and death in poverty-stricken communities.

But a study in the *Journal of the American Medical Association* found that even after controlling for all those behaviors and risk factors, higher rates of disease and death could not be explained just by these factors alone.[1]

The key, they said, was not behavior but perception of one's place in the world. The key findings that could account for the higher risk of disease and death were:

1. Lack of social relationships and social supports.
2. Personality dispositions (thinking the glass is half empty), including a lost sense of mastery, optimism, control, and self-esteem, or heightened levels of anger and hostility.
3. Chronic and acute stress in life and work, including the stress of racism, classism, and other factors related to the inequitable distribution of power and resources.

It is more than stress alone that contributes to or creates the majority of modern chronic diseases—from the epidemic of mental disorders, including depression and anxiety, to heart disease, and more.[2]

Dis-ease is a disconnection from our sense of place in the world, a loss of control and meaning as we drift from television channel to television channel looking for a program to satisfy us; consume food disconnected from its origins, processed and unidentifiable from its natural state; as our families separate, disconnect, and communicate through text messaging and e-mail. Poverty alone does not increase the prevalence of illness, morbidity, and mortality. A lost sense of culture, control, and meaning are major factors.

How do you take a pill to fix that?

Ultimately, our perceptions mediate or influence our biology in a direct and measurable way. The science of "PNEI," or psycho-neuro-endocrine-immune system, has mapped out these connections clearly and powerfully.

All our self-talk and perceptions—good or bad—work through a coordinated network or system. This system is called the HPATGG axis (hypothalamic-pituitary-adrenal-thyroid-gonadal-gut axis or network).

A big mouthful, yes, but it is simply the system that governs the bidirectional connection between your thoughts and feelings, your hormones, your immune system, and your gut (which contains all three—hormones, immune system, and nervous system).

Everything talks to everything all the time.

We have reviewed how hormones, the immune system, and the gut all talk to the brain earlier in Part II. Now we will review how the brain talks back!

Happy talk = a happy human.

Negative talk = depression, anxiety, behavioral problems, and dementia.

Let's look at how this works.

The Brain and Stress

How do thoughts, perceptions, beliefs, and attitudes affect us?

A lot of us have felt that rush of adrenaline in our lives from a near-miss car accident, or other thoughts that we are in danger. One night, a few years ago, I awoke hearing the rustling of papers and banging in my house. I grabbed the phone and called 911. My heart was racing, my breathing intensified, I could see in the dark and could hear the slightest sound.

The police came over, peered in, and saw our new puppy had escaped from his pen and was playing around in the house.

In my mind and body, I "knew" there was a burglar. That imaginary "perception" turned into real biology. My flight-or-fight response was triggered.

The stress (and relaxation) response is controlled by the brain's command and control center, called the *hypothalamus*. When I heard that "burglar," it switched on the stress response, which sends messages out to every part of the body through an automatic part of your nervous system called the *sympathetic nervous system*.

When this part of our nervous system is switched on (which is most of the time for most of us), our adrenal glands release more cortisol and the stimulating neurotransmitters epinephrine (adrenaline) and norepinephrine (or noradrenaline). These chemicals are activating and energizing.

This is a great system to have—especially when we are in trouble or danger. Think of zebras grazing in the savanna. Along comes a hungry lion and all the zebras take off acutely stressed. Then one gets killed and the rest go back to calmly grazing. Basically, your body acts like those zebras when it sets off your stress response.

According to Robert Sapolsky, of Stanford University, that is why zebras don't get ulcers.[3] They have an immediate jolt of stress, and when it's over they go back to calmly grazing. Their stress response is turned on rapidly. Then when the danger is over, it's turned off.

The problem in our culture is the chronic, unremitting, unrelenting stress and endless stressful inputs to our nervous system, including our nutrient-depleted toxic diet, environmental toxins, electropollution, and loss of a sense of control and community.

This puts us in a chronic state of alarm. In his book *The End of Stress as We Know It*, pioneering neuroscientist Bruce McEwen explains how chronic levels of stress lead to wear and tear on our systems. He calls this the "allostatic load."[4] Think of it as the sum total of all the stressors on your system over a lifetime.

All of these excess stressors—stressors we were not designed to deal with on a chronic and repetitive basis—lead to overactivation of the sympathetic nervous system and stress response, followed by burnout.

Dr. Sapolsky has mapped out the way in which this chronic stress damages the brain. High levels of cortisol, the major stress hormone, damage the hippocampus.

When considered from an adaptive point of view, when we are in dangerous or stressful situations, we want to remember everything about it. That's a good thing; it helps us avoid the situation in the future.

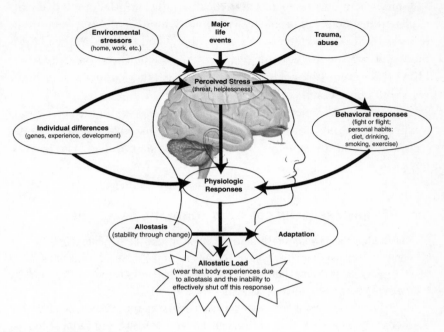

Figure 15: Allostatic load

That is why there are so many receptors for cortisol in the hippocampus, the memory center of the brain. Since we need to remember dangerous situations to avoid them in the future, our body is perfectly designed to help us do this.

However, in the modern world this system is overactivated. We don't need to remember every situation we perceive as stressful. And high levels of cortisol over the long term injure the hippocampus, leading to impaired memory,[5] dementia, and depression.[6] Sonia Lupien from McGill University has also shown how stress shrinks the memory center and has damaging effects on our brain function and cognition.[7;8]

Stress literally eats away at your brain.

The effects of stress can be seen quite clearly in those who suffer posttraumatic stress disorder (PTSD), an anxiety disorder that is the result of exposure to some traumatic event and causes the person who experienced the trauma to live in a state of hyperarousal. This condition affects about 15 percent of those who experience a major trauma such as war, violence, or abuse. It changes your brain and rewires your response to stress. Many who went through the trauma of 9/11 experienced PTSD.[9]

Chronic stress has many negative effects on the body and mind that help explain the widespread problems with obesity, health, and brain function in today's world. All the feedback from the body and the feed "down" from the brain works through the over or under activity of this important HPATGG system (the communication network that connects your brain with your entire body).

So any "stress," whether it is physical danger, a thought, perception, toxin, allergen, infection, or even abnormal gut bacteria, has negative effects throughout this system. These effects are widespread and can be very powerful.

HOW THE BRAIN CONTROLS AUTOMATIC FUNCTIONS

Your body governs your stress and relaxation responses through your autonomic nervous system. This system controls all of the automatic functions in your body, and is divided into two parts: *the sympathetic nervous system* and *the parasympathetic nervous system*.

You don't have any control over the sympathetic nervous system, and it's a good thing you don't. It controls critical bodily functions like your heartbeat and the flow of your blood. Imagine what might happen if you could stop your heartbeat or your blood flow just by thinking about it!

However, you *do* have some control over the parasympathetic nervous system. This part of your body is partially automated, but it is also responsive to your thoughts. For example, the blinking of your eyes is connected to your parasympathetic nervous system. You have some control over it (you can stop blinking your eyes for a while), but not full control over it (keep them open long enough and your eyes *will* blink).

The hypothalamus is the command and control center at the top of this entire chain of events. Its job is to control all "automatic" functions. Stress, as I mentioned above, is controlled by your sympathetic nervous system. You have control over the inputs that cause stress, but you have no control over the response itself. If you perceive stress, your body will react.

Relaxation, on the other hand, is something you *can* control. It is governed by your parasympathetic nervous system, so you can consciously engage "the relaxation response," as I will discuss below.

Chronic stress affects all of your autonomic functions negatively, but relaxation helps balance all them. These functions include:

1. Control of blood pressure and electrolyte balance.
2. Control of energy metabolism and metabolic rate.
3. Regulation of body temperature.

4. Control of reproduction and sleep cycle.

5. Regulation of the stress response (and relaxation response) via autonomic activity coordination.

What an Overactive Stress Response Does to You

Here is a short list of the effects of an overactivated stress response over the long term.[10] I list these here just to show you the extent of the research and our understanding of how stress negatively affects us and our brains. Chronic stress over time:

- Increases inflammation and inflammatory cytokines (TNF-α, IL-1, and Th1 immune response), which have all been linked to depression, bipolar disease, autism, schizophrenia, and Alzheimer's.
- Reduces the natural relaxation and anti–inflammatory calming, memory-enhancing neurotransmitter called acetylcholine.
- Increases depression and anxiety.
- Damages the hippocampus, leading to memory loss and mood disorders.
- Increases "excitotoxicity" and activation of the NMDA receptors (the on/off switch for your cells) leading to cell death.
- Reduces serotonin levels.
- Reduces BDNF (the brain's healing and repair factor necessary for the formation of new brain cells).
- Lowers growth hormone.
- Reduces slow wave sleep.
- Reduces social interactions and sexual receptivity.
- Increases abdominal fat and insulin resistance.
- Interferes with thyroid function.
- Activates pathways (BAX and p53) that lead to death of the mitochondria and loss of energy production.
- Increases the release of fats into the bloodstream.
- Raises triglycerides, lowers HDL ("good") cholesterol, and raises LDL ("bad") cholesterol.
- Increases stickiness of blood and platelet aggregation, leading to clots (which lead to heart attacks and strokes).
- Causes loss of muscle.

So, as you can see, stress is a major problem that clearly affects the health of your body and your brain. But can we do anything about it?

Is This Brain Damage Reversible?

Just reading this list of harmful events that happen as a result of a chronic stress response may make you want to join a Tibetan monastery.

But then again, you might be thrown into a gulag. So that's not the answer. What the Tibetan monks know how to do is to modulate the effects of stress. They have learned how to control something most of us have no awareness of—our vagus nerve, or the antidote to the stress response. This is our body's natural balancing system.[11]

The vagus nerve is the nerve that comes from the brain and controls the parasympathetic nervous system, which controls our relaxation response. And this nervous system uses the neurotransmitter, acetylcholine, as its main method of communication with the rest of the body.

Tibetan monks didn't do this intentionally, but engaging in practices such as meditation and the study of the nature of the mind, perception, and consciousness allowed them to move into a different state of awareness. That awareness gave them the ability to slow down their experiences, develop compassion, and break down the sense of separateness between self and others that leads to feelings of disconnection, loss of control, powerlessness, and lack of self-esteem.

Monks don't practice these ancient techniques to improve their memory, fight depression, lower blood pressure or heart rate, or boost their immune systems, although all of those things happen.

The monks practice these techniques to develop habits of mind and perception that allow them to have a different experience of their world.

But this alteration in perception isn't available only to Tibetan monks. Others have it too.

Dr. Kenneth Pelletier studied the effects of perceptions, thoughts, and beliefs on health and reviewed them in his book *Sound Mind, Sound Body*. He examined, not the sick, but the well. What are the characteristics of people who are successful in life in their work, relationships, and ability to be happy?

They did not necessarily practice stress management techniques, although practicing active relaxation is essential for health. Rather, they possessed a sense of purpose, meaning, and connection to what was important in life.

GETTING RID OF ANTS IN YOUR HEAD

Though I won't be discussing them extensively in this book, there are many techniques available to help you get the ANTS (automatic negative thoughts) out of your brain. Learning to relax and stimulate the vagus nerve (which I will discuss in a moment) helps, but there are other techniques as well, including cognitive-behavioral therapy and the new field of personal coaching. See Resources for more information on how to work on automatic negative thinking.

In Part III, I will give you specific tools you can use to turn off the stress response, turn on the relaxation response, and find your "pause" button.

Getting to Vagus: Surgery or Meditation?

There are two high-tech ways to turn off the stress response and activate the parasympathetic nervous system. You can cut out your adrenal glands. Or you can get a pacemaker that stimulates the vagus nerve. Neither of those options is too attractive.

Studies show that the hippocampus shrinks because of an adrenal (or pituitary) tumor that produces too much cortisol (Cushing's disease), which leads to depression and impaired memory and cognitive function.[12] But the researchers found that by removing the adrenal gland tumor and lowering the cortisol levels, the hippocampus increases in size[13] and memory and mood improve.[14]

While studying rats, Heather Cameron, from the National Institutes of Health, found that she could increase the rate of neurogenesis and improve cognitive function in old rats to the same level as younger rats in just a few days simply by removing their adrenal glands.[15]

You can improve your memory and learning, relieve depression, lose weight, and boost your immunity by cutting out your adrenal glands. But then you would be unable to respond to any real threat or danger. So that doesn't seem like such a great idea.

Or you can have a pacemaker implanted in your neck that stimulates the vagus nerve every few seconds. This is now being prescribed to people with treatment-resistant depression.

However, I don't think that is the major point to be taken away from the studies above.

Clearly, they tell us that stimulating the vagus nerve and reducing the amount of work your adrenal glands are doing may improve everything from memory to depression. But wouldn't it be better to learn how to activate the vagus nerve on your own.

You can, in fact, do this easily—in just a few seconds.

Right now take a deep breath into your belly to the count of five, pause for one second, then breathe out slowly to the count of five. Keep your belly soft. Put down the book and do this five times. Notice how you feel in your body and mind. Then keep reading.

You have just activated the vagus nerve, which flows from your brain through your neck, right into your chest, and through your diaphragm. So when you take a deep breath and relax and expand your diaphragm, your vagus nerve is stimulated, you instantly turn on the parasympathetic nervous system, your cortisol levels are reduced, and your brain heals.

This whole experience is called the relaxation response. The opposite of the stress response, the relaxation response is necessary for your body to heal, repair, and renew. There are *many* ways to activate the vagus nerve and turn on the relaxation response.

The Tibetan monks used meditation, which is very easy to learn (see www.ultramind.com/guide for resources), and also activates the vagus nerve. In fact the deep soft-belly breath you just did is a form of meditation that you can do almost anywhere. In Part III you will learn how to incorporate this into your daily life.

THE VAGUS NERVE AND HEART RATE VARIABILITY

Is there a way to measure your stress response? Is there a way to track the health of your autonomic nervous system and the balance between the sympathetic (or stress) response and the parasympathetic (or relaxation) response?

A few new technologies can help you do this.

Biofeedback—a technique where special devices are used to help you control bodily processes that are normally involuntary—has been used to help people learn how to control their heart rate, blood pressure, and skin temperature just by using their thoughts.

A more sophisticated form of biofeedback measures the variability of your heart rate from beat to beat. This is known as HRV (or heart rate variability), and it can be measured easily like an EKG in your doctor's office. There are at home tools *you* can use to achieve this effect. For a listing of these and other relaxation tools go to www.ultramind.com/guide and download the companion guide for this book.

The more complex your heart rate and the more variations from beat to beat, the healthier you are. The worse your heart rate is—meaning less variability—the less healthy you are. The least variable heart rate is a flat line!

The resiliency and health of your brain are directly related to the complexity and resilience of your heart rate.[16] Lower heart rate variability is a marker for increased stress and links back to all the negative effects we see with stress.

By measuring your heart rate variability, you can measure your stress response and you can increase your heart rate variability by activating the relaxation response.

Inflammation and the Vagus Nerve

The ability that the vagus nerve has to help you relax, turn off your automatic stress response, and stem the tide of cortisol in your blood is only one of the effects it has on your body.

It turns out, it also has a major impact on inflammation.

How does this work?

Remember, any type of stressor has its impact through your hypothalamus and its wide-ranging control over the autonomic nervous system's dual functions of stress or relaxation, as I discussed above.

Even the health effects of pollution register through the autonomic nervous system and can be measured by higher stress and lower heart rate variability.[17] Many of the negative effects from stress are, in part, related to increased inflammation.[18]

How does this work? Remember the key neurotransmitter, acetylcholine? This neurotransmitter is responsible for learning and memory. It is also calming and relaxing, and is the neurotransmitter your vagus nerve uses to send messages of peace and relaxation throughout your body.

It is also a major factor regulating the immune system.

As we have discussed, brain inflammation is linked to every known mood, behavior, attention, memory, or neurodegenerative disease. New research has found that acetylcholine is a major brake on inflammation in the body.[19]

Relaxing is anti-inflammatory. Stimulating your vagus nerve sends acetylcholine throughout your body, not only relaxing you but also turning down the fires of inflammation.

The body is a beautifully balanced organism working in the natural rhythm of everything in nature—day and night, yin and yang, moon and sun. Too much relaxation and you will end up in a blissful puddle. Too much stress and you will be an inflamed, aging, demented, and depressed wreck.

So activating the vagus nerve and balancing the sympathetic nervous system on a daily basis are critical to keeping your brain and body healthy.

By activating the vagus nerve you can reverse or stop all the negative effects of stress noted above.

But the good news doesn't end there. Exciting new research has linked the vagus nerve not only to improved neurogenesis, increased BDNF output (brain-derived neurotrophic factor is like super fertilizer for your brain cells) and repair of brain tissue, but to actual regeneration throughout the body.

Stem cells are directly connected to the vagus nerve. It appears that activating the vagus nerve can stimulate stem cells to produce new cells and repair and rebuild our own organs.[20] No need for placental injections, embryos, or fetal research. Just relax and you will stimulate your own stem cells to create a new you!

The Stress of Our Food

While thoughts, beliefs, and perceptions can trigger a stress response, so can any physical or chemical insult. One of the biggest stress triggers can be the food we eat.

Most of us think of food as just calories. But new findings make it clear that what you put in your body is much more than just energy. The quality and type of food directly influences your genes and the stress response.

Xenohormesis: The Attack of the Foreign Molecules in Food

In his movie *Super Size Me*, Morgan Spurlock ate three fast food meals a day for one month. Most of us recognize that eating a lot of fried, processed food, full of trans fat, high-fructose corn syrup, and calories will make us gain weight, promote heart disease and diabetes, and even give us fatty livers.

But what struck me the most was not that his cholesterol or blood sugar went up, but that his personality changed. He became aggressive, depressed, restless, foggy, and felt "good" only when he was eating the food. He became addicted to the food and felt drugged.

The explanation for this may be that our current food supply—which is genetically modified or engineered; grown in nutrient-depleted soils and fertilized with petrochemicals; shipped in boxes across thousands of miles; filled with antibiotic-, hormonally pumped livestock or farmed fish that is fed grain rather than grasses or algae, which are its native foods—can send the wrong signals to our bodies.[21]

Our cells see these foods, which are a far cry from what we evolved to eat, as foreign. "What's this?" our cells say. "Something foreign? Something dangerous? Let's get in gear by activating the stress response."

The stress response in our body created by "foreign" molecules in food is called xenohormesis. The concept of *xenohormesis*[22] describes the effect of these foreign molecules on our biology. They produce a stress response triggering the whole cascade of stress-related cellular signals that makes us sick.

This causes obesity and brain dysfunction. And it appears that there is a close connection between the obesity epidemic we are seeing and the epidemic of ADHD and behavior problems in children.[23]

Not only do we need to think of the nutrients in our food, but we also need to think about its quality. Are there "stress" molecules in our food that is raised on industrial feedlots and farms, which make us fat, depressed, and inattentive? What kind of information does the food we eat send to our bodies?

Stress Stresses Out Your Genes

Not only can stressed food cause stress in the person who eats it, but food also triggers changes in our genes that lead to more stress.

One remarkable study in the *American Journal of Clinician Nutrition* found that stress genes, inflammation genes, and insulin resistance genes were all turned on in people who ate more refined (not total) carbohydrates.[24]

The study looked at two groups of people, both with insulin resistance. They were fed two diets that were exactly the same—the same calories and the same amount of protein, carbohydrates, fat, and fiber.

The only difference was that in one group the carbohydrate source was wheat, oats, and potatoes, and in the other it was rye. Rye contains different information molecules (phytonutrients) and is absorbed and broken down more slowly than carbohydrates from wheat, oats, and potatoes.

What happened was nothing short of revolutionary in its implications.

After twelve weeks, fat biopsies were taken and changes in gene expression were measured. There was no change in weight, but the difference in gene expression was extraordinary.

In the wheat, oat, and potato group, sixty-two genes that promote inflammation, produce stress molecules and hormones, and promote insulin resistance and obesity were "turned on." In the rye group, seventy-one genes that improve insulin function and prevent cell death were "turned on."

It appears that obesity is not the only thing controlled by the information in our food. So are our stress response, mood, behavior, memory, and brain function. That is why a fresh, whole-foods, organic, real-food diet is the foundation of health and *The UltraMind Solution*.

Saying Ouch: The Pain of Thoughts, Foreign Food, Toxins, Infections, or Allergens

Remember, the body has only so many ways of saying ouch. One major way the body says "ouch" is the activation of the stress response. How can this response be turned on?

Well, it is the result of many different insults.

Taking everything personally, any negative thought or perception, or rigid beliefs or attitudes can trigger the stress response. That is how our experience of the world creates illness and damages our brain.

But every other input into your world—an imbalance in any of the other six key systems in your body—can initiate that same response.

You don't have to think bad thoughts to set the stress response in motion. Just breathe in the fumes from a coal-burning power plant, eat beef grown on a feedlot, take antibiotics, and change the ecology of your gut, which will then do the negative talking for you, or be a military recruit on a forced march and don't sleep for five days.

All these things, and anything that creates nutritional imbalances, hormonal problems, inflammation, digestive imbalances, any toxin, or anything that messes up your energy production, will all cause an activation of the stress response.

This type of thinking is foreign to medicine and difficult for most of us to grasp. We are always looking for that one thing, that one factor we can blame and say aha! That's it. But that will never happen.

We will never find the magic bullet—whether it is a new food like the acai berry, or a vitamin, or a new drug or pill that will solve our chronic health issues or the epidemic of mood, behavior, attention, and neurodegenerative disease.

The World Health Organization estimates that depression affects about 121 million people worldwide and is the leading cause of disability (as measured in years living with disability [YLDs]),[25] accounting for almost 12 percent of all disability.[26]

By the year 2025, it is estimated that major depression will be the second leading cause of medical disability in America.

A different type of thinking is necessary to solve this problem.

Everything is connected. We are one wholistic system and we need to understand the ecology of our body. We are an ecosystem connected locally and globally to everything that happens. Only by understanding and working on all the imbalances in these systems can we hope to regain our health, vitality, energy, and our clearheadedness and happiness.

That is my hope for all of you in offering the plan in *The UltraMind Solution*.

Relax Your Stressed-Out Body-Mind

The hardest part of being a doctor is helping people connect to why they want to heal. Knowing what to do comes fairly easily to me now. I have a new road map, a new way of navigating through the astounding mystery of our biology. But my challenge is always to help people to connect to meaning.

What is it they treasure? What anchors them to life? Who and what is worth living for? How can they connect to meaning and purpose? The development of a sense of place in the world, a sense of connection, belonging, and contribution must be nurtured and fed. That is the most important diet: meaning and purpose.

There begins healing. In our world, we have to be particularly vigilant to nurture connection, community, and meaning, because so many forces conspire to distract us from ourselves.

Part of the problem is the runaway stress response. Once activated, it doesn't turn itself off. This produces all the damage we explored in this chapter.

Fortunately, we can learn to turn it off and activate the relaxation response. You can turn on your vagus nerve every day and you don't need a pacemaker implanted in your neck to do it.

Learning to relax will stop the vicious cycle that keeps you from waking up and being present to your life. It will allow you to slow down long enough to consider how you might nurture compassion in your life.

In Part III (see page 285) and IV (see page 343) I will show you how to transform the effects of stress from any insult—physical or psychological. In fact, I will give you a specific plan to achieve that goal.

In Part III, you will learn the basic, six-week program for a healthy brain, a kind of owner's manual for your mind.

Then in Part IV, I will teach you how to fine-tune that plan based on *your* imbalances in the seven keys we have been exploring.

Now you have seen how all the seven keys influence your brain and biology. It is one interconnected web of problems. And because it is all connected, you can make a few simple changes that can have dramatic and life-changing effects.

Simple dietary changes, a few nutrients, a little exercise, enough sleep, and a little time each day for activating the relaxation response can transform deep-seated symptoms that show up as altered mood, behavior, attention, and memory.

Your brain can thrive. You just have to provide the right conditions.

In the rest of the book I am going to teach you those conditions.

PART III

The UltraMind Solution

THE SIX-WEEK BASIC BRAIN-BOOSTING PROGRAM FOR EVERYONE: A SIMPLE APPROACH TO OPTIMAL BRAIN FUNCTION AND HEALTH

In six short weeks you will learn more about your body and brain than you ever imagined.

You have in your hands the tools to immediately transform your health and well-being. Using the six-week brain-boosting program you are about to learn, you may:

- Feel more alert and focused
- Experience a more stable mood
- Develop a better memory
- Increase your attention
- Feel more energy
- Sleep better
- Get rid of chronic sinus and digestive problems
- Eliminate joint pains
- Wipe out headaches
- Lose weight
- Create optimal brain function

You will do this simply by changing your diet, taking a few brain-boosting supplements, and making some lifestyle changes that will not only improve your brain health but will make you feel better physically as well.

I know it's hard to believe a few simple changes can make such a difference.

So I don't want you to believe me.

Prove it to yourself.

If you can suspend your disbelief for just six weeks and follow the program I suggest in the following chapters, belief will become irrelevant. You will experience a dramatic change in your health, your mood, and your brain function. This will prove to you that change can happen now! Most of my patients who follow this approach see significant changes within the first two weeks.

If you go through the six-week program and experience no change, then you have lost nothing—except perhaps the chance to have a few cheeseburgers and Cokes.

On the other hand, if you go through the six-week program and experience the changes listed above (including weight loss), you will have gained something extraordinary—a new understanding of your mind and body and the tools and skills to achieve UltraWellness.

What I hope for all of you is that you can experience the connection between your behaviors, your choices, your habits, things you put in your mouth, and how you feel right now.

How can we know that eating wheat, or not liking fish, or eating too much blue fin sushi, or staying out of the sun and using sunblock are making us depressed, anxious, or demented? The only way is to change our habits and pay attention to what happens.

That is what this six-week program is designed to help you do.

Some of the changes you experience will happen almost immediately. If you are gluten-sensitive and you stop eating gluten, within a week your life will change. If you are B_{12}-deficient and you take B_{12}, you will improve your mood and brain function in a few weeks.

Other changes may take a little longer to achieve. If you are mercury toxic, then it may take a few years and some hard work to fully recover, but you can regain your health and renew your brain. I did.

Whatever the case, I will guide you to discovering the potential you have for a fully engaged, happy, purposeful, awake, and attentive life step-by-step in Parts III and IV.

In Part III, you will learn the brain essentials! This is just basic maintenance 101: the raw ingredients everyone needs to detoxify, repair, and renew their brain. Everyone reading this book should go on this basic six-week plan, regardless of your circumstances.

In Part IV, you can customize your six-week plan based on how you scored on the quizzes in Part II. If your score indicated a care plan that included "Self-Care" or "Medical Care" in any of the keys, simply add the steps in Part IV for each of those keys to the six-week plan to optimize it for your needs. I will teach you more about how to do this in Part IV.

If your quiz score qualified you for "Medical Care," you may need the help of a doctor trained in Functional and/or Integrative Medicine to help you navigate the testing and treatment options, particularly in the realm of hormone therapy, gut healing, treating infections, and heavy metal detoxification.

But for most of you, 70 to 80 percent of the benefits from the UltraMind Solution can be reached on your own with a few simple changes in diet, nutritional supplementation, and lifestyle.

Here's how you do it.

What Is the Six-Week Basic Brain-Boosting Program?

The six-week plan consists of four basic components. These are:

1. A healthy eating plan designed to help you heal and optimize your brain.
2. Basic supplements you need to take to balance and enhance your brain chemistry.
3. Lifestyle changes including exercise, relaxation, sleep, and "brain" or mental exercises.
4. Living clean and green to reduce your exposure to environmental toxins and support a sustainable future for us all.

It is a six-week program, with a one-week preparation phase. All four elements above are incorporated in this easy-to-follow, step-by-step system.

Let's review how it works.

The Preparation Phase—One Week Before the Program Starts

We are often locked into habits without recognizing their effect on us. Most of us are drug addicts and don't realize it. Sugar, junk food, caffeine, and alcohol all affect our ability to function, and though they temporarily make us feel better, they often deplete us in a deeper way.

Taking a "drug holiday" is an important way to discover how you really feel and give yourself the opportunity to tune into your own body's signals for hunger, sleep, and relaxation. Getting off sugar, high-fructose corn syrup, hydrogenated fats or trans fats, junk food, alcohol, and caffeine for one week, in fact, is powerful enough to totally change your health and your mind.

Take a risk and try it out. Even if you do nothing else, this will change your life.

The Six-Week Plan: Developing an UltraMind

Once you are finished with the preparation week, you will move into the six-week program for healing and optimizing your brain.

The key component of the program is cleaning up your diet. Getting rid of garbage foods, moving toward a diet of whole, unprocessed foods, and eliminating foods that you may have sensitivities or delayed allergies to will help you start the process of healing your brain.

I recommend everyone take a six-week holiday from gluten and dairy. Gluten and dairy are the two major food allergens that most often lead to brain dysfunction, and eliminating them for six weeks (as you will during this program) may cause remarkable improvements in the health of your brain (not to mention your body).

You will also eliminate sugar, processed and toxic foods, and you will introduce whole, healing foods into your diet. The purpose of doing so is to show you just how great you can feel by simply changing what you eat.

Part of the healing occurs because of all the junk you are eliminating, but most occurs because you introduce delicious, whole real foods. Doing so will help rebuild the very structure and function of your brain.

SPECIAL NOTE FOR THOSE WHO ARE VERY INFLAMED

For those who scored high on the inflammation quiz in chapter 8, I recommend a more comprehensive food allergy elimination program in Part IV that may help cure more dramatic brain problems caused by inflammation.

During the program you will start to reeducate your body-mind and reprogram your brain with improved mood, attention, memory, and behavior. By doing so you will build the foundation for lifelong healthy brain function and balanced moods, and prevent most of the age-related brain conditions such as Alzheimer's and Parkinson's disease.

At the end of the six weeks you will stick to the whole foods healthy-eating plan, I hope, for life. However, you can reintegrate gluten and dairy systematically once the program is done to test for sensitivities you may have to them. I will explain how to do that in chapter 20.

By reintroducing these foods the way I describe, you can monitor their effects on your health. (If you get a stomachache or your nose stuffs up when you eat dairy, or you feel tired and depressed if you eat gluten, it is best to stay away from them.)

The six-week program is really just a start for the rest of your life. Variety, fun, nourishment, pleasure, color, and wholeness are essential for making this way of eating your way of eating for life.

Feel free to improvise and adapt—just stick with whole real foods and you will have difficulty getting into trouble.

By the end of seven weeks (one week preparation, six weeks of the UltraMind program) you may have more energy, feel more emotionally balanced, more alert, focused, and mentally sharper. UltraWellness is now yours.

The next few chapters will give you an overview of the healthy-eating plan, supplements, and lifestyle changes you need to make during the program. They will also tell you how to set the stage for success, and teach you how to stay on the program.

Read through them. Then simply follow the guidelines and checklists in chapter 19 to take advantage of the UltraMind Solution.

EATING RIGHT FOR YOUR BRAIN: A SCIENCE-BASED, WHOLE-FOODS APPROACH TO EATING—FOOD AS MEDICINE

The most powerful tool you have to transform your health and improve your mood, mind, and metabolism is your fork! Use it well and you will thrive. Choose poorly and you will suffer.

The varied components of a whole-foods diet not only taste better, make you feel better, and prevent disease, but they are literally medicine. Mounting scientific evidence points to the power of food as medicine. These "medicinal" foods are simply the foods our bodies evolved eating— fresh, unadulterated, slow-burning, high-fiber, vitamin- and mineral-rich, omega-3 plentiful, and phytonutrient-dense foods.

That is why we can treat and prevent most chronic illnesses with a whole, organic, real, unprocessed diet of fresh fruits and vegetables, whole grains, beans, nuts, and seeds, small omega-3–containing fish like sardines and herring, and lean animal protein. It is a one-stop shopping method for dealing with everything.

In fact, all nutritional science is converging on a few basic concepts, which everyone agrees on. These are the principles the six-week Ultra-Mind Solution is based on:

1. Eat whole, real, fresh, organic, unprocessed food.
2. Eat a lot of fruit and vegetables full of colorful phytonutrients.
3. Eat foods with plenty of fiber.
4. Eat foods containing omega-3 fats.

If you follow these four principles, then you are doing 90 percent of what you need to do to stay healthy and heal your brain. The rest are small refinements and details.

You will automatically be eating this way as long as you follow the eating plan in this program. I will discuss more about what kinds of foods to include in a moment.

But keep in mind that what is omitted is just as important as what's included.

If you want to realize the full potential of the UltraMind Solution to transform your health and your brain in six weeks, the first step is to temporarily stop all factors that have been shown to cause brain damage.

Stopping the Brain Damage: Foods to Avoid on the UltraMind Solution

Give your brain a break for six weeks from known brain-damaging substances. If you think there will be nothing left to eat, then you will have the biggest gains to achieve in making a change. Please avoid foods in any of the following categories.

Sugars in Any Form

- High-fructose corn syrup
- Sugar-laden foods
  - Candy, cookies, cereals, pastries, pies, etc., including honey, maple syrup, or molasses
- Flour products, all types of flour
  - Bagels, breads, rolls, wraps, pastas, etc.
- Liquid sugar
  - Processed fruit juices, which are often loaded with sugars. Try juicing your own carrots, celery, and beets instead, or other fruit and vegetable combinations
  - Sodas or any type of canned or bottled drinks with any type of sugar or sweetener
- Artificial sweeteners
  - Equal; aspartame—NutraSweet; saccharin-Sweet N' Low; sucralose-Splenda; acesulfame-K-Sunette, Sweet-n-Safe, Sweet One; neotame
- Stevia (a natural plant-based sweetner, yes, but it still tricks your body into craving more and eating more)
- Sugar alcohols
  - Polyols such as mannitol, sorbitol, lactitol, malitol, xylitol, etc. These can cause significant gas and bloating.

Toxic Fats

❖ Trans or hydrogenated fats (found in most crackers, chips, cakes, candies, cookies, doughnuts, and processed cheese)
❖ Processed oils such as corn, safflower, sunflower, peanut, and canola
❖ Fat substitutes (Olean and Salatrim/Benefat)
❖ Fried foods

Food Additives and Chemicals

❖ Any food in a box, can, or package; in other words, if it has a label don't eat it
❖ Artificial colorings
❖ Any food additives
  ❖ Potassium bromate, propyl gallate, sodium nitrite, sodium nitrate, monosodium glutamate, etc.

Check out the Center for Science in the Public Interest's website for further information and updates: www.cspinet.org/reports/chemcuisine.htm.

Toxin Rich Foods

❖ Red meats (unless organic or grass-fed) and organ meats (liver, thymus or sweetbreads, and kidneys)
❖ Large predatory fish and river fish, including swordfish, tuna, tilefish, and shark, which contain mercury and other contaminants in unacceptable amounts.
❖ Avoid the fruits and vegetables with the highest toxin load. Here are the ten worst offenders: peaches, apples, sweet bell peppers, celery, nectarines, strawberries, cherries, lettuce, grapes, and pears. (See www.foodnews.org for a list of low- and high-pesticide containing foods.) Choose only organic versions of the fruits and vegetables noted above, as their conventionally farmed counterparts have the highest toxic burden.

Addictions

❖ Caffeine (sodas, coffee, tea)
❖ Alcohol

These are the primary foods you will avoid during the program. However, there is another critically important group of foods you will avoid as well. These are the foods that are most likely giving you brain allergies.

Brain "Allergies": How the Six-Week Plan Will Help Clear Your Head

The stresses of our modern, toxic, genetically altered, nutrient-depleted diet; the stress of our lives; and the overuse of antibiotics and other gut-damaging stresses have led many modern humans to suffer from delayed or hidden food allergies. This is the result of a leaky gut. (See chapters 8 and 9 for a refresher on food allergies.)

A leaky gut leads to brain "allergies."[1] Clearing up these brain allergies can dramatically impact your mood, attention, and behavior, and may resolve a laundry list of symptoms, including digestive, allergic, autoimmune, and neurological symptoms.

The only way to know what you are allergic to (aside from medical IgE and IgG allergy testing) is to eliminate certain substances from your diet and then systematically add them back in. This is called an elimination/reintroduction diet, and it is a critical part of the UltraMind Solution.

The concept is simple. If you get rid of the foods that commonly cause bad reactions, you may feel better and you can heal. If you add them back and you get sick, you know you have a problem with them.

The most common and most serious undiagnosed immune or toxic reactions are to gluten and dairy (especially the casein, and not so much the whey component, of dairy). These are also the main allergens and foods that cause bad brain reactions. Stopping these foods can be life changing for the majority with brain or mood problems.

The inflammation and toxic effects of these otherwise harmless and often healthful foods are so powerful in derailing our brain function that they can lead to everything from brain fog, to depression, to ADHD, autism, and dementia.

That is why I recommend a short holiday from these two worst offenders, which are unfortunately the staples in our diet. During the six-week program you will eliminate the following foods in addition to those listed above:

❖ Gluten (from wheat, barley, rye, spelt, kamut, triticale, and oats)
❖ And dairy (milk, cheese, yogurt, sour cream, ice cream)

This means a complete 100 percent elimination of all gluten, no exceptions (not even a crumb), and all dairy foods (not even a drop in your tea) for a full six weeks.

That is enough time to feel better, and notice a change. And it is long enough that when you add it back, you will immediately see how you react to it.

At the end of the program, I will teach you how to systematically reintegrate gluten and dairy and test for reactions to see if they are contributing to your mental and brain problems.

But be warned: gluten and dairy (or other hidden allergens) may not cause symptoms for up to three days after eating them. That is why careful reintroduction of these foods and monitoring how you feel for three days is necessary.

In some cases, you may have to eliminate some foods you are sensitive to for a longer period of time or avoid them altogether if you want to maintain an UltraMind. I will explain all of this in more detail later, when I talk about food reintroduction.

The beauty of an elimination/reintroduction diet is that it gives you the power of knowledge—the power to know whether these items are contributing to your mental-health problems. Then you can make choices about what you eat and what you avoid based on your experience with food and how it affects you.

THE TOP FOOD ALLERGENS

While gluten and dairy are the most important allergens that lead to brain problems, there are a few other common allergens that may contribute to your health problems as well.

However, since these are not the most important or as common in creating brain problems, I have not addressed them in this program.

For an in-depth discussion of delayed food allergies and a comprehensive elimination diet, see *The UltraSimple Diet.* The following list constitutes the staples of the American diet. It is also what we typically become allergic to if we have leaky gut lining.

If you do not experience relief by following the six-week program in this book just eliminating gluten and dairy from your diet, there may be other hidden culprits. Blood testing for IgG food allergens (www.immunolabs.com and other labs) may help you identify more uncommon foods that are responsible for symptoms. Or you can go on a more comprehensive elimination/reintroduction diet like the one outlined in *The UltraSimple Diet* to help you.

The top food allergens are:

- Gluten (barley, rye, oats, spelt, kamut, wheat, triticale—see www.celiac.com for a complete list of foods containing gluten, as well as often surprising and hidden sources of gluten—salad dressing, soup, beer, etc.)
- Dairy (milk, cheese, butter, yogurt)
- Eggs
- Yeasted products (wine, vinegar, breads)
- Corn
- Peanuts
- Nightshades (tomatoes, eggplants, peppers, potatoes)
- Citrus fruits (oranges, grapefruits, etc.)
- Soy

A few others deserve honorable mention but are not as common. They are chocolate, tree nuts, vinegar, and shellfish.

What Should I Eat and How Should I Eat? The Principles of the UltraMind Solution

Now you know what *not* to eat and what foods you are going to avoid for the six-week program. The next step is to understand what you *are* going to eat and how you are going to eat it.

In the sections that follow I have outlined the basic principles of what to eat on the six-week program. These are important eating guidelines you will want to integrate for a lifetime if you are going to achieve UltraWellness. As long as you follow these guidelines, you will work through the six weeks without a problem.

Keep in mind these are just the principles. I have developed a full six-week eating plan complete with lists of foods you can include on the program, tips on how to cook, shopping lists, and a set of delicious recipes in

The UltraMind Solution Companion Guide. If you want to make your experience on the program even easier, go to www.ultramind.com/guide and download the guide for the complete eating plan.

Food Quality: Feed Your Brain Right

If food is information and your brain runs on the right information, then clearly just getting enough calories in a day is not enough. The quality of those calories will determine the quality of your mind.

Remember your health is also connected to the health of the planet. You can reduce the "carbon footprint" of your diet and transform your health at the same time. What you put on your fork has broad impact not only on your health but on agriculture, energy consumption, the environment, politics, and the economy.

Here are the principles of choosing quality food. They are in order of importance:

- **Real**—Choose real, whole, unprocessed fresh foods in as close to their natural state as possible—fresh vegetables, fruit, whole grains, beans, nuts, seeds, lean animal protein such as small fish, chicken, and eggs.
- **Clean**—Choose grass-fed,★ antibiotic-, hormone-, and pesticide-free animal products.
- **Organic**—Choose organic fruits and vegetables to reduce the toxic effects of pesticides on your brain, and also your thyroid and your sex hormones, which are very sensitive to the effects of low-level toxins.
- **Local**—Eat local foods that are in season. Frequent your local farmers' market or consider joining your local community-supported agriculture projects. Learn more at www.localharvest .org/csa.

These are the principles I used when I designed the six-week eating plan in *The UltraMind Solution Companion Guide.* Go to www.ultramind.com/ guide to download the free guide.

★ *Grass-fed* means that the animals you eat spend their lives roaming and eating grass in a pasture, as they evolved doing. Grass-fed animals are not closed up in a stockyard, which means they have much less need for antibiotics. In addition, they move and eat a healthier, more natural diet, which means they are leaner. And they eat grass, which leads to higher amounts of omega-3 fats, vitamins, and minerals in the meat than grain-fed animals.

When Should I Eat? The Importance of Meal Timing

Controlling insulin and balancing your blood sugar are critical for balancing your mood, focusing, having energy, and preventing all the age-related brain diseases such as Alzheimer's.

It is not very hard. Besides avoiding flour and sugar products, eating smaller, more frequent meals keeps your blood sugar even and prevents swings in energy, mood, and appetite. Not only will your anxiety and depression improve, but you will also automatically lose weight.

Meal Timing

- For breakfast every day eat protein such as whole omega-3 eggs, soy or rice protein shakes, and nut butters. (See www.ultramind .com/guide for recipe ideas.) Beside controlling your appetite and helping you lose weight, protein in the morning provides the amino acids necessary to produce all the neurotransmitters needed for optimal brain function.
- Eat something every four hours to keep your insulin and glucose levels normal.
- Eat a small protein snack in the morning and afternoon such as a handful of almonds.
- When possible, avoid eating during the two to three hours before you go to bed. If you have a snack earlier in the day, you won't be as hungry and eat as much later in the day.

The daily eating plan and checklists in chapter 19 that lay out the six-week program follow this schedule step-by-step. As long as you follow that plan, you will be eating your meals when you should for optimal brain and body health.

How Should I Eat? The Importance of Meal Composition

Composing the perfect meal is essential. To do that, just choose something from each of the whole-food categories below—carbohydrates, fats, and protein.

Or you can go to www.ultramind.com/guide and download *The Ultra-Mind Solution Companion Guide* for a complete six-week eating plan, including recipes that are composed based on the standards outlined below.

Becoming a Fat Head

Omega-3 fats are the most important building blocks for a healthy brain and cells. It can take a year to rebuild and remake all your cells and tissues with the right fats.

- ✣ Cold-water fish such as wild salmon, sardines, herring, small halibut, and sable (black cod) contain an abundance of beneficial omega-3 essential fatty acids that reduce inflammation. A great source of smaller, wild Alaskan salmon, sable, and halibut (all high in omega-3 fats and low in toxins) is available from www.vital choice.com.
- ✣ Canned wild salmon, sardines, or herring (kippers) are great emergency foods full of safe omega-3 fats and choline for your brain.
- ✣ Eat omega-3 eggs, which contain a safe form of DHA. You can enjoy up to eight eggs a week. Eggs also are a rich source of choline for your brain.
- ✣ Use extra-virgin olive oil, which contains anti-inflammatory and antioxidant phytochemicals. It should be your main oil except for high-temperature cooking.
- ✣ Use unrefined or expeller pressed sesame oil for high-temperature cooking.

Protein for Brain Power

To make neurotransmitters you need amino acids. And amino acids come from the protein you eat.

Research, including T. Colin Campbell's China Study,[2,3] points to the risks of too much animal protein. Each person is different and thrives on different types of food. Some do fantastic as vegans, others wither. Some thrive on animal protein, some are sluggish and sick. Find the right balance for you by experimenting.

But it is essential to choose protein at each meal. Choose from these high-quality safe sources of protein.

- ✣ Beans or legumes, including whole, traditional soy products such as edamame, tofu, and tempeh
- ✣ Nuts (almonds, walnuts, macadamia nuts, pecans)
- ✣ Seeds (pumpkin, sunflower, flax, chia, etc.)
- ✣ Omega-3 eggs

❖ Safe, mercury-free fish as above

❖ Organic, grass-fed, hormone-, antibiotic-, and pesticide-free poultry

❖ Small amounts of lean, organic grass-fed, hormone-, and antibiotic-free lamb or beef (or try buffalo, venison, or ostrich, which are leaner) no more than once or twice a week and no more than four to six ounces per serving

❖ Avoid excessive quantities of meat. Use lean, organic, or grass-fed (when possible) animal products—eggs, beef, chicken, lamb, buffalo, ostrich, etc. There are good sources at Whole Foods or other local health-food stores. (Also see the mail-order resources in *The UltraMind Solution Companion Guide*. You can access it by going to www.ultramind.com/guide.)

Brain Food: The Right Carbs

Carbohydrates are the most essential part of your diet for long-term health and brain function. But not the doughnuts, bagels, and sweets we typically think of as carbs. These are highly processed foods, stripped of their nutrients and fiber.

When I say carbohydrates, I mean real, whole plant foods containing all the vitamins, minerals, fiber, and phytonutrients that create health.

❖ Create meals high in low-glycemic legumes such as lentils, chickpeas, and soybeans (try edamame, the Japanese soybeans in a pod, quickly steamed with a little salt, as a snack). These foods slow the release of sugars into the bloodstream, helping to prevent excess insulin release leading to insulin resistance and its related health concerns, including dementia, depression, poor heart health, obesity, high blood pressure, high LDL or "bad" cholesterol, and low HDL or "good" cholesterol.

❖ Eat a cornucopia of fresh fruits and vegetables teeming with phytonutrients—carotenoids, flavonoids, and polyphenols— associated with a lower incidence of nearly all health problems, including dementia, obesity, and aging.

❖ Use more slow-burning, low-glycemic vegetables such as asparagus, broccoli, kale, spinach, cabbage, and Brussels sprouts.

❖ Berries, cherries, peaches, plums, rhubarb, pears, and apples are optimal fruits; cantaloupes and melons, grapes and kiwifruit are suitable; however, they contain more sugar. Organic frozen berries (from Cascadian Farms) can be used if you make protein shakes (this is a good way to get protein in the morning).

✤ A diet high in fiber further helps to stabilize blood sugar by slowing the absorption of carbohydrates and supports a healthy digestive tract. Try to gradually increase fiber to 30 to 50 gm a day and use predominantly soluble or viscous fiber (legumes, nuts, seeds, whole grains, vegetables, and fruit), which slows sugar absorption from the gut

✤ Minimize starchy, high-glycemic cooked vegetables, such as potatoes, corn, and root vegetables, such as rutabagas, parsnips, and turnips.

CONTROLLING YOUR GLYCEMIC LOAD

The glycemic load of a food or meal is defined as the total effect that food or meal has on your blood sugar. The food or meals you eat can have either a high glycemic load or a low glycemic load.

Controlling the glycemic load of your meals is essential. It is easy to do. Simply combine adequate protein, fats, and whole-food carbohydrates from vegetables, legumes, nuts, seeds, and fruit at every meal or snack. It is most important to avoid eating quickly absorbed carbohydrates alone, as they raise your sugar and insulin levels. And any large meal will raise your blood sugar, so smaller meals help keep your blood sugar even.

Phytonutrients—Hidden Brain Protectors: Healing Anti-inflammatory, Antioxidant, and Detoxifying Foods

Healing chemicals in foods may, in the end, be more important than the protein, fat, carbohydrates, vitamins, and minerals they contain.

Practically the only thing *everyone* agrees about in nutrition is that eating five to nine servings of fruits and vegetables a day can reduce your risk from almost every known disease of our "modern" civilization, including heart disease, stroke, Alzheimer's, cancer, and all of the brain and mood disorders so many suffer from.

One of the reasons phytonutrients are so powerful has to do with their anti-inflammatory, antioxidant, and detoxifying properties. To get enough phytonutrients in your diet, try the following:

✤ Focus on anti-inflammatory foods, including wild fish and other sources of omega-3 fats, red and purple berries (these are rich in polyphenols), dark green leafy vegetables, orange sweet potatoes, and nuts.

❖ Eat more antioxidant-rich and energy-boosting foods, including orange and yellow vegetables, dark green leafy vegetables (kale, collards, spinach, etc.), anthocyanidins (berries, beets, grapes, pomegranate), purple grapes containing trans-resveratrol, blueberries, bilberries, cranberries, and cherries. In fact, antioxidants are in all colorful fruits and vegetables.

❖ Include detoxifying foods in your diet such as cruciferous vegetables (broccoli, kale, collards, brocollini, broccoli rabe, Brussels sprouts, cauliflower, bok choy, Chinese cabbage, Chinese broccoli), green tea, watercress, dandelion greens, cilantro, artichokes, garlic, citrus peels, pomegranate, and even cocoa.

❖ Use hormone-balancing foods such as whole soy foods and ground flaxseeds.

❖ Use herbs such as turmeric, rosemary, and ginger, which are powerful antioxidants, anti-inflammatories, and detoxifiers.

❖ Eat garlic and onions, noted for their cholesterol blood-pressure-lowering and antioxidant effects. They are also anti-inflammatory and enhance detoxification.

❖ Drink green tea, which contains abundant amounts of anti-inflammatory, detoxifying, and antioxidant phytonutrients.

❖ And yes . . . chocolate, only the darkest, most luxurious kind and only one to two ounces a day. It should be 70 percent cocoa.

> Sticking to these eating principles every day for six weeks will take you a long way toward building an UltraMind. However, if you want to be sure you follow the program, go to www.ultramind.com/guide and download the companion guide for this book, where you will find an easy-to-follow, six-week eating plan based on these guidelines. It's an easy way to stick to the program, and a delicious way to heal your brain.

Now that you understand the basic underpinnings of the diet itself, next we need to discuss the supplementation you will need to create optimal brain function. We will do that in the next chapter.

CHAPTER 15

TUNING UP YOUR BRAIN CHEMISTRY WITH SUPPLEMENTS

Think of nutrients as fertilizer for your brain. Think of them as little helpers that improve communications and connections.

In a perfect world, no one would need supplements. But given the stress of our modern life, the poor quality of our food supply, and the high load of toxins on our brains and bodies, we clearly need a basic daily supply of the raw materials for all our enzymes and biochemistry to run as designed.

In Part II we reviewed the research and the importance of nutrients for optimal brain function. If your doctor asks for evidence about the importance of nutritional supplementation, have him read the scientific review "Vitamins, Minerals and Mood,"[1] which summarizes only 126 of the best scientific papers and the rationale for using nutrients to support mood.

That doesn't even cover the data on autism, ADHD, or any of the neurodegenerative diseases.[2,3]

Remember, studying one nutrient alone as a drug to treat one disease will often fail. That is because nutrients work as a team.

And there is a basic workhorse team needed for everyone. Additional supplements may help people with specific imbalances. You have identified these imbalances by taking the quizzes in Part II. I will show you how to incorporate these additional supplements in Part IV.

In this chapter, I want to focus on the basic supplements everyone needs for good brain health. These supplements are an important part of the basic six-week plan. In chapter 19, where I give you a full outline of the program, I will show you how to incorporate them into your daily routine.

Here are the basic raw materials needed for everyone who wants to keep their brain healthy.

1. A high-quality, high-potency, highly bioavailable broad spectrum multivitamin, which contains all the basic essential vitamins and minerals

2. Calcium and magnesium
3. Vitamin D_3
4. Omega–3 fatty acids (EPA and DHA)
5. Methylation factors: folate, B_6, and B_{12}. Often special activated forms of these nutrients are needed to be most effective for brain health.
6. Probiotics or beneficial bacteria to improve your digestion, reduce food allergies, and reduce gut inflammation

Not All Supplements Are Created Equal

Over the last fifteen years researching and treating thousands of patients, I have learned much about how to find safe, high-quality, and effective nutritional supplement products.

Finding the best products to support health has always been the most difficult part of my job, as it is for any practitioner of Functional Medicine. The lack of adequate government regulations, the dizzying number of products on the market, and the large variations in quality all create a minefield of obstacles for anyone trying to find the right supplement, vitamin, or herb.

Be aware that all brands are not created equal. Quality is up to the manufacturer because of limited regulations regarding manufacturing. Certain companies are more careful about quality, sourcing of raw materials, consistency of dose from batch to batch, the use of active forms of nutrients, not using fillers, additives, colorings, etc.

When choosing supplements it is important that you choose quality products. While I do not officially endorse or have any consulting or employee relationship with any supplement companies, I do believe a few have risen to the top of the supplement industry and can be safely used to help support and enhance your health. When choosing supplements, make sure to consider the following factors:

- Manufacturers who use GMP (good manufacturing practices) for drug or supplement standards from an outside certifying body
- Third-party analysis for independent verification of active ingredients and contaminants
- Products that have some basis in basic science, clinical trials, or have a long history of use and safety
- Use clean products, free of preservatives, fillers, binders, excipients, flow agents, shellacs, coloring agents, gluten, yeast, lactose, and other allergens.

Each person must be cautious and evaluate companies and products for themselves. Be sure to pick quality supplements as you acquire the list of vitamins outlined below. It is optimal to work with a trained dietitian, nutritionist, or nutrionally oriented physician or health-care practitioner to select the best products.

Basic Nutritional Support for the Brain

Ninety-two percent of Americans are deficient in one or more essential vitamins and minerals, 80 percent are deficient in vitamin D, and over 99 percent are deficient in the essential omega-3 fatty acids.

Therefore, I recommend that *all* people take a basic multivitamin and mineral, as well as calcium and magnesium, extra vitamin D, omega-3 fats, and probiotics as the foundation for good health, as well as a healthy brain. Because methylation is so important for the brain and nearly every other function of the body, I recommend methylation nutrients (B_6, B_{12}, and folate) in addition to what is in your multivitamin as outlined below.

These vitamins are to be taken *daily*.

Here is a guide to get started on a comprehensive brain-supportive-supplement regimen:

Multivitamin and Mineral

A good multivitamin and mineral generally contains the following:

- Mixed carotenes (alpha, beta, cryptoxanthin, zeaxanthin, and lutein), 15,000 to 25,000 IU
- Vitamin A, 1,000–2,000 IU preformed retinol
- Vitamin D_3, 400 IU to 800 IU
- Mixed tocopherols (vitamin E, including d-alpha, gamma, and delta), 400 IU
- Vitamin C (as mixed buffered mineral ascorbates), 500 to 1,000 mg
- Vitamin K_1, 30 mcg
- B_1 thiamine, 25 to 50 mg
- B_2 riboflavin, 25 to 50 mg
- B_3 niacin, 50 to 100 mg
- B_6 pyridoxine, 25 to 50 mg (ideally including pyridoxyl-5-phosphate)
- Folic acid (ideally as mixed folic acid and methyl-folate), 800 mcg

- B_{12}, 500 to 1,000 mcg (ideally as methylcobalamin)
- Biotin, 150 mcg to 1,000 mcg
- Pantothenic acid, 100 to 500 mg
- Iodine, 25 to 75 mcg
- Zinc (as amino acid chelate), 10 to 30 mg
- Selenium, 100 to 200 mcg (ideally as selenomethionine)
- Copper, 1 mg (should be avoided if you have autism or ADHD)
- Manganese, 5 mg
- Chromium (ideally as chromium polynicotinate), 100 to 200 mcg
- Molybdenum, 25 to 75 mcg
- Potassium, 50 to 100 mg
- Boron, 1 mg
- Vanadium, 50 mcg
- Inositol, 25 to 50 mg
- Choline, 100 to 200 mg
- Iron (as chelate), 8 to 12 mg (only for menstruating women)

Keep in mind that this usually requires the intake of two to six capsules or tablets a day to obtain adequate amounts. Some people may have unique needs for much higher doses that need to be prescribed by a trained nutritionist or Functional Medicine physician.

You may not get exactly these amounts, forms, or ratios of ingredients in your multivitamin. Remember these are optimal guidelines and the exact forms and amounts of nutrients in a vitamin depend on the company that formulates it. So don't be rigid. These are overall guidelines.

If you have problems swallowing supplements, you can try capsules instead of tablets. Or you can crush them, open them, and sprinkle them in food, or put them in shakes. There are also powdered and liquid forms of nutrients. Some nutrients can even be given as topical creams, such as magnesium or zinc.

There is something for everyone, even infants and children.

Balanced Absorbable Calcium and Magnesium

In addition to a multivitamin and mineral you will need to consider taking additional calcium and magnesium supplements. The amounts noted are the total daily requirements. What you will need depends on what is in your multivitamin. If your multivitamin contains 500 mg of calcium and 250 mg of magnesium, then you will need less from your calcium and magnesium supplement.

I recommend the following:

- ❖ Calcium citrate, 600 to 800 mg
- ❖ Magnesium amino acid chelate (aspartate, glycinate, ascorbate, taurate, or citrate), 400 to 600 mg

Special Considerations for Calcium and Magnesium

- ❖ There are risks associated with too much calcium from supplements, so don't go over the amount recommended. It is optimal to obtain most of your calcium (1,200 to 1,500 mg a day) from your diet (greens, sardines with bones, sesame seed tahini). You should limit your calcium supplements to no more than 600 to 800 mg a day. The amount often quoted by doctors of 1,500 mg a day is the *total* requirement, not that to be taken in supplements.
- ❖ Some with severe magnesium deficiency may need more. Some may need less. If you are concerned you may be severely deficient, discuss the details with your doctor.
- ❖ Diarrhea is often a sign that you are getting a little too much magnesium. If this occurs, just back off on the dose. This can also be avoided if you switch to magnesium glycinate.
- ❖ Avoid magnesium carbonate, sulfate, gluconate, or oxide. They are poorly absorbed (and the cheapest and most common forms found in supplements).
- ❖ People with kidney disease or severe heart disease should take magnesium only under a doctor's supervision.

Vitamin D$_3$

Vitamin D deficiency is epidemic, with up to 80 percent of modern humans being deficient or suboptimal in their intake and blood levels. Therefore, you should consider taking additional vitamin D to what is in your multivitamin.

For maintenance I recommend:

- ❖ Vitamin D$_3$, 2,000 IU (This is *in addition* to what is in your multivitamin, because so many people are significantly vitamin D–deficient.)

However, there are many things to keep in mind as you take vitamin D.

Special Considerations for Vitamin D

1. Take the right type of vitamin D.
- Take only vitamin D_3 in the active form (cholecalciferol). Look for this type.
- Many vitamins and prescriptions of vitamin D have vitamin D_2, which is not biologically active.

2. For deficiencies you may need more vitamin D.
- For correcting deficiency you can safely take 5,000 to 10,000 IU a day for three months, but only under a doctor's supervision. Some people may need higher doses than my daily recommendations over the long run to maintain optimal levels because of genetic differences in vitamin D receptors, living in northern latitudes, indoor living, or skin pigmentation.

3. Monitor your vitamin D status.
- Monitoring your vitamin D blood level (25 OH vitamin D) is necessary to be sure you are not on too little or too much. It should be part of every checkup with your doctor.
- The ideal range is 50 to 80 ng/ml.
- If you are taking high doses (10,000 IU a day) your doctor must do a blood test to check your calcium, phosphorous, and parathyroid hormone levels every three months.

4. Give Time to Fill Up Your Tank
- It takes up to six to ten months to fill up the tank for vitamin D if you are deficient. As mentioned above, you may need 5,000 to 10,000 IU a day to get to this level. Don't do this without your doctor's supervision.
- Once you are at optimal levels you can lower the dose to 2,000 IU a day for maintenance.

Omega-3 Fatty Acid Supplement

I recommend that everyone supplement his or her dietary intake of omega-3 fatty acids. These brain-building essential nutrients are difficult to come by in our modern diet, and many of the good sources such as fish are con-

taminated with toxins. The data support the benefits for everyone young or
old. Try the following:

 ∻ Fish oil, 1,000 mg twice a day containing a ratio of EPA/DHA
   300/200, once in the morning and once in the evening. (This
   must be from a reputable company that certifies purity from
   heavy metals and pesticides.)

Mighty Methylators and the B Complex Vitamins

Among the most important ingredients for healthy mood and improved
behavior, cognitive function, and memory are the nutrients needed for
methylation. That is why I usually recommend additional methylation supplementation to those already in a multivitamin for people with brain disorders.

These nutrients can be obtained in an additional high-quality B complex vitamin or taken individually. Our B vitamins are quickly depleted
from any type of stress. And all play one role or another in our brain
function.

I generally recommend special active forms of folate, B_6, and B_{12}. I believe they are needed because of our genes, our lifestyle, medication use,
and our unique biochemistry.

For most, the following list of additional methylation vitamins will do
just fine. The exact dose needed will vary from person to person, but these
general guidelines apply to most.

 ∻ Folate (also referred to as folic acid), 800 mcg with at least 400
   mcg coming from the active form or 5-MTHF (or L-methyl-
   folate)
 ∻ B_6 or pyridoxine, 50 mg
 ∻ B_{12}, 1,000 mcg with at least half coming in the form of
   methylcobalamin.

Special Considerations for B Complex Vitamins

 ∻ Some people may need up to 250 mg of B_6 or even a special
   "active" B_5 called pyridoxyl-5-phosphate to be most effective.
 ∻ Absorption of B_{12} can be impaired with aging, digestive
   disorders, and common medications (acid blockers), so
   occasionally B_{12} shots may be required.

- ❖ Sublingual or under-the-tongue forms of B_{12} may also be effective.
- ❖ These nutrients are often found together in special supplements for homocysteine or methylation.

Probiotics

These are essential, necessary ingredients for support of intestinal health. Our poor-quality diet, overuse of medication, and stress all alter our normal, healthy intestinal flora or bacteria.

I recommend at least a six-week course of probiotics to restore normal symbiosis (or ecological balance). That means using them the whole time you are on the UltraMind Solution.

However, these can be used for long-term health as well. In fact, I believe that given all the stresses on our guts, probiotics should be a part of our basic supplementation program for long-term health.

There are many different strains and varieties of probiotics. Some have extensive research behind them, others years of clinical experience. The key things to look for are:

1. What strains of organisms are there in the supplement you choose?
2. How many CFU or organisms per dose?
3. Are they fresh?

Here are my recommendations:

- ❖ 10 to 20 billion organisms taken on an empty stomach or with food twice a day, once in the morning and once in the evening.

Special Considerations for Probiotics

- ❖ Preparations include freeze-dried bacteria packaged in powders, tablets, or capsule forms.
- ❖ It is important to take a combination product with multiple species of organisms.
- ❖ If you are dairy-sensitive, seek out dairy-free brands.

Special Guidelines for Taking Supplements

When taking all of these supplements, there are a few things to keep in mind.

1. The dosages outlined are the *maximum* total daily amount I recommend taking without a doctor's supervision (with the exception of vitamin D). That means if you are getting B_{12} from several sources (your multivitamin and a separate B_{12} tablet), the total you should take every day from all sources is 1,000 mcg—no more.

2. Generally take all your vitamins with food—optimally with the meal or just before. People who take them after a meal may find they just sit on top of their food and upset their stomach. If you still have an upset stomach when taking your supplements, find a doctor who can help to correct any digestive problems, which are often the source of intolerance.

3. Take fish oil just before meals to prevent any fish taste from coming up, or freeze the capsules. If you swallow them frozen, they will be in your intestines before they dissolve.

These supplements and the guidelines in this chapter are critical if you want to obtain optimal brain health and move toward an UltraMind. To make it as easy as possible to keep track of the supplements you are taking, I have included a "Supplement Checklist" in *The UltraMind Solution Companion Guide*. Please go to www.ultramind.com/guide and download the guide to acquire that checklist.

The next part of the program we need to discuss are the lifestyle changes that are an important part of the UltraMind Solution.

CHAPTER 16

THE ULTRAMIND LIFESTYLE

Exercise, Relax, Sleep, and Train Your Brain

In addition to the dietary changes and supplements you take on the UltraMind Solution, there are four basic lifestyle changes I recommend you integrate as well. These are:

1. Exercise
2. Relaxation
3. Improved sleep patterns
4. Brain exercises

Each of these has been scientifically proven to improve mood and all brain functions.

In the checklists in chapter 19, I will outline when you should exercise, relax, and do your brain exercises.

When you do, choose from the options in this chapter to integrate these changes into your life.

In addition, you should institute the sleep program I have outlined here every day for the rest of your life. Sleep is your body's and brain's time to rebuild cells and recharge. Without optimal sleep you will have a dull, anxious, unhealthy brain and body.

While diet and supplementation are the heart of the program and the key to acquiring the nutrients you need for a healthy life, each one of these lifestyle changes is important as well. They are critical factors in obtaining an UltraMind.

Exercise Is Better than Prozac: The Benefits of Exercise for Your Brain

---

While most of us accept the benefits of exercise on our bodies, perhaps its most powerful effect is on our brains. It helps rewire our circuits and improve learning, memory, concentration, and focus. And it is the best anti-depressant and antianxiety therapy available.

If it were in a pill it would be the biggest blockbuster drug of all time. Yet all you need to take advantage of it is a pair of shoes and not even that if you live near a beach.

Exercise and Your Brain: The Benefits

Here is what exercise will do for your brain:

- *Strengthens your cardiovascular system.* Here the vascular part in-cludes the blood vessels, which supply your brain. In fact, the most common source of cognitive decline as we age is not Alzheimer's but hardening of the brain arteries, called vascular dementia.
- *Corrects and prevents insulin resistance.* This is how to stop the major source of brain aging, which occurs through blood sugar and insulin imbalances.
- *Erases the effects of stress* and improves your resistance to stress.
- *Improves mood and balances neurotransmitter function.* It is better than Prozac for depression. It increases GABA (the antianxiety neurotransmitter), serotonin (the happy neurotransmitter), and dopamine (the energizing neurotransmitter), and helps keep all the neurotransmitters in balance.
- *Reduces inflammation* and improves immune function.
- *Reduces pain* through increased endorphins, your body's natural painkillers.
- *Boosts overall motivation* and the ability to be fully engaged in life.
- *Increases neuroplasticity and neurogenesis.* It improves existing connections, makes new ones, and helps stimulate the production of new brain cells.
- It does this through naturally *increasing BDNF,* or brain-derived neurotrophic factor. This is super fertilizer for the brain. It improves the function of neurons, helps them grow and sprout new connections, and protects them against cell death. It is the key link between thoughts, emotions, and movement.
- *Balances hormones,* including boosting testosterone and growth hormone, and balances swings related to estrogen and progesterone, which cause symptoms of PMS or menopause.

❖ *Prevents cancer.*
❖ *Prevents dementia.*

What Do You Need to Do?

Something.

For the six-week program I ask you to commit to this: walk vigorously for thirty minutes every day. That is the only exercise you need to do for the UltraMind Solution.

More is better. But anything is better than nothing, which is the habit of about half of Americans. About 40 percent never exercise, about 30 percent exercise only sporadically and only 12 percent do regular vigorous exercise. That means that 88 percent of Americans are not getting enough exercise.

Exercise is necessary for our brains to work properly. And the side effects are great—weight loss, increased energy, better sleep, and happier mood (not to mention better sex).

I personally hate to exercise.

But I love to play.

If you don't like going to the gym, there are many ways you can exercise without really "exercising." You don't have to go to the gym, run on a treadmill, and pump iron to stay in shape. Just start moving around more.

Go for walks with your friends or family. Go out and do some gardening. Play Frisbee in the park with your kids. Pick up a tennis racket and just knock a tennis ball around. You don't even have to play a real match if you don't want to.

Anything you can do to get out and move your body can be considered exercise. So don't think that you absolutely have to go to the gym to get fit. Just use your body more.

A fun way to check in with how much you are exercising is to get a step counter. These devices are relatively inexpensive and they are a great way to get a sense for how much you move around every day. If you buy one, see if you can get up to ten thousand steps per day. (See Resources in *The UltraMind Solution Companion Guide* for information on where you can purchase a step counter.)

Whatever you do, just get moving!

Keeping physically fit is essential for keeping mentally fit.

On the six-week program I recommend you walk for thirty minutes a day every day. This is what you need to do to get your brain and body to start thriving again. That's it. Just do that—thirty minutes of vigorous walking a day.

SPECIAL NOTE
GUIDELINES FOR A COMPREHENSIVE EXERCISE PROGRAM

In *The UltraMind Solution Companion Guide* (www.ultramind.com/guide), I have provided a more comprehensive exercise program including further guidelines for aerobic conditioning, a special energy-boosting type of aerobic exercise called interval training, muscle building or strength training, and a stretching program.

In the long term, building your exercise program around aerobic cardiovascular fitness, stretching, and flexibility will provide the greatest benefits to your health and brain, but are not essential to the six-week UltraMind Solution.

Using the Mind-Body Effect with the Body-Mind Effect Maximizing Benefits

Each of us must find a way to bring meaning, purpose, peace, and serenity into our lives in an active and deliberate way. Stress will find you. Don't worry. Relaxation is more elusive . . .

The odd paradox is that you must "actively" relax (and that doesn't mean sitting on the sofa with a bowl of chips or ice cream watching TV). Remember the stress response is automatic and designed to protect us from danger. But deep relaxation does not happen automatically. You have to work at it.

There are hundreds of ways to turn on the relaxation response, and no one way is right or wrong. But to thrive, protect your brain, and heal the damage from a chronically activated stress response, you must find the antidote. Most of us don't need any help finding our alarm button. That button gets pushed dozens of times a day. But we *do* need help finding the pause button.

Here are a few recommendations on how you can do that. You will find many more in *The UltraMind Solution Companion Guide*, which you can access by going to www.ultramind.com/guide.

Finding the Pause Button

Where is your pause button? Do you know how to find it? Most of us don't. It is not something we ever learn.

Healing, repair, renewal, and regeneration all occur in a state of relaxation. So how do we find the pause button and activate the parasympathetic nervous system, otherwise known as the relaxation response?[1]

Dr. Herbert Benson, of Harvard's Institute for Mind Body Medicine, calls it "remembered wellness." Studying Tibetan monks with decades of meditation experience, he found that their brains were different,[2] and they could quickly slow down their physiology, breathing, heart rate, and blood pressure, and produce calming brain waves.

This is something ancient and familiar to all cultures—except ours. The relaxation response or deep relaxation is activated with human connection, community, love, sex, prayer, celebration, music, dancing, chanting, and meditation,[3] even laughter.

The simplest is often the best.

Soft-Belly Breathing

James Gordon, M.D., of the Center for Mind–Body Medicine (www .cmbm.org), has used this simple and ancient technique to transform trauma and build connections in war- and disaster-torn areas such as Kosovo, the Middle East, and New Orleans.[4] It is called "soft belly." You can do it anywhere, anytime.

During the program try doing it five times a day. Do it when you wake up, before you go to bed, and when you sit down to each meal. Your life will change.

Here is how to do soft-belly breathing:

1. Put your hand on your belly and allow your abdomen to relax.
2. Close your eyes or soften your focus, looking at the floor a few feet in front of you.
3. Inhale through your nose and exhale through your mouth.
4. Breath deeply into your abdomen and feel it expand to the count of five.
5. Pause for a count of one.
6. Exhale slowly to a count of five, allowing your body to relax and release tension.
7. Repeat for five breaths or until you feel relaxed.

The UltraBath

My next favorite way to push the pause button is the *UltraBath*. I like it because it is passive. Just fill a bath with hot water, two cups of Epsom salt, a half cup of baking soda, and ten drops of lavender oil. Then get in and soak for twenty minutes. If you want to enhance your experience, light a candle and put on some quiet rhythmic music. It is helpful for both relaxation and detoxification.

You need to do nothing more to push the pause button.

But you *can* do more, if you choose to.

Many Ways to Push the Pause Button

Personally, I find I like variety, and I have found many ways to activate the pause button. My favorites are exercise, massage, yoga, saunas, journaling, deep breathing, and the UltraBath.

We each may have a different route to achieving the same thing. The route we take may be spiritual, emotional, intellectual or physical, but all lead to the same results. Find the pause button and heal your brain.

The key is to do something every day—even if it is just for five minutes. Profound, deep relaxation for thirty minutes a day will transform your life.

There are more resources and suggestions for activating the pause button in *The UltraMind Solution Companion Guide*. Go to www.ultramind.com/guide and download the guide for more ideas.

Sleep for a Sound Mind

Sleep is one of those things we take for granted—until we can't.

The good news is that everything that is good for your brain is good for sleep. Correcting imbalances in all the seven keys helps restore normal sleep. If your blood sugar swings up and down giving you night sweats, or your thyroid is out of balance, you have food allergies or are magnesium-deficient, or you have mercury poisoning, you won't be able to sleep well.

If you have sleep apnea you will need to see a specialist who can treat you, but for most other types of sleep disorders, getting to the roots of systemic balance will take care of the problem.

In addition to restoring balance in all your body's core systems, there are many habits we engage in, including caffeine, alcohol, late-night Internet surfing, and TV in the bedroom, which impair our ability to get or stay asleep and alter our natural biological rhythms. They also negatively affect the quality of our sleep.

The other big obstacle to getting enough good quality sleep is your thoughts and emotions. Working with imagery and deep relaxation tools can be very helpful.

If you are having trouble falling asleep, staying asleep, or getting enough sleep, try to change your relationship to sleep. Think of it as a sacred, precious, healing part of your day and prepare for it carefully.

How to Get a Good Night's Sleep

So what are we to do about our sleep problems?

1. For those who can sleep, getting more sleep (around seven to nine hours depending on the person) can have a dramatic benefit for your health and weight.
2. For those who snore or have sleep apnea, get tested and treated as soon as possible. Ask your doctor to order an overnight sleep study done in a sleep lab if this is a concern for you.
3. For those who have trouble sleeping, here are a few tips I use to help my patients get and stay asleep. This is what is often called practicing good sleep hygiene.

Avoid Substances That Interfere with Sleep

- Avoid substances that affect sleep, including caffeine, sugar, and alcohol.
- Avoid medications that interfere with sleep.
  - Sedatives (these are used to treat insomnia, but ultimately lead to dependence and disruption of normal sleep rhythms and architecture)
  - Antihistamines
  - Stimulants (like Ritalin)
  - Cold medication (pseudephedrine, phenylephrine)
  - Steroids (prednisone)
  - Headache medication containing caffeine (Floricet), etc.

Get Back in Rhythm

- Avoid any stimulating activities—such as watching TV, using the Internet, and answering e-mails—for two hours before bed.
- Go to bed and wake up at the same time every day (and try to be in bed before 10 to 11 P.M.).
- Exercise daily for thirty minutes before dinnertime.
- Don't exercise vigorously after dinner (an evening walk is fine).

✣ Get regular exposure to daylight for at least twenty minutes, preferably first thing in the morning. The light from the sun enters our eyes and triggers our brain to release specific chemicals and hormones, like melatonin, that are vital to healthy sleep, mood, and aging.

✣ Eat no later than three hours before bed. Eating a heavy meal prior to bed will lead to a bad night's sleep.

Create a Sleepy Environment

✣ Use the bed only for sleep and sex.

✣ Keep your bedroom very dark or use eyeshades.

✣ If you have a noisy environment, block out sound by using earplugs (the soft silicone ones work the best).

✣ Make the room a comfortable temperature for sleep—not too hot or cold.

✣ Create an aesthetic environment helpful for sleeping by using serene and restful colors and eliminating clutter and distraction.

Calm and Clear Your Mind

✣ Write your worries down. One hour before bed, write down the things that are causing you anxiety and make plans for what you might do the next day to reduce your worry. It will free up your mind and energy to move into deep and restful sleep.

✣ Get a guided imagery or relaxation CD to help you get to sleep.

Relax Your Body

✣ Take an UltraBath. Raising your body temperature before bed helps to induce sleep. A hot bath relaxes your muscles and reduces tension physically and psychically. The UltraBath also gives you the benefits of magnesium absorbed through your skin, the alkaline balancing effects of the baking soda, and the cortisol-lowering effects of lavender, all of which help with sleep.

✣ Get a massage, stretch, or do a ten-minute yoga routine before bed.

✣ Use a hot water bottle on your solar plexus (or snuggle next to a warm body). Warming your middle raises your core temperature.

This helps trigger the proper chemistry for sleep. Either a hot water bottle, a heating pad, or a warm body can do the trick.

Nutrients and Herbs for Sleep

- ✢ Take an extra 200 to 400 mg of magnesium citrate or glycinate before bed in addition to what is on the basic supplement program. This relaxes the nervous system and muscles.
- ✢ Try 1 to 2 mg of melatonin thirty minutes before bedtime.

If you are still having trouble sleeping, make sure all of the keys outlined in Part IV are in balance.

Exercises for Your Mind and Brain

What's the point of having a healthy brain if you don't use it to engage more fully in life? The joy of life is in all the things we humans get to experience—love, learning, discovery, connection, understanding, wisdom, and curiosity.

You can eat well, exercise, learn to relax, and sleep well, all of which will nourish your brain. But then what do you do with it?

Engage fully with your life. In work. In play. In love.

But to do that you must keep your brain active. The mental decline we commonly see with aging is very much due to imbalance in nutrition, hormones, immune and digestive function, damage to our energy metabolism, toxins, and stress.

But some of it is also from lack of use. Just like your muscles—you need to use it or you lose it. Brain fitness is a real phenomenon. In a study of over 450 adults over seventy-five years old it was shown that just reading books, doing crossword puzzles, playing cards and board games, playing a musical instrument, or dancing can all reduce the risk of Alzheimer's disease.[5]

So mental workouts also are needed. That is, doing something new, different, and challenging with your brain. You want to sprout new neural connections and wake up sleeping parts of your brain.

In college, I learned two thousand Chinese characters, which I think helped me get through all the memorization of medical school. I started playing basketball at forty and tennis at forty-five. And I spend a lot of time trying to understand the mysterious, complicated world of genes and molecules. You must find what works for you.

What follows are some ideas that can get you started. I also recommend

Dr. Gary Small's book *The Memory Prescription*, Dr. David Perlmutter's *The Better Brain Book*, and *The Healthy Brain Kit* by Drs. Andrew Weil and Gary Small. There are many other helpful tools available for mental aerobics. The important thing is to keep your mind and brain engaged and active.

- Be creative—write in a journal, paint, make music, or dance.
- Seek out new ideas through attending lectures or local classes.
- Try a new hobby.
- Do math in your head instead of on a calculator.
- Memorize all your friends' phone numbers, and all your credit card numbers.
- Travel and explore new places.
- Play word games, do crossword puzzles or Sudoku.
- Join a study group, a book club, or start a "conversation" dinner club where you pick a topic and everyone has to engage and share.
- Practice mental aerobics (see Resources for more recommendations on products you can use).

CHAPTER 17

LIVING CLEAN AND GREEN

Our brains are exquisitely sensitive to environmental toxins and stresses. That is why I have included living clean and green as an essential part of the UltraMind Solution.

Here are my suggestions for how to take care of your own health and the planet at the same time. There is an intimate connection between the sustainability of our own health and that of the planet. Small everyday choices lead to big changes over time for our communities, our planet, and ourselves.

Living clean and green involves four steps.

1. Drink clean water.
2. Limit your exposure to chemicals and metals.
3. Keep your body fluids moving.
4. Reduce your exposure to electropollution or electromagnetic radiation.

Drink Clean Water

You should drink a minimum of six to eight 8-ounce glasses of clean filtered water every day you are on the program (and every day for the rest of your life for that matter). One of the reasons drinking this much water every day is important has to do with detoxification.

Toxins are ultimately excreted through your stool and urine. When you don't drink enough water, you become constipated, have darker urine, and urinate less frequently. These are signs that your detoxification system is not operating optimally and your health and mind will suffer as a consequence.

Drinking water will also help you reduce withdrawal symptoms from addictive substances and food allergens you may experience on the program, especially during the preparation week. I will explain more about these symptoms in chapter 18, where I discuss the preparation week.

Unfortunately much of our water supply is contaminated with microbes, pesticides, plastics, metals, chlorine, fluoride[1] (yes, fluoride), and other toxins. So drinking water out of the tap is less than ideal.

The best water to drink is water that has been passed through a filtering process. Common and inexpensive filters, such as carbon filters like the ones Brita makes, are available. See *The UltraMind Solution Companion Guide* for water-filter suggestions.

The best filter is a reverse osmosis filter that puts the water through a multistep process to remove microbes, pesticides, metals, and other toxins. This can be installed under the sink. It's a great filtering system (and it's cheaper over the long run).

Water in plastic bottles contains phthalates or bisphenol A, toxic petrochemicals. So avoid them if you can. Mineral water or still water in glass bottles is acceptable to drink.

Limit Exposure to Chemicals and Metals

While doing all the things in the following list is neither practical nor realistic, it is unfortunately what is optimal for our health. Incorporate the things you can. Find alternatives to the water you drink, get an air filter, or get rid of molds and other sources of indoor air pollution (the garden or household chemicals you use, and artificial lighting).

- Avoid water from plastic bottles, which contains phthalates. Drink water that comes in glass bottles or just filter your tap water as I explained above.
- Avoid excess exposure to environmental petrochemicals and toxins (garden chemicals, dry cleaning, car exhaust, secondhand smoke).
- Avoid charbroiled foods that contain cancer-causing polycyclic aromatic hydrocarbons.
- Avoid microwaved food, which produces more AGEs or advanced glycation end products in the food and creates more oxidative stress and inflammation.[2]
- Use HEPA/ULPA filters and ionizers to reduce dust, molds, volatile organic compounds (off-gassing from synthetic carpets, furniture, and paints), and other sources of indoor air pollution.

- Have house plants, which help detoxify the air.
- Reduce heavy metal exposure by reducing intake or exposure to large predatory and river fish, water, lead paint, thimerosal-containing products, silver fillings.
- Clean and monitor heating systems for release of carbon monoxide—the most common cause of death by poisoning in America.
- Reduce or eliminate the use of toxic household and personal care products (aluminum-containing underarm deodorants, antacids, petrochemical-/and toxin-containing creams and cosmetics, and pots and pans.
- Avoid or minimize exposure to bright and fluorescent lit areas. Use subdued full-spectrum/natural incandescent bulbs or candlelight as much as possible.

Get Your Fluids Moving

In addition to exercise, which is a powerful natural detoxifier, you can include the following in your UltraMind program. Remember the only way toxins have to get out of your body is through urine, stool, and sweat.

- Facilitate excretory functions:
  - Have one to two bowel movements a day.
  - Drink six to eight glasses of water a day to have clear urine.
  - Sweat regularly and profusely with exercise and the use of exercise, steam baths, or saunas. You can also use the UltraBath (see page 317).
- Learn and practice deep breathing using the soft-belly technique (see page 317).

Minimize Your EMR (Electromagnetic Radiation) Exposure

We do not live in an ideal world. And it is impossible to eliminate exposure to electromagnetic radiation. Debate still rages. The research on harm from EMR is not as extensive as it should be. *Yet the absence of evidence is not evidence of absence.*

Just because we have not proved beyond a doubt that EMR is harmful, neither is there any evidence that it is safe. Until we have clear evidence of safety I recommend erring on the side of caution, rather than waiting for forty years like we did with cigarettes before it was clear there was harm.

Here are things you can do to minimize your risk from EMR. Do what you can.

- Try to minimize your exposure and usage of wireless communication devices, including cell phones, cordless phones, and WiFi devices.
- Turn your cell phone off when not in use and sleeping. Do not keep it near your head or use it to play games, movies, etc.
- Try to keep your cell phone at least six to seven inches away from your body while it is on, or when you are talking, texting, or downloading.
- Use air-tube headsets or speaker mode when talking. Wireless and wired headsets may still conduct radiation.
- Do not keep your cell phone in your pocket or on your hip all day. The bone marrow in your hip produces 80 percent of the body's red blood cells and is especially vulnerable to EMR damage. The proximity to your genitals may also affect fertility.
- Children and pregnant women should avoid talking on cell phones.
- Replace as many cordless and WiFi items as you can with wired, corded lines (phones, Internet, games, appliances, devices, etc.).
- Minimize or space out your computer use. Sit as far back from the screen as possible; flat screens are preferable. Use wired Internet connections, not WiFi—especially for laptops.
- Keep a low-EMR sleep, home, and personal zone.
  - Move your alarm clock radio at least three feet from your head or use battery-powered ones; six feet is the recommended distance from all electronic devices during sleep.
  - Avoid water beds, electric blankets, and metal frames, which attract electromagnetic frequencies.
  - Futons and wood-framed beds are better than metal-coiled mattresses and box springs.
  - When using electric stoves, cook on back burners instead of front as much as possible.
  - Metals attract EMR: keep them away from and off the body.
- Measure EMR from wireless and wired devices with appropriate meters (see www.safewireless.org).

❖ To decrease exposures, consider installing EMR filters and pre-
ventive technologies to electrical circuits, devices, and appliances.
These may help, although human studies are limited.

I have now outlined the major principles of the UltraMind Solution.
These revolve around diet, supplements, lifestyle changes, and living clean
and green. Now it's time start doing the program. In the next two chapters
I will outline what to do for the preparation week and what to do every day
you are on the six-week UltraMind Solution.

CHAPTER 18

THE PREPARATION WEEK

Preparing Your Body and Mind for the Goodness to Come

One week before you start the six-week program, prepare your body for all the goodness to come by shedding habits that interfere with your brain. By eliminating items from your diet in a systematic way you will make your transition into the program simple and painless.

Items to Eliminate

Over the course of the next week you should eliminate these items from your diet entirely. Remember, in some cases they are hidden in places you may not expect. Be as vigilant as you can about reading labels and making sure the foods you eat do not contain the following:

- ❖ *Caffeine*—Cut your daily dose in half each day over the course of a week until you are off it. If you have four cups of coffee, go to two cups, then one cup, then one-half cup, then stop.
- ❖ *Processed and refined carbohydrates and sugar*—This includes all flour-based products (like bread and pasta) and all forms of sugar.
- ❖ *High-fructose corn syrup*—Go cold turkey and read EVERY label. High-fructose corn syrup is in places you don't expect.
- ❖ *Hydrogenated fats or trans fats*—Found in baked goods, chips, fries, in fact, in almost every packaged food. Read labels for ingredients and look for the word "hydrogenated" even if it says zero trans fats, because if it has less than half a gram per serving the government allows the food industry to deceptively say "zero" trans fats.
- ❖ *Processed and packaged foods*—This means anything that comes in a box, bag, package, or can.
- ❖ *Alcohol.*

If you are concerned about reading labels correctly, go to www.ultra mind.com/guide and download the companion guide for this book where I have included a set of tips on what to look for on labels.

Common Symptoms in the First Few Days

The following symptoms are very common at the beginning of the preparation phase and may continue through the first few days of the six-week program as you eliminate gluten and dairy. Don't worry, these symptoms are indicative that your body is eliminating toxins and are a good sign!

- Bad breath
- Constipation (If this is a problem for you, it should be addressed rather aggressively. I give a complete program for doing so in *The UltraMind Solution Companion Guide*—www.ultramind.com/ guide.)
- Achy, flulike feeling
- Fatigue
- Headaches
- Hunger
- Irritability
- Itchy skin
- Nausea
- Offensive body odor
- Sleep difficulties (too much or too little)

These symptoms can occur for a number of reasons.

First, eliminating food allergens like gluten and dairy often cause a withdrawal reaction, much like withdrawal from other addictive substances like caffeine, alcohol, nicotine, cocaine, or heroin. We are often most addicted to the foods we are allergic to. This causes an allergy-addiction cycle. Getting off those allergens can cause a brief, flulike achy syndrome that may last one to three days.

Second, toxins in our digestive tract may make us feel ill if we don't eliminate them. That is why it is important to address and prevent constipation if this is a problem for you.

The last major cause of symptoms is caffeine withdrawal (which you will be dealing with in this preparation phase). This may cause a predictable headache, fatigue, and an achy feeling the afternoon after you give it up.

If you experience any of these symptoms either during the preparation week or during the six-week program, I provide a specific set of recommendations that will ease your withdrawal symptoms, and make your transitions into the UltraMind Solution much easier.

Unfortunately, we don't have the space to publish those recommendations here.

However, I give all the details in *The UltraMind Solution Companion Guide*. If you suffer from withdrawal symptoms, or are concerned about this possibility before you begin, I strongly encourage you to go to www.ultra mind.com/guide and download the companion guide to this book.

It's a big help on your road to an UltraMind.

Once you have completed your preparation week, it is time to begin the six-week program. In the next chapter I will explain how the program works and give you all the tools you need to make it as simple and enjoyable as possible.

CHAPTER 19

THE ULTRAMIND SOLUTION

Boosting Your Brain Power for Life

The six-week program is designed to remove all the processed, high-sugar foods from your diet as well as the two main allergens (gluten and dairy) that lead to your "broken brain" and replace them with an unprocessed, real, natural, whole-foods diet. The foods you need to avoid are outlined in detail in chapter 14.

Instead of these toxic and inflammatory foods, you will eat the foods outlined in chapter 14 that are rich in healthy fats; slowly released, low-glycemic load, high-fiber carbohydrates; plant proteins; and minimal lean animal products; as well as disease- and weight-fighting anti-inflammatory, detoxifying, and antioxidant chemicals and phytonutrients. These foods give your body and brain the raw materials they need to heal and function optimally.

No restriction is put on the *amount* of food you eat, because counting calories, carbs, or fat grams is not necessary. If you eat whole fresh foods, your body self-regulates. The emphasis is on cleansing, renewal, revitalization, and optimizing your body and your brain so they work as originally designed.

Over the course of the diet pay attention to how your body and brain feel to find out what works for you. You may be more like the Greenland Inuit and feel satisfied with more healthful fats in your diet, or perhaps you are more like the Pima Indians and find that more fiber-rich carbohydrates work better for you. The same result can be obtained as long as you follow the basic nutritional wisdom that is the foundation of *The UltraMind Solution*.

By committing to this diet for six weeks, these principles will become second nature to you. The foods on this program will speak to your genes in new ways and your genes will say *yes!*

Once your genes begin to say *yes*, you will be on your way to a lifetime of UltraWellness and the improvements you have experienced in your mind and mood will become permanent.

After the six weeks are over, you can begin to reintroduce gluten and dairy if you choose to. I will teach you how to do that systematically so you find out if you are allergic to them (in the next chapter).

But remember, it is only by eliminating gluten and dairy in the first place that you can tune back into your body and develop a realistic picture of how they have been affecting your health and your brain.

Before you even begin the program I *strongly* encourage you to get the free *UltraMind Solution Companion Guide* (download at www.ultramind .com/guide), where I have included a six-week eating program, shopping lists, foods to enjoy, and foods to avoid, as well as many delicious recipes and other resources to guide you through the program.

Supplements and Lifestyle Changes During the UltraMind Solution

In addition to the dietary changes you will experience during the Ultra-Mind Solution, taking the basic supplement regimen I outlined in chapter 15, exercising, relaxing, and doing brain exercises are all critical parts of the program.

In the checklist at the end of this chapter I have outlined when you should integrate exercise, relaxation, and brain exercises into your day. I have also explained when to take your supplements.

Remember, you should at minimum walk for thirty minutes a day, every day, on the program. If you can manage it, it's even better to do vigorous aerobic exercise four to five times a week (an interval training program where you regularly vary your heart rate is ideal). You can also include a strength-training regimen two to three times a week if you wish, but this is not absolutely necessary. See *The UltraMind Solution Companion Guide* (www.ultramind.com/guide) for specific suggestions on how to exercise.

You should also practice active relaxation as I explained in chapter 16. I recommend you do the soft-belly breathing exercise immediately when you wake up, before each of your meals, and before you go to sleep. It's a simple, quick way to initiate the relaxation response, so don't forget it.

In addition, I recommend you try one more relaxation exercise of your choosing (my favorite is the UltraBath) in the evening before you go to bed. This is a wonderful way to end your day and sets the stage for excellent sleep at the same time.

Don't underestimate the power of relaxation. Give yourself this gift for six weeks and watch how your life is transformed.

Finally I suggest you engage in some of the brain exercises outlined in chapter 16 every day you are on the program if possible. If you can't manage that, do a brain exercise of some kind two to three times a week. It's fun, and it will work out your mind in new and interesting ways.

In terms of daily supplements—they are daily, and you should take them every day for the rest of your life. I have given you reminders in the checklist at the end of the chapter as to when to take your supplements. However, you will find you remember naturally after a few days of doing it.

In *The UltraMind Solution Companion Guide* I have provided a simple supplement chart to help you know what, when, and how to take your basic supplements as well as any additional supplements you may need based on the imbalances in any of the keys which you will learn about in Part IV. Download the guide at www.ultramind.com/guide.

Living Clean and Green During the UltraMind Solution

I also encourage you to incorporate the recommendations for living clean and green in chapter 17 during the six-week program. Every one of us is affected by environmental toxins, and they impact brain and body health in serious ways. Give yourself a break from this toxic exposure. You may find it becomes a way of life for you—one that not only makes you healthier but heals our planet as well.

The Daily Plan

To make the UltraMind Solution simple, I recommend you stick to a ritualized daily schedule as much as you can. This means doing the same things (like waking up, eating, exercising, relaxing, and sleeping) at the same times every day. You don't *have* to do this. But it makes the program easier and has several biological advantages like balancing your blood-sugar levels and reestablishing normal sleep rhythms.

The schedule outlined in the checklist below is what I recommend you do every day on the program. Just follow the steps on the checklist every day, keep to the foods-to-eat and foods-to-avoid lists, and use the allergy-free brain food recipes found in *The UltraMind Solution Companion Guide* at www.ultramind.com/guide and you will automatically stay on the program. *The UltraMetabolism Cookbook* also contains many gluten and dairy-free whole-foods recipes.

You don't have to do this perfectly. I know many people have schedules that vary quite a bit, and six weeks is a long time to do the same thing without interruption. Just stick to it the best you can and tune in to what your body is telling you about what works for you.

Daily Checklist for the Six-Week Program

Use the following checklist every day you are on the program. Make photocopies, and check off each item as you go through your day. You can also find this checklist in *The UltraMind Solution Companion Guide*. Go to www.ultramind.com/guide, download the guide, and you can print out a copy.

DAILY ACTION ITEMS

Wake up ninety minutes before you need to leave the house. ☐

MORNING RITUAL

Do soft-belly breathing upon waking. ☐

Engage in physical exercise, relaxation, or a brain exercise during this time (yoga is perfect in the morning). ☐

Drink one cup of decaf or caffeinated green tea that has been steeped in hot water for five minutes. (You may also have green tea later in the day. Limit your intake to two cups.) ☐

BREAKFAST (7 TO 9 A.M.)

Take the first dose of your multivitamin, calcium/magnesium, vitamin D, omega-3 fats, and methylation supplements with your breakfast. (Other than the vitamin D, it is best to take your supplements in two daily doses.) ☐

Do soft-belly breathing. ☐

Eat breakfast. ☐

A few possible options are:

- ❖ Omega-3 eggs
- ❖ A protein shake
- ❖ Gluten-free, whole-grain toast with nut butter and fruit

MORNING SNACK (10 TO 11 A.M.)

Eating snacks is an important way to stay in balance. Protein is   ☐
particularly helpful. Possible snacks include:
        ☐

⁘ A handful of nuts (almonds, macadamia nuts, walnuts,
  or pecans), seeds (pumpkin seeds)
⁘ Fresh fruit

LUNCH (12 TO 1 P.M.)

Do soft-belly breathing.   ☐
Eat lunch.   ☐
While there are many lunch options, one option that I like is:

⁘ Two cups of steamed or sautéed vegetables
⁘ One-half cup of brown rice
⁘ Sautéed fish—if you don't have time to cook at lunch, canned
  salmon is also an excellent option (see Resources for clean
  sources).

AFTERNOON SNACK (2 TO 3 P.M.)

Any of the morning snack options are excellent, or, if you are really
hungry, you could try another protein shake.   ☐

BEFORE DINNER

Walk for thirty minutes, or do your aerobic-exercise training.   ☐
Do soft-belly breathing.   ☐

DINNER (5 TO 7 P.M.)

Take the second dose of your multivitamin, calcium/magnesium,
omega-3 fats and methylation supplements with your dinner.
(Remember, you do not need to take vitamin D again here.)   ☐
Eat dinner—again, there are *many* possibilities here. However, one
fast and delicious option is: ☐

⁘ Two cups steamed or sautéed vegetables
⁘ Four to six ounces of baked or sautéed chicken (try seasoning
  with salt, pepper, lemon, and a little rosemary or thyme)
⁘ One-half cup of brown rice or other whole grain

(continued)

BEDTIME OR EVENING RITUAL

Twenty to thirty minutes of relaxation. I suggest an UltraBath. (It is not
only relaxing, but helps you detoxify.) ☐
Do soft-belly breathing before falling asleep. ☐

---

* Caffeinated green tea has so many health benefits and so little caffeine that it is safe
to drink on the program. You can also choose decaffeinated green tea.

Remember, you can find delicious recipes for all your meals and snacks, recommendations on how to exercise, more tools for relaxation, a complete supplements checklist, and much more in *The UltraMind Solution Companion Guide*. Go to www.ultramind.com/guide and download the free guide to help you make the program as simple as possible.

Summary of the Six-Week Program

Before we move on, let me quickly summarize the principles of the six-week program for you. Remember, it revolves around a handful of simple principles. These are:

1. *Eat Healthy.* The key to the whole program is eating a diet rich in healthy fats; slowly released, low-glycemic load, high-fiber carbohydrates; plant proteins; and minimal lean animal products; as well as disease- and weight-fighting anti-inflammatory, detoxifying, and antioxidant chemicals and phytonutrients.
2. *Take Supplements.* The daily supplements outlined in chapter 15 are critical for optimal health, and *everyone* should take them *every day* to achieve an UltraMind.
3. *Exercise.* Its effects on your mind and body have been proven beyond the shadow of a doubt. Our bodies evolved at a time when we used them to survive. Enjoy your body and learn about the pleasures exercise can bring, mentally and physically.
4. *Relax.* Stress kills you. Relaxation correlates with long-term health. If you think you don't have the time to relax, think again. You can't afford *not* to. Your brain and body will thank you for it.
5. *Live Green.* Toxins are ruining your health and destroying our planet. We all need to make a concerted effort to live clean and

green for ourselves, for future generations, and for the health of
the earth.

6. *Sleep.* Get out of the habit of sleeping too little and then "supplementing" with coffee to keep going. Sleep restores and regener-
ates your body. It's the time your cells heal. Give your brain a
chance to recuperate. It needs a rest and so do you.

You now have all the tools you need to do the six-week UltraMind program. In the next chapter I will explain what to do when the six weeks are
over.

CHAPTER 20

WHAT TO DO WHEN THE SIX WEEKS ARE OVER

Achieve an UltraMind for Life

Once you are finished with the six-week UltraMind Solution, I encourage you to transition out of it slowly to savor its full benefits.

The temptation will be to splurge or reward yourself for your hard work, but resist that temptation. Overloading your system with foods that are bad for the health of your brain and body can often cause severe reactions.

On the other hand, if you want to see for yourself the power of food to affect how you feel—indulge in all your old bad habits for one day and see just how bad you feel. That might be the best teacher for you, although take heed, you may not be able to function at all that day.

Take it slowly, and choose what you really want carefully. Think about what was just a bad habit. Your body has wisdom that will awaken during your experience on the program. Listen to the wisdom of your body when creating your life after it has ended. Go slowly and monitor your responses.

What to Do When the Program Is Over

When the six-week program is over you can (and should) continue many of the healthy habits you learned on it. At this point you have two options.

Option 1: Continue the Program

You may choose to stay off gluten and dairy for as long as you wish. In fact, you can keep following the program for a lifetime.

If this way of eating and living feels right for your body and mind, then perhaps it is the way you will choose to continue living. If so, you are already well on your way to UltraWellness.

Within the parameters of the program there is almost infinite flexibility—Asian, Mediterranean, Indian, traditional Mexican, and Middle Eastern cooking are all options you can explore if you choose to.

Learning how to eat real food is a discovery process. Because these foods have more fiber and nutrients, they are more filling and satisfying. Over time, you will learn to adjust portion sizes to your needs, and you will find foods that truly make your brain and body thrive.

Once you have reset your metabolism and you have established a pattern of eating and self-care that nourishes you, flexibility is important. Eating any food with great relish and delight—whether it is a decadent chocolate cake or the richest ice cream—is good for the soul and the senses.

While some people may have trigger foods, like the first drink for an alcoholic, most of us can enjoy treats once in a while. Your body will tell you what feels good and what doesn't.

Once you have reestablished a relationship with your body and brain, you will be drawn to those foods that make you feel good, and from time to time that may include almost anything. Staying in balance and finding a rhythm are the keys to lifelong health and a healthy metabolism.

Moderation in all things is still great advice, and that includes moderation in moderation. Enjoy yourself. I wish you all endless health and happiness.

Option 2: Reintegrate Dairy and Gluten

If you choose, you may begin integrating dairy and gluten into your diet once the six weeks are over.

Actually, it can be good to reintegrate dairy and gluten into your diet. This allows you to test it and find out whether or not it was contributing to your mood, behavior, attention, and memory problems, or other health issues such as headaches, joint pain, sinus problems, irritable bowel syndrome, and even weight gain.

To reintegrate dairy and gluten into your diet, follow these guidelines.

Reintroducing Gluten and Dairy When the Six Weeks Are Over

At the end of the six-week program you may reintroduce gluten and dairy to see if they contribute to your brain problems. You need to be aware of what is going on in your body and mind as you do.

You may not have been aware that gluten or dairy was triggering problems for you. When you eliminated it during the six weeks you may have unknowingly eliminated the very core of your psychiatric or neurological disorders. That means you need to be careful as you bring it back into your diet to find out whether or not it was truly the cause of your problems.

Reintroducing gluten and dairy (and any other foods you are sensitive or allergic to) can trigger many symptoms, including:

- Brain fog
- Difficulty remembering things
- Mood problems (depression, anxiety, or anger)
- Nasal congestion
- Chest congestion
- Headaches
- Sleep problems
- Joint aches
- Muscle aches
- Pain
- Fatigue
- Changes in your skin (acne)
- Changes in digestion or bowel function

When you reintroduce foods you are sensitive to (like gluten and dairy), eat them at least two to three times a day for **three** days to see if you notice a reaction (unless, of course, you notice a problem right away, then stop immediately). But be sure to leave three days between the time you introduce each food. For example, if you introduce gluten on Monday, don't add dairy until Thursday.

Symptoms can occur from a few minutes to seventy-two hours later. If you have a reaction, note the food and eliminate it for ninety days. This will give your immune system a chance to cool off and your gut a chance to heal. In turn, this makes it more likely you will be able to tolerate more foods in the long run. However, you may find it best to eat them only occasionally (not more than once every three to four days) to keep the immune system cooled off.

If you still react after eliminating the food from your diet for twelve weeks, you should stay off it for the long term, or see a physician, dietitian, or nutritionist skilled in managing food allergies.

Keep a log of any symptoms that you experience when you reintroduce different food groups. Tracking your symptoms should guide you to which foods trigger allergic reactions in your system.

Using a food log to track your symptoms and monitor your progress is an excellent way to identify what foods you can tolerate and what foods you are allergic to.

There is not enough room here to print a sample; however, I have included one in *The UltraMind Solution Companion Guide* at www.ultramind .com/guide. It is a very detailed food log that you can use to track your symptoms.

Keeping a food log helps create the connection between your daily food choices, activities, stress management, and how you feel. A journal will record your continuing sense of well-being, energy level, and weight loss. Having a written record is a more practical and accessible way to keep track of what is going on for you than simply trying to remember it.

You can use this same system to reintegrate other foods not allowed on the program as well. However, always keep in mind the foods you should permanently avoid, and be wary of falling back into addictive patterns like eating sugar, flour products, or consuming too much caffeine (more than one cup a day) or alcohol (more than three drinks per week).

While you may want to reintegrate some of these foods, there are other habits you learned on the program you will definitely want to adhere to from now on.

The basic supplement plan is one of them. As I have said throughout this book, using the basic supplement plan I outline is critical for long-term health.

Exercise and relaxation is another. Exercise and stress reduction are among the few things that always correlate with long-term health in the scientific research. Don't stop moving your body, and always take the time to relax. These are critical to finding UltraWellness.

The single biggest gift you can give yourself at the end of this program is identifying which foods you are sensitive to, which were causing you brain problems, and which you can eat and enjoy safely.

That is why I focus on eliminating the two main foods that lead to mood problems and cognitive disorders and then reintegrate them systematically. It is the best way to find out which foods harm you and which help you.

Your fork is your key to a healthy body and mind. Listen to your body's wisdom—sometimes it is smarter than your mind.

Now you have learned the basic maintenance program that will take care of 70 to 80 percent of problems with your mood, behavior, attention, cognitive function, and memory.

If you follow the basic plan as I have outlined here, you will discover improvement not only in mood, focus, and memory, but also in energy, weight, metabolism, and many other chronic health problems.

However, some of us need a little extra help. We suffer from deeper imbalances that require a little more fine-tuning. Since you have taken all the quizzes in Part II, you should know what areas you need to focus on.

In Part IV, I will guide you in going deeper. What supplements and other treatments are available that help correct these imbalances? This and more you will learn in Part IV. We are all unique and different. In the next part you will learn how to personalize the UltraMind Solution.

Balancing the Seven Keys and Optimizing the Plan

CHAPTER 21

CREATING AN ULTRAMIND

Balance the Seven Keys to UltraWellness and Optimize the Six-Week Plan

My deepest wish for each of you is to find and work with a Func-
tional/Integrative Medicine practitioner, someone who will help
you fine-tune and personalize the UltraMind Solution.

However, I know that is not possible, because there are not enough
around. I am working with the Institute for Functional Medicine (www
.functionalmedicine.org) to create curriculums for medical schools, resi-
dencies, and certification programs to train more doctors in practice. In ten
to twenty years, I believe, all physicians will be trained in and practice the
principles of Functional Medicine, because it is the medicine of the future.

Fortunately, for 80 percent of you it may not be necessary to work with
a physician or Functional Medicine practitioner if you follow the six-week
plan for an UltraMind.

I also believe that, by using the quizzes in Part II to identify which keys
are out of balance, you can customize the UltraMind Solution for yourself
by adding the suggestions I will provide in the chapters that follow.

The quizzes in Part II offer three options to fix your broken brain and
optimize your health. These are:

1. The UltraMind Solution
   ❖ Follow the basic six-week plan for an UltraMind in Part III.
2. Self-Care
   ❖ Add the recommendations for specific foods, lifestyle suggestions, and supplements in the chapters that follow to optimize
   the keys that are out of balance for you.
3. Medical Care
   ❖ If you have a severe imbalance in any of the keys I advise you to
   seek the assistance of a practitioner of Functional or Integrative
   Medicine. In addition to the suggestions for optimizing the keys,

I will give you recommendations for tests or treatments you should discuss with your physician in the chapters that follow.

In each quiz your score will put you in one of the three groups:

1. If your score qualifies you for the UltraMind Solution, simply follow the basic plan in Part III.
2. If your score qualifies you for Self-Care, then integrate the additional suggestions here in Part IV into your six-week plan.
3. If your score qualifies you for Medical Care, follow the Ultra-Mind Solution with the additional recommendations for Self-Care for six weeks. Then retake the quizzes. Many of you will then no longer qualify for Medical Care. If you still do, then seek out a practitioner of Functional or Integrative Medicine to request the necessary tests and treatments.

I have kept to a few suggestions in each key that I have found to be the most effective and important interventions to optimize your body's core systems. There are, of course, many other options that are available to normalize function in each key; however, they are best applied with an experienced practitioner.

Personalizing the UltraMind Solution: Self-Care and Medical Care

Each of us is unique, genetically, developmentally, environmentally, psychologically, and spiritually. Each of us has areas of weakness and strength. Finding those and adapting your health practices and treatment to that uniqueness is essential if you are to regain full health and vitality.

The practice of Functional Medicine, the art of creating UltraWellness for my patients, is so very different from the process I learned in medical school. Yet it is a much better map for the territory of illness. And ultimately it is quite simple. It involves two simple principles:

1. Get rid of the bad stuff.
2. Add the good stuff.

That's it.

The amazing healing powers of the body for regeneration and repair show up if we simply find what's not agreeing with you and remove it, and then provide the missing ingredients your body needs to thrive.

This is the process I have done thousands of times with my patients and I have had extraordinary success.

In this part of the book, I will use these same principles to guide you toward optimizing key areas that may be out of balance for you. I will also explain how you can integrate these steps into the six-week plan outlined in Part III, so you can take full advantage of the UltraMind Solution. There are a few simple steps to follow.

For all the seven keys to UltraWellness that help you create an Ultra-Mind there is a short list of things that create imbalances and a short list of things that are needed to create optimal function.

Here is the list of the bad stuff and the good stuff. It's not a long list really, and it is enough to address nearly any medical problem. This is the different map. And it will get you to where you want to go—optimal, vigorous, resilient, and robust health—or, more simply, the state of UltraWellness.

The Bad Stuff

These are the things in your diet, lifestyle, and environment that are sending your body out of balance. These five factors are, in fact, the cause of *all* disease.

1. Poor diet (nutrient poor, calorie dense)
2. Stress (physical or psychological)
3. Toxins (chemicals, metals, biological, and internal metabolic toxins)
4. Allergens (foods, molds, dust, pollens, and chemicals)
5. Microbes or bugs (bacteria, yeast, parasites, viruses, prions, etc.)

The Good Stuff

This is what you need to add to your diet, lifestyle, and environment to rebalance your systems.

1. High-quality food (proteins, fats, carbohydrates, fiber, phytonutrients)
2. Vitamins, minerals, and conditionally essential nutrients (and occasionally bioidentical hormones)
3. Water, air, and light
4. Exercise/movement
5. Sleep
6. Deep relaxation

7. Rhythm

8. Love, community, connection, meaning, and purpose

Much of this is incorporated into the basic six-week UltraMind Solution outlined in Part III. In fact, it is remarkable that by simply eating whole fresh foods, taking a few essential supplements, and getting some exercise, restful sleep, and deep relaxation, the core systems of the body can reset, recover, repair, and heal.

In the six-week plan, most of the bad stuff is removed and nearly all of the good stuff is recommended. The body's wisdom then rebalances your whole system.

Occasionally, a few additional steps are necessary to correct more serious problems such as intestinal infections or heavy metal poisoning. But up to 80 percent of your problems may be taken care of by the basic six-week UltraMind Solution.

In some cases, when key systems are really out of balance, it's necessary to add these few additional steps. That is what I am going to teach you to do here. In each chapter you will find:

The Self-Care Plan

1. *Foods*—A list of additional foods you should focus on integrating into your diet to help optimize each key (I have included this only in cases where there are specific foods you should incorporate *in addition* to what is on the six-week program).

2. *Supplements*—Supplements you can add to help you optimize each key. **Note:** If you are out of balance in several keys, it may seem like there are a lot of supplements to take. However, it isn't as overwhelming as it seems. I have created a special checklist for supplements that makes it very easy to understand what to take. It is in *The UltraMind Solution Companion Guide* at www.ultramind.com/guide.

3. *Lifestyle Changes*—Lifestyle changes that may assist you in key optimization.

The Medical Care Plan

1. *Doctor Actions*—A list of action items you can take with your doctor's assistance.

2. *Doctor Guidelines*—Guidelines on specific treatments that your doctor may use, such as hormones or metal detoxification.

Go back to your quiz scores and identify which keys you need to work through. Then simply follow the Self-Care or the Medical Care plans, depending on how you scored.

(You can find printable copies of all the quizzes in *The UltraMind Solution Companion Guide.* Go to www.ultramind.com/guide for more information.)

Many people will score high in several key areas. This is because your body is one ecosystem—when one system goes out of balance it can send the others out of balance as well.

If you score high in several keys, start the six-week program and integrate steps to optimize each key in the following order:

1. Fix your digestion—it's amazing how many problems can be resolved by fixing your gut. Start here and you may witness miraculous changes in your health.
2. Cool off inflammation—this key is intimately related to the gut and the next natural step to take.
3. Optimize nutrition.
4. Enhance detoxification.
5. Balance your hormones.
6. Boost energy metabolism.
7. Calm your mind.

Wait three days to begin working on a new key. For example, if you scored high on the "Fatty Acids" quiz, the "Insulin" quiz, and the "Gut" quiz, you would start the six-week program and begin working in the steps in chapter 25 to fix your digestion. After three days, you could begin integrating the steps in chapter 22 to enhance your phospholipids. Then, after three more days, you could begin integrating the steps in chapter 23 to improve your insulin balance.

A SPECIAL NOTE ON MEDICAL CARE AND TESTING

Up to 80 percent of people will recover and thrive by following the six-week UltraMind Solution in Part III with a few additional steps for Self-Care in Part IV. However, the other 20 percent will need further care.

(continued)

If you don't get significantly better following the UltraMind Solution and the Self-Care plan in this section, then you may need some laboratory tests and further medical treatment. I have outlined this in *The UltraMind Solution Companion Guide* (www.ultramind.com/guide). To do those tests and get the treatment you need, you will need to find an experienced practitioner of Functional or Integrative Medicine. I will offer some options in the Resources, or you can visit our team at **The UltraWellness Center** in Lenox, Massachusetts (www.ultrawellnesscenter.com).

Most tests I recommend in my practice are available through conventional large commercial labs such as Quest Diagnostics or LabCorp. Others are small, specialty labs that specialize in metabolic, immune, nutritional, or functional testing.

There is still great controversy in conventional medical circles about the utility of these laboratory tests, but I have used them successfully for over twenty years in treating patients.

I have used these tests on thousands of patients to help me navigate this new medical territory with great success. They are often imperfect and may not always give clear yes or no answers.

Rather, many of these tests identify disturbances in function, not pathology. In other words, you may not have anemia from lack of folate, but you might have any number of important pathways that are jammed because you don't have enough folate for you—leading to depression, dementia, autism, or ADHD.

The tests I recommend can often help me identify patterns and guide me in choosing the best therapies to help my patients regain balance. I think they can help you and your doctor the same way.

While testing isn't always necessary, it can be very helpful in honing in on specific imbalances in your biochemistry that are creating problems for you.

In the guide I explain exactly which tests to use to identify deeper imbalances in each of the seven keys. They will help you work with your physician to find the cause of your problems.

Practicing Self-Care

I believe in self-care. Take back your health from the medical system. Leave your diseases to the "disease care" system. Most health problems can be addressed without the help of a trained health professional. If you work on taking out the bad stuff and putting in the good stuff, 80 percent of problems will heal.

For the other 20 percent you need the help of a trained professional in

Functional or Integrative Medicine, or a conventional medical specialist, depending on the problem.

Part IV of the UltraMind Solution is designed to help you regain control of your health and your health care. I know I can help you achieve that goal.

CHAPTER 22

KEY #1: OPTIMIZE NUTRITION

Hippocrates said thousands of years ago that doctors should "leave their potions in the chemist's crucible if they heal their patients with food." Because of our widespread nutrient deficiencies, I would add ". . . heal their patients with food *and* nutrients."

By far, the most powerful tool I have to help my patients heal—more powerful than any medication—is food (and nutritional therapy).

Remember . . .

1. You must all have essential fats—DHA, EPA, and PC and PS for your brain and every one of your 100 trillion cells to function well.
2. Amino acids are the building blocks of moods, thought, and memory—get them tuned up.
3. Keep the methylation and sulfation trains running with the right types and amounts of folate, B_{12}, B_6, and betaine, and sources of sulfur in the diet and supplements (see chapter 6).
4. Most of us are vitamin D–deficient. Getting enough on board will help your brain and prevent many diseases.
5. Magnesium is the major relaxation mineral.
6. Zinc and selenium are absolutely critical for a happy, healthy brain and body.

Using the basic program, you can take care of most of your needs. However, in some cases people need additional support, especially with phospholipids and neurotransmitters.

Self-Care Plan

The Self-Care plan for nutrition is quite simple. It involves just a few additional suggestions.

Supplementation for Phospholipid Membrane Support

If you scored over 5 on the "Fatty Acids" quiz on page 85, increase your intake of phospholipids by taking the following:

- ❖ PS (phosphatidylserine), 200 mg twice a day with meals for two months, after two months reduce to 100 mg twice a day with meals.
- ❖ GPC (glycerophosphocholine) or CDP-choline, 1,200 mg three times a day with meals for two months, after two months reduce to 400 mg three times a day with meals

Supplementation with Amino Acids to Optimize Neurotransmitters

Remember that all of your neurotransmitters are built out of amino acids, the building blocks of protein. Eating protein with each meal helps supply adequate amino acids for you to make all your neurotransmitters. Supplementing these amino acids can, in many cases, help you overcome the neurotransmitter deficiencies that may be leading to your mood problems and brain dysfunction.

You should start by supporting one neurotransmitter at a time. Start with the neurotransmitter you scored highest on in the quizzes.

For example, if you scored highest on the serotonin deficiency quiz, start with serotonin support. You can slowly add support for each additional neurotransmitter if your symptoms persist. Try the support for one neurotransmitter for one week, and then add support for the next one the following week (while continuing your previous regimen) until you have achieved the balance you desire.

SPECIAL CONSIDERATIONS FOR AMINO-ACID THERAPY

1. Since many neurotransmitters are often out of balance, multiple supplements are often necessary.
2. Start with one neurotransmitter support program at a time. Give each new neurotransmitter support program one week to work before adding the next.

(continued)

3. It is best to start with the inhibitory neurotransmitter support (serotonin and GABA) and then after a week or two move to the excitatory support (dopamine and acetylcholine).

4. Amino-acid therapy can usually safely be used with psychiatric medication with one exception—monoamine oxidase inhibitors (Parnate, Nardil, Marplan). However, combining medication with amino-acid therapy should be done with the supervision of a physician who understands amino acids and psychotropic medications.

5. Using amino acids helps prevent the depletion of neurotransmitters and can often help people wean off medications.

6. Amino-acid therapy often works quickly and you may notice effects within days to weeks.

7. You should continue the therapy for a total of six months before slowly weaning yourself off the amino acids. You may not need them after that.

Serotonin Support

You can either take 5-HTP or tryptophan to support your serotonin level. Try:

❖ 5-HTP (5-hydroxytryptophan), 50 mg twice a day, once in the afternoon and once before bed. Add an additional 50 mg in the afternoon and at bedtime every three days until you get to a maximum dose of 150 mg once in the afternoon and once before bed.

Or,

❖ Take tryptophan, 500 mg once in the afternoon and once before bed.

❖ Take these on an empty stomach (one hour before or two hours after meals).

Remember, use either 5-HTP or tryptophan, not both. *If you are taking an SSRI or antidepressant, check with your health-care provider before taking 5-HTP or tryptophan.*

To help you sleep, you can also try:

❖ 1 to 3 mg of melatonin before bed to help with sleep if needed.

GABA Support

❖ Take GABA, 500 mg once mid–afternoon and once before bed.
❖ Take theanine, 200 mg once in the morning and once before bed. (This is the amino acid from green tea.)
❖ GABA and Theanine complement each other.

Dopamine Support

❖ Take L–tyrosine, 500 mg once before breakfast, once mid-morning, and once mid–afternoon. After three days increase to 1,000 mg before breakfast, mid–morning, and mid–afternoon.
❖ After one week add I-phenylalanine, 500 mg once before break-fast, once mid-morning, and once mid–afternoon. After three days increase to 1,000 mg before breakfast, mid–morning, and mid-afternoon.

These should be taken on an empty stomach.

Acetylcholine Support

❖ See page 353 for GPC support. Acetylcholine is made from choline; you should get a sufficient amount with the supplementation recommendations above.

MEDICAL CARE PLAN

❖ Testing for amino acids and neurotransmitters can help identify your particular imbalances more accurately.
❖ Further customization of amino-acid therapy is possible based on testing and your symptoms.
❖ Testing for omega-3 fats, vitamin D, magnesium, zinc, and selenium can be helpful in identifying the need for additional supplementation.
❖ Testing for methylation problems with homocysteine and methylmalonic acid is often very helpful in optimizing doses of folate, B_{12}, and B_6.
❖ Occasionally medication may be necessary as a short-term treatment while you are balancing the seven keys to UltraWellness.

CHAPTER 23

KEY #2: BALANCE YOUR HORMONES

B alance is the key to staying healthy, and nowhere is this truer than in the world of hormones. It is important not to think of them separately but as interconnected parts of a whole that all affect each other.

Hormones are influenced by imbalances in all the seven keys. Our body is one whole system where everything is linked to everything else. So improving your nutrition, or reducing inflammation, fixing your gut, and getting rid of toxins all support normalization of hormone function, which translates into better mood, more focus, and better brain function.

The quizzes in Part II may have alerted you to focus on imbalances that lead to problems with insulin, your thyroid, or sex hormones. Balancing your hormones is relatively easy. Follow these guidelines.

Optimizing Insulin Balance: Self-Care Plan

The key to insulin balance is eating the diet in the six-week program.

However, if you scored over 9 on the "Insulin" quiz, you may also need to integrate the following supplements.

Supplementation for Insulin Resistance

There are many blood-sugar balancing nutrients often found in combinations.

In addition to what you will get in your basic supplement plan, these nutrients can be used to help balance blood sugar and insulin.

- Chromium, 500 mcg twice a day
- Glucomannan fiber, polyglycoplex (PGX), or konjac root, four capsules five to ten minutes before meals with a glass of water

(Note: This is one of the most powerful treatments for insulin problems and weight.)

OPTIMIZING INSULIN BALANCE: MEDICAL CARE PLAN

1. Additional testing may be necessary, including:
   a. A two-hour glucose-tolerance test measuring both insulin and glucose.
   b. Cholesterol profile measuring the size of cholesterol particles, which are smaller in insulin resistance and more prone to clog your arteries.
   c. C-reactive protein, which measures inflammation that is associated with insulin resistance.
   d. Liver function tests with GGT that identify the fatty liver associated with insulin resistance.
2. Additional supplements that are often helpful include alpha lipoic acid, biotin, vanadium, N-acetylcysteine.
3. Herbs may also be helpful, including extracts of hops, acacia bark, ginseng, green tea, fenugreek, cinnamon, gymnena sylvestre, bitter melon, and garlic.
4. Medications such as glucophage (metformin) or Actos are occasionally helpful as a bridge in balancing your blood sugar.

Support Your Thyroid: Self-Care Plan

The production of thyroid hormones requires iodine and omega-3 fatty acids; converting the inactive T4 to the active T3 requires selenium, the binding of T3 to the receptor on the nucleus, and switching it on requires vitamins A, D, and zinc. All of these elements are found in a good whole foods diet and your basic supplements.

However, there are a few food items you should concentrate on integrating into the program to support your thyroid.

Foods for Thyroid Support

These foods are particularly good for thyroid problems:

- Seaweed or sea vegetables have iodine.
- Fish has iodine, omega-3 fats, and vitamin D (especially sardines and wild salmon).

❖ Dandelion greens have vitamin A.

❖ Smelt, herring, scallops, and Brazil nuts have selenium.

Also make sure you eliminate the cause of thyroid problems. The following may be contributing to your problems:

❖ Soy foods and the broccoli family (broccoli, cabbage, kale, Brussels sprouts, collard greens) have all been said to cause thyroid dysfunction, but they also have many other health *benefits*. Human studies have shown no significant effect when whole traditional soy (tofu, tempeh, miso, edamame) is consumed in normal quantities.[1] I don't recommend avoiding any of these foods, because the benefits are so great and the potential risk is questionable or negligible. However I would avoid all processed soy foods such as burgers, cheese, and bars—these have harmful health effects.

❖ Gluten sensitivity or hidden allergy to wheat, barley, rye, oats, spelt, kamut, and triticale are the most common dietary cause of thyroid problems. (Eliminating these is already part of the UltraMind Solution, but I wanted to emphasize that gluten can be a significant factor in thyroid problems.)

❖ Avoid fluoride (avoid toothpaste with fluoride and filter your water).[2] It has been linked to thyroid problems.

SUPPORT YOUR THYROID: MEDICAL-CARE PLAN

TESTING FOR THYROID PROBLEMS

1. Testing should include all the thyroid hormones (TSH, free T3, and free T4) and thyroid antibodies (TPO and antithyroglobulin antibodies). Most doctors just check TSH, which is inadequate to identify mild problems.
2. Further testing may be necessary and is described in *The UltraMind Solution Companion Guide*.

(continued)

CHOOSING THE RIGHT THYROID HORMONE REPLACEMENT

To properly balance a thyroid that is severely out of balance, you may need to go on some type of thyroid hormone–replacement therapy. There are certain things you can do by altering your diet and your lifestyle, but if your thyroid isn't functioning properly you may need to have some additional thyroid hormones to supplement its output. Knowing what's available and what to ask about can empower you to make better decisions about your health.

A combination of experience, testing, and trial and error are necessary to get it just right. However, I have found that the majority of my patients benefit from a combination hormone treatment including T4 and T3.

Synthroid, the most commonly prescribed thyroid hormone, is just T4, the inactive hormone. Most doctors assume that the body will convert it to T3 and all will be well. Unfortunately, pesticides, stress, mercury, infections, allergies, and selenium deficiencies can block that process. Since 100 percent of us have stored pesticides in our bodies, we will all likely have some problem with Synthroid.

The most common treatment I use is Armour thyroid,[3] a whole combination of thyroid hormones including T4, T3, and T2[4] (a little-known product of thyroid metabolism that actually may be very important).

Armour is a prescription drug made from desiccated or dried porcine thyroid. It contains the full spectrum of thyroid hormones, including T4, T3, and T2. It seems paradoxical that taking a pig hormone can make your brain better, but it does. The right dose ranges from 15 to 180 mg, depending on the person.

Many doctors still hold the outdated belief that the preparation is unstable and the dosages difficult to monitor. That was true with the old preparation of Armour, not the new one. (See www.armourthyroid.com for more information.)

Sometimes the only way to find out if you have a thyroid problem is a short trial of something like Armour thyroid for three months. If you feel better, your symptoms disappear, your mood, memory, and behavior improve, you have more energy, and you lose weight (assuming this a problem for you, which it is for many people with a thyroid deficiency), it's the right choice. Occasionally, further customization of thyroid hormones is necessary using various combinations of T4 and T3 in prescription or compounded forms.

Once started, it doesn't have to be taken for life (a common misperception). Once all the factors that disturb your thyroid have been corrected, you may be able to reduce or discontinue the dose.

(continued)

As with any treatment, always work with an experienced physician in using medications for your thyroid. Careful monitoring is essential. Taking too much thyroid hormone, or taking it when you don't need it, can lead to undesirable side effects including anxiety, insomnia, palpitations, and over the long-term, bone loss.

WARNING

If your adrenal glands are burned out from long-term stress, treating the thyroid without supporting the adrenal glands through relaxation and the adaptogenic herbs (like ginseng, rhodiola, or Siberian ginseng) can actually make people feel worse. Your Functional Medicine practitioner will know how to balance your adrenals before treating your thyroid with medication.

Rebalance Your Sex Hormones: Self-Care Plan

These two hormone–balancing foods should be included in your diet:

- ❖ Whole traditional soy foods such as tofu, tempeh, miso, natto, and edamame
- ❖ Ground flaxseeds, two tablespoons a day

Supplements for Sex-Hormone Balance

In addition to your basic supplement plan, this essential anti–inflammatory omega–6 fat (GLA or gamma linoleic acid) can help balance sex hormones:

- ❖ Evening primrose oil, 1,000 mg twice a day

Herbs and Phytonutrients

The following herbs and phytonutrients can be particularly helpful for women coping with PMS or menopause.

For PMS

- *Chasteberry Fruit Extract* (Vitex Agnus-astus) can help balance the hormones released by the pituitary gland that control your overall hormone function. Studies of over five thousand women found it effective. Take 100 mg twice a day of a 10:1 extract.
- *DIM* (diindolylmethane) is a metabolite of indole-3-carbinol (I3C). Both are found naturally in cruciferous vegetables like broccoli, kale, and Brussels sprouts and help improve the detoxification of your sex hormones. Take 100 mg twice a day with food.

For Menopause

- Black cohosh (*Cimicifuga racemosa*): Black cohosh has been shown to significantly reduce hot flashes, night sweats, mood swings, irritability, and related occasional sleeplessness. Take 20 mg of black cohosh extract (root and rhizome) twice a day, once in the morning and once in the evening.

REBALANCE YOUR SEX HORMONES: MEDICAL-CARE PLAN

TESTING YOUR SEX HORMONES

Testing of blood, urine, or saliva can often be helpful in identifying hormonal imbalances such as too much or too little of various hormones. This can guide a doctor's therapy.

BIOIDENTICAL HORMONE REPLACEMENT

Hormones interact directly with the brain and affect mood and cognition. Occasionally, despite lifestyle therapies, diet, exercise, stress reduction, nutrient supplementation, and herbs, hormone therapy can be lifesaving (as well as mood- and brain-saving).

(continued)

Only a physician knowledgeable and experienced with bioidentical hormone therapy should prescribe them. The *only* hormones that should be used are ones that are identical to those made by your body. They have very specific actions when they bind to their hormone receptors on your cells. Synthetic or animal hormones typically have unwanted side effects and dangers.

For menopause your doctor may try:

- Topical combinations of estradiol, estriol, progesterone, and testosterone, which are prepared by compounding pharmacies (see Resources for recommendations on how to find a doctor).
- My approach is to use the lowest dose possible to relieve symptoms, to use only bioidentical hormones, and to use them topically (vaginal, skin, under the tongue).
- Oral hormones should be used with as low a dose as possible and only when topical hormones are not effective.
- DHEA supplementation (see information on adrenal support in chapter 28).

For severe cases of PMS not improved by diet, lifestyle, or supplements, your doctor may try:

- Topical, natural, bioidentical progesterone in the last two weeks of the menstrual cycle. The usual dose is one-half teaspoon (20 to 40 mg) applied at night to thin skin areas of your body for the last two weeks of the menstrual cycle.

For men's hormone balance your doctor may use:

- Testosterone—topical is ideal after measurement of your hormone levels and with ongoing monitoring of testosterone and PSA levels.
- DHEA supplementation (see adrenal support in chapter 28).

CHAPTER 24

KEY #3: COOL OFF INFLAMMATION

If you have a sore throat, a swollen joint, or a rash, you know you are inflamed, but if your brain is inflamed you feel nothing. Nothing, that is, besides being depressed, unfocused, or worse, autistic or demented.

If your score on the "Inflammation" quiz in chapter 8 rated you for Self-Care or Medical Care, you need to focus on finding and getting rid of the causes of inflammation.

The list of causes is, thankfully, short: an inflammatory, high-sugar, processed-food diet; a sedentary and stressful lifestyle; toxins; infections; and allergens. That's it.

Since most of our inflammation is from diet and lifestyle, the treatment for inflammation comes on your plate and in your shoes. What you eat and how much you exercise are the most important factors governing inflammation.

Finding the causes of inflammation is not always easy. The most common and obvious causes are our diet and being sedentary. But there are many factors, and at times specialized testing is needed to find hidden causes.

+ **The two most common sources of inflammation in the twenty-first century are sugar (and refined carbohydrates) and hidden food allergens (perhaps most important, gluten).**

Common, but often unrecognized, inflammation comes from hidden food allergies—especially gluten. Eliminating gluten and other delayed IgG food allergens is one of the most powerful treatments I use in my practice.

You do this as part of the six-week program.

Other, often overlooked, sources of inflammation are mold in your surroundings in damp basements or moldy bathrooms, or hidden in the walls of your house: environmental allergies, a hidden infection such as a virus, parasite, or bacteria that doesn't cause immediately obvious symptoms; or a medication you are taking, and even toxins such as mercury or pesticides.

Stress may also make you inflamed.

And while just sitting around doing nothing also causes inflammation, regular exercise is one of the best-known anti-inflammatories on the planet.[1]

Multivitamins are also a great natural inflammation-fighting tool.[2]

Sometimes locating and eliminating the sources of inflammation requires detective work, testing, and working with an experienced doctor, but the results for your brain, your weight, and your health will be worth the effort.

Self-Care Plan

Cooling off inflammation requires only a few basic steps

Eat an Anti-Inflammatory Diet

The six-week plan is designed to be anti-inflammatory, but be sure to add extra anti-inflammatory herbs in your cooking:

❖ Add anti-inflammatory herbs, including turmeric (a source of curcumin), ginger, and rosemary, to your diet daily.

Get Rid of Hidden Food Allergies

Many people suffer needlessly with hidden food sensitivities and allergies. The most powerful, immediate, and dramatic results you can achieve for reducing systemic inflammation is to eliminate the most common food allergens in your diet: gluten, dairy, eggs, yeast, corn, peanuts, citrus, and occasionally soy.

In the six-week plan in Part III, I have provided you a method for eliminating the top two allergens—gluten and dairy—from your diet. This is because these are the most common allergens that affect the brain and benefit almost everyone.

However, for some people the other food allergens mentioned above may be a problem. If you still experience problems with inflammation after the six-week program is over, you may need to go on a more rigorous elimination and reintroduction program.

The UltraSimple Diet provides all the guidance, tools, and resources for you to do this successfully. If you follow the UltraMind Solution and the Self-Care program for six weeks and don't get the results you expect, I strongly suggest you do the program outlined in *The UltraSimple Diet* for two weeks, then reintroduce foods slowly to identify the connection between what you are eating and how you feel.

For most of you, eliminating gluten and dairy (by far the worst culprits) will give you significant anti-inflammatory benefit without having to do *The UltraSimple Diet*.

Special Note: Sugar and Refined Carbohydrates

The biggest cause of inflammation in our culture is belly fat resulting from insulin resistance. Too much sugar promotes high insulin levels, which trigger a domino effect leading to system-wide damage, including inflammation.

Fixing insulin resistance by following the recommendations for healthy eating in Part III will take care of much of the inflammation we see from our diet other than hidden food allergies.

Supplements to Reduce Inflammation

The nutritional supplement recommendation in Part III, including a multivitamin, omega-3 fats, and vitamin D, all have powerful anti-inflammatory benefits. Here are some additional anti-inflammatory supplements that can be helpful:

- Turmeric—the yellow spice found in curry is the best anti-inflammatory. Take 200 mg twice a day with food.
- A well-researched combination of anti-inflammatory herbs (including turmeric, ginger, and rosemary) can be used. Take one softgel of Zyflamend by New Chapter twice a day with meals.
- Enzymes, four capsules twice a day between meals for six weeks (bromelain and other proteolytic enzymes).

MEDICAL CARE PLAN

1. Testing for inflammation may include C-reactive protein (a generalized marker for inflammation), autoimmune markers (ESR, anti-CCP, TPO, ANA), or food allergies (IgG or IgE), and celiac- or gluten-testing. Testing for hidden infections, including viruses, bacteria, parasites, and yeast, may also be helpful.
2. Specific treatments for infections or more aggressive treatments for autoimmunity and allergies may be needed.

CHAPTER 25

KEY #4: FIX YOUR DIGESTION

One of the most powerful things you can do to fix your brain is fix your gut. The link is clear, and the results are often immediate and dramatic. Clear out the bad bugs, eliminate food allergens, support digestion with enzymes, add in healthy bacteria or probiotics, prebiotics (fiber fertilizer for probiotics), healing nutrients, and learn to find the pause button so your second brain can relax too.

This is an easy, clear, and simple process that, if followed, can achieve dramatic results quickly, not only for your brain and mood, but also for your overall health and well-being.

Once your gut is healthy you can keep toxins and allergens out, cool off inflammation, and digest and absorb all the nutrients you need to run your body and your brain at top performance.

Self-Care Plan

Often you can heal your gut by taking the few simple steps I describe below.

A Gut-Healing Diet

- ❖ The whole, real, fresh-food eating plan in Part III that includes the elimination of dairy and gluten, sugars, and sugar alcohols may by itself do much to heal your gut.
- ❖ If you scored in the Self-Care section on the "Gut" quiz or if you always feel bloated after eating, follow the UltraMind Solution (Part III) *and* eliminate all grains and beans from your diet for six weeks (these foods are easily fermented and feed yeast and bacteria). This may "starve" the yeast or bacteria, and

may be enough for many to heal the gut without antibiotics or antifungals that clear out the bad bugs.

Lifestyle Factors and Your Gut

In addition to the dietary factors above, the following lifestyle changes can also help you heal your gut:

+ Chew each mouthful of food twenty-five to fifty times—or at least try! This releases EGF (epithelial growth factor), needed for repair and healing of the digestive lining.
+ Eat slowly and do not do anything else while eating. Remember, it takes twenty minutes for the brain to get the message that the stomach is full.
+ Never eat standing up.

Gut-Healing Supplements

In addition to taking the probiotics included in the six-week UltraMind Solution, taking digestive enzymes and hydrochloric acid at the onset of a gut-healing program is very effective. The enzymes help break down the food and prevent food allergies and the harmful effects of partially digested food products, which trigger allergy. The overgrowth of bacteria in your gut can ferment these half-digested starches and cause more havoc, such as bloating and gas.

Here is what I suggest.

Enzymes

You should take a good, plant-based, broad-spectrum digestive enzyme. This should contain enzymes that break down proteins (proteases), fats (lipases), and carbohydrates (amylases). There is also an important enzyme found to be particularly helpful in addressing neurological issues that result from partially digested gluten and dairy. It is called DPP IV. Anyone who scored high enough to work the steps in this chapter should:

+ Take two capsules of broad-spectrum enzymes containing proteases, lipases, and amylases with each meal for at least six months while your gut is healing.

Hydrochloric Acid Support

Many of us think that too much stomach acid is our problem, and for some it may be. But often, digestive problems occur because of weak stomach acid, which actually can, in some cases, be the cause of reflux and heartburn. Acid-blocking medications often compound the problem. Adequate stomach acid is needed to break down food and activate digestive enzymes.

Betaine or hydrochloric-acid supplements must be used carefully and usually under the supervision of a health-care practitioner. But they can often be very helpful while your gut is healing.

❖ Start with one capsule or tablet at the beginning of each meal. Increase the dose by one capsule per meal until you have a warm feeling in your stomach. Then drop back down to the dose just before the warm feeling occurred.

A Special Probiotic: Yeast against Yeast

A basic probiotic supplement is necessary for the six-week UltraMind Solution. But there is a unique and often helpful probiotic that many find counterintuitive—why would we take one strain of yeast to kill other yeasts? It has profound benefits in controlling diarrhea, fighting other yeasts in the gut, controlling bad bugs such as Clostridia, improving gut immunity, improving digestive enzyme function, reducing inflammation, and improving overall gut function. I find it is one of the mainstays of my gut-repair program. Take:

❖ Saccharomyces boulardii, 150 mg to 250 mg (3 billion to 5 billion CFUs) one or two times a day on an empty stomach.

Gut Repair: Healing Nutrients and Herbs

Specialized gut-support products and nutrients are often necessary for gut healing and repair. These are the final tools for correcting digestive problems, healing a leaky gut, and reducing relapse or recurrence of digestive, immune, and brain problems.

The following should be taken for three months, depending on the severity of symptoms and response to treatment. Add a few other supplements at the repair stage (after removing the bad bugs, allergens, and toxins). These compounds needed for gut repair can be divided into two main categories:

Gut Food

✢ Glutamine, 2,500 mg twice a day
  ✢ You can use the powder or capsule form.
  ✢ This is a nonessential amino acid that is the preferred fuel for the lining of the small intestine and can greatly facilitate healing. It can be taken for one to two months. It generally comes in powder form and is often combined with other compounds that facilitate gut repair.

Gut Anti-inflammatories

✢ Quercitin, 500 mg twice a day with food and other bioflavonoids
  ✢ This potent anti-inflammatory is helpful in restoring balance in the gut.

MEDICAL CARE PLAN

Very often some simple dietary changes and supplements can help overcome years of digestive problems and help improve the secondary mood and brain dysfunction that results. However, this is an area where it is often helpful to have some testing and to work with a doctor of Functional Medicine who knows how to address and work with digestive problems.

The healing process takes four main steps, which have to be done in the right order for you to get the best results. This is often referred to as the 4R program.

1. Remove any offending factors, including potential food allergens; overgrowth of bacteria, yeast, parasites; and toxins such as heavy metals (see chapters 10 and 26 on detoxification).
2. Replace missing or weakened enzymes, acid, and fiber or prebiotics to help fertilize the healthy bacteria.
3. Reinnoculate with probiotics or beneficial bacteria.
4. Repair the intestinal lining with healing nutrients.

Eliminating allergens and taking enzymes, prebiotics, probiotics, and healing nutrients can be done without medical care, *except* if you have a significant overgrowth of bacteria in your small intestine, yeast overgrowth, infestation with parasites, or heavy metal toxicity.

Testing is often needed to identify these problems. Then medication is often needed for adequate treatment. Sometimes herbs can be helpful as well in reducing the bad bugs. So you can try working through fixing your gut on your own, but if things don't improve it may be time for testing and medication with your doctor's help.

Remember, if you are standing on a tack it takes a lot of aspirin to feel better. If you have too much bacteria, yeast, or a parasite, you can eliminate all the foods you like or add all the healthy bacteria, but it may be an uphill battle unless you fully address any imbalances or infections with bugs in the gut.

SPECIAL NOTE: TREATING BUGS

Bugs that affect the gut come in three main varieties.

1. Bacteria
2. Yeast
3. Parasites

Each type of bug needs different treatment. Testing can identify which bug or bugs are a problem for you.

Herbal therapies can often be helpful, but most of the time a short course of curative medication is necessary and dramatically effective.

Guidance from a trained practitioner is often necessary to test for and treat these problems. You can also get more information and a detailed guide for testing and treatment of bad bugs in your gut by going to www.ultramind.com/guide and downloading the companion guide for this book. It includes not only additional information on healing your gut but also many other tips and tools to make this program more powerful and easier to follow.

CHAPTER 26

KEY #5: ENHANCE DETOXIFICATION

The sustainability of our environment is directly connected to the sustainability of our health. Identifying if and how we are toxic, and addressing it directly by changing our habits, our choices, and our purchases in the marketplace, can have a global effect.

The connection between toxins and their effects on our brains are well established. The link between our addiction to energy, industrialization, and the millions of pounds of chemicals and heavy metals released every year into our environment, and the epidemics of autism, ADHD, Alzheimer's, Parkinson's, and mood disorders, as well as heart disease, obesity, and cancer, should make us all stop and think about how we live.

Small choices can make a big difference. Imagine if one day everyone shifted to organic food, or as they did in Europe, to non-GMO food (genetically modified organisms). It would change the agriculture industry overnight.

That is why I believe it is important for everyone to live clean and green.

In most cases, the techniques for limiting your exposure to environmental toxins I outlined in Part III will help you detoxify and stay free of toxic substances.

Unfortunately, in some cases people have already been exposed to so much toxic material they need a little extra help. If you scored over 6 on the "Toxins" quiz, this may apply to you.

In this case, learning how your body's own detoxification system works, and how to optimize its function, is key to achieving and maintaining optimal health. There is no great mystery on how do to this.

There are a few simple things you can do to boost your detoxification system.

Dietary Support for Detoxification

Thankfully, plants have evolved many protective defenses against pests and infection, called phytonutrients. Many of these also help human biology to function better—especially in the realm of detoxification.

These defenses are better developed in organic foods because they have to work harder to survive. Eating organic food provides higher concentrations of these protective detoxifying, antioxidant, and anti-inflammatory compounds. These compounds may outweigh the benefits we can get from other nutritional supplements in their overall effects on our health.

And they taste better!

The Detox Powerhouses

While I recommend these healing foods as part of the basic eating plan in Part III of the UltraMind Solution, it is worth emphasizing how important they are, and ensuring that you include these in your daily diet. There are many others that help in detoxification, including cilantro, celery, parsley, dandelion greens, citrus peels, and rosemary, but these are the ones I want you to be sure to include in your diet as often as possible—even daily.

- Cruciferous vegetables (cabbage, broccoli, collards, kale, Brussels sprouts, Chinese cabbage, bok choy, arugula, radish, wasabi, watercress, kohlrabi, mustard greens, rutabaga, turnips). Eat at least one to two cups, cooked, daily.
- Curcuminoids (turmeric and curry)
- One to two cups of green tea a day boosts liver detoxification (increases GST or glutathione enzymes).
- High-quality sulfur-containing proteins or foods—eggs, garlic (a few cloves a day), onions

Supplements to Enhance Detoxification

There are many detoxification pathways—or routes for toxins to get out of the body. But these pathways require many helpers. Vitamins, minerals, amino acids, special nutrients, and a whole range of phytonutrients from the foods noted above are needed for our detox system to function day in and day out.

As I explained in chapter 10, the most important factor for our detoxification system is keeping our glutathione levels up. Glutathione is the main detoxifier in the body (an antioxidant and immune booster). Our body needs to regenerate it all the time. That is why we need to keep the sulfation train and the methylation train running smoothly. Our brains and our health depend on it.

The main nutrients helpful in boosting glutathione are all the methylation nutrients, zinc, and selenium that are part of your basic supplement program.

In fact, as far as my personal supplement program goes, besides taking a multivitamin and fish oil, supporting my glutathione levels is the most important thing I do every day for my health.

Here are some additional supplements you can take to do that:

- N-acetylcysteine or NAC, 500 mg twice a day
  - This is a special amino acid that dramatically increases glutathione. It is even used in the emergency room to treat liver failure from Tylenol overdose.
- Buffered ascorbic acid (vitamin C), 1,000 mg twice a day *in addition to what is in your basic multivitamin*
  - Buffered vitamin C with mineral ascorbates in powder, capsule, or tablets during periods of increased detoxification is especially useful.
  - Too much vitamin C may cause diarrhea. Simply reduce the dose.
- Milk thistle (silymarin), 140 mg twice a day of a standardized extract
  - This herb has long been used in liver disease and helps boost glutathione levels.

Hyperthermic Therapy or Heat Therapy (Saunas)

Saunas and heat therapies are an ancient method of cleansing. The Native American sweat lodge was a tool for physical and spiritual purification. Today, the Environmental Protection Agency has shown that sauna therapy increases excretion of heavy metals (lead, mercury, cadmium, and fat-soluble chemicals—PCBs, PBBs, and HCBs). It seems science has finally caught up with these historical practices for maintaining health.

The process of liberating fat-stored toxins through sweating must be done carefully and sometimes under a doctor's supervision to prevent complications.

Follow these guidelines for safe detoxification.

Saunas or Steam Baths

- Find a health club or gym near you that has a sauna or steam room.
- Drink at least sixteen ounces of purified water before entering the sauna.
- Drink during the treatment if you can, and at least sixteen ounces after the therapy to help flush the mobilized toxins through your kidneys and circulation. Drink more if you are thirsty.
- If you are generally healthy, start with ten minutes and increase by five minutes daily to a maximum of thirty to forty-five minutes. You should take cold dips or rinses in the shower every ten minutes.
- If you are chronically ill, or take medication, be sure to get your doctor's permission and start with five minutes and increase gradually as tolerated.
- Sauna temperatures should be no higher than 140 to 150 degrees Farenheit for those with environmental illness or a history of increased toxic exposures.
- Far infrared saunas are used at lower temperatures and may be more easily tolerated than regular saunas for liberating stored toxins. They may also be more effective at helping you get rid of stored toxins. (See Resources for suggestions.)
- Shower thoroughly with soap after the sauna to remove the liberated toxins from your skin.

✢ For those needing an intensive detoxification program, daily saunas for six weeks can be dramatically helpful with once-a-week maintenance therapy afterward.

✢ Some people have symptoms from the release of toxins, including skin rashes, headaches, fatigue, nausea, irritable bowel, and confusion or memory problems. If you experience these side effects, take buffered vitamin C or get the help of a Functional Medicine practitioner.

MEDICAL CARE PLAN

In a medically supervised detoxification program, many other nutrients, herbs, and phytonutrients may be used, including alpha lipoic acid, bioactive whey protein, amino acids such as taurine, glycine, glutamine, calcium-D-glucarate, and methionine.

Specialized tests, which assess your body's detoxification system, including genetic testing for detoxification enzymes, and tests for heavy metals, including tests of blood, urine, and hair, may be necessary.

Detoxifying from heavy metals is an important step on the road to health for many and needs to be done with an experienced and qualified health-care practitioner.

SPECIAL NOTE: DETOXIFYING FROM HEAVY METALS

Aside from addressing hidden food allergens and helping people balance their blood sugar and consume a whole-foods diet, one of the most powerful ways to correct many chronic health problems is a medically supervised heavy-metal detoxification program.

Proper testing, preparation, and care are needed in order for safe and effective heavy-metal detoxification. Below you will find the steps I often recommend just to prepare my patients for heavy-metal detoxification. I will also outline options available for treatment.

I want to reinforce that this *must* be done with a qualified health-care practitioner.

Below I describe the most important steps to help prepare you for safe metal removal. Once you have improved your health and optimized your detoxification system, you can begin working to remove metals from your body through various approaches, including safe amalgam removal (see www.iaomt .org) and the use of chelating agents such as DMSA, which is a prescription medication designed and approved for lead removal in children, but also effective for mercury and many other toxic metals.

While there needs to be more research in this area, the current body of evidence, my experience, and the experience of thousands of other doctors and patients make it clear to me that this can be a critical part of the process of healing for chronic illness, including mood, behavior, and neurodegenerative diseases such as autism, ADHD, and dementia.

For an excellent consensus position paper on heavy-metal detoxification developed by the group involved with autism treatment called DAN! see www.autism.com/triggers/vaccine/heavymetals.pdf.

GETTING READY FOR DETOXIFICATION

These are the general guidelines I use with my patients for you to follow with your doctor. They should generally be done in collaboration with your health-care practioner and may take a few months.

1. *Optimize Gut Function*—First optimize your gut function by eliminating the common food allergens and taking probiotics and enzymes for one to two months before detoxifying.
2. *Optimize Your Nutritional Status for Detoxification*—You can do this by using healthy fats (omega-3 fats, olive oil, and flax oil), the amino acids found in plants and lean animal proteins (which boost your liver's detoxification capacity), and minerals, particularly zinc and selenium (which help your body detoxify metals).
3. *Enhance Your Liver's Detoxification Pathways*—Especially the sulfation and methylation pathways—by taking folate, B_{12}, and B_6, and eating foods that contain sulfur, such as broccoli, collards, kale, daikon radish, garlic, onions, and omega-3 eggs, as well as supplements such as alpha lipoic acid and n-acetylcysteine.
4. *Use Herbal Support for Heavy-Metal Detoxification*—Include alginate, cilantro, garlic, and milk thistle.
5. *Start Sauna Therapy*—Make sure you take adequate electrolyte and mineral replacement to prevent dehydration and mineral loss from the sweat.
6. *Optimize Elimination Routes for Metals*—This includes your urine, stool, and sweat by drinking plenty of clean pure water, eating a diet high in plant fibers, and taking daily saunas for thirty minutes.

CHAPTER 27

KEY #6: BOOST ENERGY METABOLISM

Energy is something we lose with age. But it can also be lost because of anything that triggers more free radicals and oxidative stress or damage to our mitochondria.

Even as we are learning how mitochondrial injury is a final common pathway in so many neurological and psychiatric disorders, fortunately we are also learning how to protect and defend ourselves.

Getting a metabolic tune-up is not only possible, but also necessary for most of us. This is especially true for those whose score indicates either Self-Care or Medical Care in the quiz in chapter 11.

Thankfully, by eating a plant-based diet, reducing toxic exposures, and supplementing with mitochondrial protective and antioxidant compounds, we can protect and restore our energy metabolism to optimal function.

Self-Care Plan

Here is what you need to do to boost your energy metabolism.

Dietary Changes to Boost and Improve Energy Production

The dietary factors that boost your energy metabolism are already built into the UltraMind Solution. Just be sure to focus on antioxidant-rich foods such as yellow and orange fruits and vegetables, blueberries, red grapes, spinach, green tea, and the herbs turmeric, ginger, and garlic. The darker and richer the color, the more potent the antioxidants and energy boosters are in food.

Supplements to Boost Energy and Reduce Oxidative Stress

The super nutrients that fire up your energy factories or mitochondria include:

Super Mitochondrial-Boosting Nutrients

There are a number of special nutrients that are not "essential" but become essential under conditions of stress, toxicity, and aging and can dramatically improve energy production, improve mitochondrial function, and protect the mitochondria from damage. The most important are:

- Acetyl-L-carnitine, 500 mg twice a day
- Alpha lipoic acid, 100 mg twice a day
- Coenzyme Q10, 100 mg a day
- D-ribose, 5 gm a day in powder
- NADH, 10 mg a day
  - This energy booster is taken as a tablet that dissolves under your tongue.

Lifestyle Changes for Boosting Energy

The most important lifestyle factor for supporting your mitochondria and increasing your energy is exercise. In Part III, I have outlined some exercise options for you to follow. If you don't exercise and you scored high in this key, you need to get moving.

I particularly recommend using an interval training program. It will give you an excellent aerobic workout and it will save you time.

I have outlined a complete interval training program in *The UltraMind Solution Companion Guide*. Please go to www.ultramind.com/guide and download this free guide if you want to learn more.

MEDICAL CARE PLAN

1. There are a number of tests, including those of organic acids and cardiometabolic stress testing as well as tests for oxidative stress (8 OHDG, or lipid peroxides), that help your doctor personalize treatment and monitor your progress.

(continued)

2. Additional supplements, including creatine, NAC, sulfate, and reduced glutathione, may also be recommended.

3. Resveratrol derivatives or extracts are powerful mitochondrial energy boosters and are in drug development now (Sirtris was just purchased by GlaxoSmithKline).

4. Your doctor may prescribe additional energy-boosting treatments and exercises such as interval training.

CHAPTER 28

KEY #7: CALM YOUR MIND

Most of us were never trained to calm ourselves. Unless, of course, we do it with a big jelly doughnut or a glass of chardonnay. A runaway stress response has become a part of our daily lives, but most of us are unaware that we are in a perpetual state of alarm. It is just how we are.

Our bodies and brains react to stress immediately and constantly. Unrelieved stress triggers biological responses that become worn into deep grooves in our moods and brain function.

Of course, we know that stress can result from psychological causes—feeling powerless and helpless at work or in our relationships—in other words, toxic thoughts, beliefs, and attitudes. But toxic foods, environmental toxins, digestive problems, and even infections can also trigger the same biological stress response.

That is why each of us must find a way to push our pause button on a daily basis. Most of us don't even know where it is. But we must learn how to identify the ways in which we are stressed, try to minimize them, and then actively learn to engage the relaxation response or the pause button. This is key to long-term brain health. We have to make it part of our daily lives.

Identifying what is stressing you out and learning to press the pause button are critically important, especially when you are out of balance in this key. If you scored over 7 on the "Adrenal Dysfunction" quiz, the following steps may help you find balance again.

Self-Care Plan

Practicing Self-Care to calm your mind is relatively easy.

Identify and Reduce the Causes of Stress

Looking closely at the habits of our life—both what we do and how we think—is not something most of us do on a regular basis. We often don't connect the choices we make in our diet, in our relationships, or in our work with how we feel every day. Nor do we equate the way we feel with the use of brain-altering substances like sugar, caffeine, and alcohol.

There is a big disconnect for many in understanding that the way we live our lives makes us sick and leads to trouble focusing, thinking, remembering, or just feeling happy and alive.

Eating junk food, drinking six cups of coffee a day, having those two cocktails at night to calm down, watching four hours of television a day, doing work we hate, or being stuck in relationships that don't give us peace or joy—we tend to accept these without too much thought about how they drive our moods and brain function.

We cannot eliminate all the causes of stress, but we can take an inventory—a close examination of our life—and consider which things we can let go of that are triggering stress and which things we can add that help us heal and thrive.

Consider which things give you energy and which things deplete it. Take a piece of paper, and in one column write down all those things that rob you of energy. Beside it, in another column, write down all the things that give it to you.

Make an agreement with yourself to eliminate at least one thing this week that robs you of energy and add one thing to your life that gives you energy. Do this once a week during the six-week program.

For those things you cannot eliminate, you can transform your way of thinking about them. You can move from your ordinary thinking to extraordinary thinking about your life, from thinking that creates "dis-ease" to thinking that creates well-being for you.

For now, make a list of your own stressors. I have included a simple form to do this in *The UltraMind Solution Companion Guide*. Go to www .ultramind.com/guide to download the guide.

Social or Psychosocial Stressors

- ❖ Thoughts and beliefs about ourselves
- ❖ Jobs
- ❖ Relationships

✛ Financial situation
✛ Kids
✛ Psychological disorders (i.e., depression, anxiety, etc.)
✛ Low self-esteem
✛ The state of the world (i.e., the international political situation, problems in your neighborhood, etc.)

Physical Stressors

✛ Overweight or obesity
✛ Chronic illness
✛ Allergens
✛ Toxins
✛ Sugar and high-fructose corn syrup
✛ Saturated and trans fats
✛ Processed foods
✛ Chronic infections
✛ Alcohol, tobacco, drugs

Once you have made a list of your various stressors, try to think of ways that you might eliminate them. In some cases, this is easy. For example, if you are sitting watching four hours of television a day or drinking half a bottle of wine every night, these might be physical stressors for you. Instead of watching TV you can take an hour to move your body or do something else that gives you energy. Instead of drinking half a bottle of wine every night, you can choose to drink less.

In other cases, it may be more difficult. If you are dealing with chronic psychological or health issues, for example, it will probably take some energy to get them worked out.

But always remember you *can* take some action to reduce the amount of stress in your life.

Find the Pause Button: Learning Life Skills for Thriving

My three favorite tools for pushing my pause button are described in Part III and in other keys. They are:

1. Soft-Belly Breathing (the UltraMind Solution)
2. The UltraBath (the UltraMind Solution)
3. Hyperthermic or Sauna Therapy (Enhance Detoxification)

You need to find your own favorites: try to incorporate a few of these during your six-week program.

Other Pause Button Pushers

- *Yoga* is a wonderful way to increase fitness and flexibility, calm your mind, and deeply relax. There are classes in almost every town. My favorite yogic technique is called yogic sleep or yoga "nidra." See the Resources for recommendations on CDs, videos, and DVDs for yoga and relaxation.
- *Massage.* Learn massage and use it on your partner or friends. And then exchange. Or get a massage as often as you can.
- *Tense and relax.* By slowly tensing and relaxing your whole body (all at once or moving progressively from one muscle group to the next—face, neck and shoulders, arms, legs) and then relaxing your whole body (or each muscle group progressively), you will shift the stress response and enter into deep relaxation.
- *Use biofeedback.* There are some wonderful computer-simulated tools and devices that can lead you through various mental and physical exercises that will activate the stress response. See the Resources for some options. Just load it into your computer, put three little sensors on your fingers that measure your heart rate variability, and take a journey into deep relaxation.
- *Learn meditation.* Mindfulness meditation is a powerful, well-researched tool developed by Buddhists, but now practiced and used all over the world, thanks to the work of Jon Kabat Zinn, Ph.D., of the University of Massachusetts, in many hospitals and medical centers. Read his book *Wherever You Go, There You Are* to learn basic meditation techniques or attend a local class on meditation.
- *Pray, chant, dance, and celebrate.* All these are ancient tools for healing and all help you deeply relax. Just pull down the shades, turn on the music, and dance in your living room.
- *Practice tai qi quan or qi gong.* These are ancient, energy-balancing tools that can help restore your health and calm your nervous system.
- *Writing away stress.* Journaling is a well studied and powerful tool to help improve mood and become more intimate with yourself. Studies show how it boosts immunity and improves mood.[1]

Daily journaling for twenty minutes can be helpful.

You can also try this well-researched tool, which can create immediate benefits: Set aside twenty minutes four days a week to write in your journal. Write nonstop about the most upsetting or traumatic experience of your life. Don't worry about spelling or grammar. Write about all your emotions and thoughts, as many details as you can remember, and any insights you have.

❖ *Be in nature.* A walk in the woods, or on the beach, a hike up a mountain, and watching a sunset all have soothing effects on us and help us push that pause button.

❖ *Listen to music.* Certain types of music have soothing effects on our nervous system. Listen to Bach, Chopin, Mozart, Pachelbel, and Vivaldi. Or to traditional types of music such as Benedictine monks chanting or Sanskrit chants.

❖ *Be artful.* Painting, drawing, sculpting, or participating in any of the arts engages our brains and minds, creating a soothing and calming effect.

Use Stress-Reducing Supplements and Herbs

Nutrients help regulate and control all the hormones and neurotransmitters involved in brain function and in the stress and relaxation responses. Stress can also quickly deplete the very nutrients needed for deep relaxation of the nervous system, including magnesium, the B vitamins, and vitamin C. These stress-reducing supplements are included in the basic recommendations for long-term supplements in Part III.

Herbs to Help You Adapt and Respond to Stress

Certain herbs help you adapt better to stress. If you want to add another dimension to your stress reduction program, try these herbal remedies alone or in combinations. You can reduce the overactivity and increase the resilience of the system by using adaptogenic (named that way because they may help you adapt to stress) or balancing herbs such as:

❖ Asian Ginseng Root Extract (*Panax ginseng*)—standardized to 8 percent (16 mg) ginsenosides—200 mg twice a day

❖ Rhodiola Root Extract (*Rhodiola rosea*)—standardized to 1 percent (0.5 mg) salidroside—100 mg twice a day

✛ Siberian Ginseng (*Eleuthrococcus senticosus*)—root, standardized to contain 0.8 percent eleutherosides—250 mg twice a day

---

MEDICAL CARE PLAN

1. Your doctor may recommend testing for stress hormones or heart rate variability.
2. Occasionally hormonal treatment with DHEA or low-dose cortisone can be helpful if you have adrenal burnout.

SPECIAL CONSIDERATIONS

In addition to the steps outlined in the six-week program and the keys, there are a few special considerations I would like to address before I close.

Sometimes it is not a toxin, allergen, infection, or nutrient-poor diet that makes us depressed or mentally ill. Sometimes it is just life itself—a divorce, childhood trauma, the death of a loved one, a crazy boss, or a major trauma.

During those times in life, seeking help from a trained psychotherapist, a social worker, or even a personal coach can be lifesaving and may help guide you through troubled times.

In traditional cultures, the family and social structure provided a container and meaning for all life's events. Today, unfortunately, many of us are left alone to struggle through life's transitions and questions. Getting support can help you heal and recover along with the UltraMind Solution.

As a former emergency room physician, I recognize that extreme times call for extreme measures. I use and support the intelligent, appropriate use of medication, including psychotropic medications when needed. They can often be helpful as a bridge for recovery from all the stresses and toxins that affect our brain and mind.

It may take months or years to heal from damage that has occurred over a lifetime. In extreme cases, the damage may be so deep that full recovery is not possible using the UltraMind Solution (although most see remarkable results in a few weeks). In some cases, combining medication with the tools of the UltraMind Solution can give people their lives back.

Working with an experienced psychopharmacologist who welcomes the integration of nutrition, supplements, exercise, and mind–body therapies is sometimes a necessary step to recovering a whole life.

Many times medications can be reduced or eliminated after applying the principles found in the UltraMind Solution.

I would caution you that psychotropic medications offer only partial solutions, often packaged with side effects. Tread intelligently, expect bumps on the road, and seek to find the causes of your suffering, which may be found in the stories of your life, on your plate, in your lifestyle, or in your toxic environment. You will rarely find the solution to your problems in a prescription bottle.

If you need to, use medication without guilt just as you would any other tool to rebuild your life. And do not be afraid to put it down when you have rebuilt your health and your world.

Special Herbs for the Brain

A few other herbs and nutrients deserve special mention. I often find these beneficial in patients with mood or memory problems. I encourage you to work with your health-care practitioner when you use these herbs and nutrients. They can be used safely and effectively for many.

Memory-Enhancing Herbs

Huperzine A

Huperzine A is derived from Chinese club moss and has shown significant benefits in dementia with few side effects. Clinical trials have shown that huperzine A is comparably effective to the drugs currently on the market, and may even be a bit safer in terms of side effects. It works by increasing acetylcholine in the brain, in a similar way to the current medications for Alzheimer's.

Currently, the National Institute on Aging is conducting a Phase II clinical trial to evaluate the safety and efficiency of huperzine A in the treatment of Alzheimer's disease in a randomized controlled trial of its effect on cognitive function.

The recommended dose is 100 mcg twice a day.

Vinpocetine

Vinpocetine is an extract of the periwinkle plant. More than fifty studies have found it effective in improving blood flow to the brain, improving energy production in the brain, and preventing blood clots.

The recommended dose is 5 to 10 mg twice a day.

If you are taking blood-thinning medicine, do not take this herb.

Ginkgo biloba

Ginkgo biloba is a powerful brain antioxidant and improves circulation. It has been used for thousands of years in traditional Chinese medicine for memory and mental health.

Take Ginkgo Leaf Extract 80 to 160 mg twice a day (*Ginkgo biloba*)—standardized to 24 percent ginkgoflavonglycosides and 6 percent terpene lactones.

Mood-Enhancing Herbs and Supplements

St. John's Wort

St. John's Wort contains many phytonutrients, called hypericins, that are helpful in the treatment of depression. It can be helpful in those with serotonin deficiency or with anxiety or sleep problems. Do not combine this with any other antidepressants or psychotropic medication (such as MAO inhibitors).

The therapeutic dose is 300 to 450 mg twice a day.

SAMe

SAMe is an amino acid that is formed as part of your methylation cycle. It has been researched extensively and found effective for depression.

Start with a dose of 400 mg four times a day, or 800 mg twice a day.

A response usually occurs within three weeks and you can then reduce the dose to 400 mg twice a day.

Use with your methylation supplement and magnesium.

If you have bipolar disorder, use this amino acid only with your doctor's supervision.

CONCLUSION

The Future of Medicine

You will observe with concern how long a useful truth may be known and exist, before it is generally received and practiced upon.

—BENJAMIN FRANKLIN

Many of my patients know intuitively that their various complaints must be related in some fashion. They don't know exactly what's wrong or how to find the answers, but they know that it is not in the type of medical care we have now. They understand that a health-care system focused on specialization and pharmacologic treatments of specific "diseases" often misses the underlying story of the origins and the reasons for their suffering.

They intuitively know that a new approach to medicine, one in which we treat the underlying systems that cause disease when they are out of balance, would work better than the paradigm we are currently stuck in. They know this even if they have never heard the terms Functional Medicine or "systems biology."

Nonetheless, I, like almost every other doctor in the country, was trained to be a clinical pharmacologist, not a clinical physiologist, biochemist, geneticist, or practitioner of Functional Medicine. I was trained to dispense medication. I was not trained to process or understand biological information systems, or to make sense of patterns and relationships and connections in biological systems. I was not trained to see how everything communicates with everything else.

However, by treating thousands of patients like Clayton (whom you learned about in Part I) and all the others you have learned about in this book for more than twenty years, and by studying the rich medical literature that explains, in detail, the way the underlying systems in our body create health or illness, I have been able to develop a whole new way of understanding medicine, one that is radically different than the method of diagnosis and treatment I was trained in.

We are in the middle of an information revolution—not just in technology but also in biology. What I have studied and learned about for more than a decade now is the future of medicine. Functional Medicine and systems biology are the wave of the future, and it is what you just learned while you read *The UltraMind Solution*.

Looking in the Wrong Place for Answers

Could it be that we are looking in the wrong place for the answers to our epidemic of neurological and psychiatric disorders? Could it be that the medications we use for mood and brain disorders attempt to control the smoke while ignoring the fire?

Could it be that these are, in fact, not primary brain disorders at all, but systemic disorders that affect the brain? And could it be that therapies primarily aimed at altering brain function through antidepressants, stimulants, antipsychotics, and seizure medications may miss the primary mechanisms or disturbances that show up as behavioral, mood, or neurological symptoms?

New research shows clearly that the communication between the brain and the body is bidirectional. Even though Mind-Body Medicine has been studied and accepted as legitimate,[1] it provides only a one-dimensional view of the interaction between the brain and the body.[2]

The conclusion from the science is irrefutable and must be heeded to effectively address the epidemic of "broken brains"—mood disorders, attention deficit disorder, autism, psychoses, Alzheimer's, Parkinson's, and other neurodegenerative disorders.

Unless we focus on the metabolic, nutritional, and environmental influences that exert their effects on the brain *through the body,* we will not succeed in our efforts to promote mental and cognitive well-being.

The next frontier in medicine is to define how "body" dysfunction or imbalances lead to abnormal brain chemistry and communication between brain cells, altered behavior, mood, and neurodegeneration.

Today there is a new model of thinking in medical science. It is called Functional Medicine. It provides a new road map for navigating the mysteries of how the body works together as a whole system.

Science is by nature reductionistic, breaking things into smaller and smaller parts and learning what each of them do separately. But what is missing in science is synthesis and integration. Putting the pieces of the puzzle back together. There are millions of bits of data and information, and yet for most practitioners of medicine they are strewn about the floor like a million puzzle pieces.

Until we put the pieces of the puzzle together, we cannot see what picture it forms, or what story it tells us about the mystery of how the body works, and how the mind, brain, and body are all connected and intertwined.

Functional Medicine is a method of putting those pieces together so we can see the picture of the whole clearly. It is not a new treatment or test or a new alternative method. It is just a way of putting together the pieces of the puzzle of chronic disease in a new way so we can truly see what is going on. It is a practical method of approaching each patient as an individual.

The era of treating all depressed or anxious or ADHD or autistic or demented people the same way is over. There may be dozens of causes of depression or autism or dementia or ADHD. *Finding the right cause and treatment for each individual will require a different way of practicing medicine.*

This is a radical shift from our conventional training where we use symptoms to make a diagnosis and then match a drug to that diagnosis. The science of genomics and molecular biology is forcing us to radically redefine disease. Could it be that many different "diseases" show up as the same symptoms? For example, can a nutritional deficiency, or a toxic level of mercury, or a food allergy all cause memory problems, attention deficit disorder, or depression?

Today we know that they can.

The symptoms may be exactly the same for people with the same label or "disease," but the causes and treatment are completely different. The body (or brain) has only so many ways of saying ouch—sadness, happiness, anxiousness, forgetfulness, trouble with attention—but the reasons each person has that experience may be completely different.

So how can we find a new model that gets to the root of the problem?

This model already exists. This new medical paradigm has been laid out in detail in *The Textbook of Functional Medicine* (to which I contributed two chapters). It is a story of how all the pieces of the puzzle that create disease and promote health fit together. It is based on excellent science. There are about twenty thousand scientific references, and contributions from scientific giants.

This model is the medicine of the future, but it is available to you today. It is what the seven keys to UltraWellness and the UltraMind Solution are based on, and it is what you have already begun to learn about in the pages of this book.

But this road map is focused mostly on basic research. The practical application of this thinking is not being explored directly. But people do not need to wait twenty years to take advantage of this thinking. It is available now and it is the approach of Functional Medicine, or what I call Ultra-Wellness (www.ultrawellness.com).

It is only by teasing apart how each of these fundamental physiological processes alters brain function and studying how correcting them can restore normal function that a new model of psychiatry, neurology, and clinical neuroscience can emerge; one that provides more satisfactory answers than only partially effective pharmacologic treatments.

The paradox is that in the detail of any one pattern or system of physiologic imbalance, the answer will not be found. It is only by putting together all the pieces of the puzzle, by assessing and treating all the imbalanced systems (nutritional, hormonal, inflammatory, immune, digestive, toxic, energy metabolism and oxidative stress, and mind-body) simultaneously that true advances can occur.

Single drugs or methods are destined to fail. The nature of biology is that of a system, one whole, interdependent, interconnected system.

In order to make real progress we must understand how our genes are affected by environment and lifestyle and how that leads to disturbances in cellular communication, physiology, and biochemistry, which are responsible for much of the accelerating rate of psychiatric and neurological disease in the twenty-first century.

This new thinking will provide relief for millions if applied deliberately and carefully.

Mark Hyman, M.D.
West Stockbridge, Massachusetts
June 2008

ACKNOWLEDGMENTS

The opportunity to write a book is both a gift and a burden. Its virtues are more often borrowed, and its errors entirely my own. It is a journey supported by the vast community I find myself living in and exploring with wonder.

The community that wrote this book through me includes all the scientists who worked thanklessly to understand the mysteries of the human body and brain, and made all the puzzle pieces I put together in this story. It also includes all my patients who trusted me, then worked with me to find the answers to their health and struggles with broken bodies and broken brains. They taught me more than they realized.

My agent Richard Pine, with patience, clarity, insight, and an uncommon directness, has guided this book from the beginning, as usual in his understated loving way. Beth Wareham, my editor; Susan Moldow, my publisher; and all my friends and supporters at Simon & Schuster have supported me from the beginning to the end, over and over again believing in and making possible the birth of sometimes radical and often unexpected ideas. Sandi Mendelson, my publicist, and her team chip away at the noise in the media to get the truth to break through. Marc Stockman just "gets it" like no one else. He took scribblings on a napkin and helped me create a world of good from a naked hope for change. It was a good day when you showed up. Jeff Radich, who creates beauty and mini-miracles from my too often rough work. And Jessica Cerretani, who takes the edges off my writing and makes it go down easier. Liana Baum for her help making ideas into pictures. And Spencer Smith, my comrade in words who has given more than his mind to this book. He has given his heart and soul often when there was little left. Thank you!!!

The community that helped me write this book extends to well over a hundred people, all of whom I unfortunately can't name here. You know who you are—thank you, thank you, and thank you. I must mention a few special people who have inspired, helped, and supported me—Jeffrey Bland, who cracked open my world twelve years ago and it has never been the same; Sidney Baker, one of the greatest unrecognized and original thinkers of our time—in medicine and in life; my friends at the Institute for Functional Medicine—Laurie, David, Bethany, Robert, Jennifer, Joe, and Susan, and the many unnamed who just make it happen at IFM. And all those who have supported me from the beginning with their time and money to launch the future of medicine: John Bitzer, Stephen and Sandy Muss, Maja Hoffmann and Stanley Buchthal, Adelaide Gomer, Alicia Wittink, Ritchie Scaife, Jerry and Emy Lou Baldridge, Donna Karan, Daphne Barak, and so many more, including those who have yet to know how great a difference they can make with so little.

And without friendship and my whole community I couldn't do what I do—thank you for being there even when I am not—and for those unnamed, you who all know who you are: Marc David, David and Zea Piver, Jonathan and Michelle Kalman, Dan and Ditte Ruderman, Paul and Andrea DeBotton, Andy and Lisa Corn, Davidi and Ruth Gilo, David Ludwig, and the list goes on and on. I want to especially thank my good friend Damon Giglio, a generous and passionate soul who has given of himself over and over to be a catalyst for transformation and good in the world. And of course, there are all my cocreators of medicine's transformation who have touched me and taught personally, and each continue to create seismic shifts in our way of thinking and living. Thank you for supporting me and trusting me and guiding me: Dean Ornish, Mehmet C. Oz, James Gordon, Andrew Weil, Jon Kabat Zinn, Leo Galland, David Perlmutter, Frank Lipman, Jay Lombard, Patrick Hanaway, Robert Hedaya, Joel Evans, Catherine Willner, David Eisenberg, Bethany Hayes, David Jones, Tracy Gaudet, Kirk Daffner, Kenneth Pelletier, Peter Libby, and Martha Herbert.

My whole life would have taken a different turn if not for Kathie Swift, my nutritionist, and coconspirator who first inspired me to ask the questions that ultimately led to this book. Her tireless hours of assistance, work, dedication to our patients, to food, and to our work to change health care, in more ways than I can count, are essential to my life. Thank you. Without the support of my team at the UltraWellness Center, where I do my real work of seeing patients, I couldn't begin to do half of everything else. You are all my foundation and at the core of my life. Your contributions wash over me daily, thank you for showing up and believing. Thank you Donna, Liz, Deb, Heather, Maggie, Pam, Sarah, and Erica. And Nina—you are the glue that makes everything stick together and the balm that gets our patients well when nothing else has.

Last, and most important, my family has put up with the dangers of my passion (early mornings, late nights, and too many absences to remember). I could not have done this without all your love and belief in what I am doing. Thank you Pier, Rachel, Misha, Thor, Ace, Ruth, Richard, Saul, Jesse, Carrie, Michael, Ben, Sarah, Paul, Lauren, Jake, and Zachary. It is for you and because of you that I wake up every day grateful and joyful.

Mark Hyman, M.D.: Learning More
UltraWellness
www.ultrawellness.com/blog

The UltraWellness Blog is written by Mark Hyman, M.D., a leader in the emerging field of Functional Medicine. If you have faced chronic illness, struggle to overcome weight issues, have a lack of energy, problems sleeping, bad skin, or any other health issues, then you will want to read this to find out how you too can achieve UltraWellness—your key to lifelong vibrant health and vitality. UltraWellness promises to help you fix the core, underlying health problems for good, instead of simply dealing with the symptoms of those problems as other medical approaches do.

Sign up now to receive alerts when new blogs are posted.

The UltraWellness Center

45 Walker Street
Lenox, MA 01240
(413) 637-9991
www.ultrawellnesscenter.com

Lifelong health and vitality are our birthright. Few of us know why we lose them or how to get them back. At the UltraWellness Center, our team of doctors, nutritionists, nurses, and health coaches is committed to helping you reach optimal health by identifying the unique underlying causes of disease and treating them. Diet and lifestyle modifications in combination with nutritional and specialized testing, nutritional supplementation, and medications are used to address your individual needs, from creating wellness to treating chronic, complex medical problems.

Other Books and Resources by Mark Hyman, M.D.

Ultraprevention: The Six-Week Plan That Will Make You Healthy for Life (Scribner, 2003)
The Detox Box: A Program for Greater Health and Vitality (Sounds True, 2004)
The 5 Forces of Wellness: The Ultraprevention System for Living an Active, Age-Defying, Disease-Free Life (an audio program by Nightingale-Conant, 2006)
UltraMetabolism: The Simple Plan for Automatic Weight Loss (Scribner, 2006)

The UltraSimple Diet (Pocket Books, 2007)
The UltraMetabolism Cookbook (Scribner, 2007)

The UltraMind Solution Online Guide and Other Online Resources at www.ultramind.com

I have created a dynamic online resource guide to provide you with all the tools and links you need to be successful in finding your way back to health and an UltraMind. In the companion guide, you will find many tools and information to support you, including:

Real Food Resources

In the guide there are links to the best resources for eating whole, real, fresh food.

- Organic food
- Produce
- Grass-fed meat, poultry, dairy and eggs
- Healthy fish
- Wild foods
- Bean and legumes
- Grains
- Nuts, seeds, and oils
- Non-dairy beverages
- Spices, seasonings, sauces, soups
- Organic tea

I have also included links for:

- Therapeutic supplements for health and treatment
- Laboratories for specialized testing
- Safe personal-care products
- Further reading and favorite books

Integrative and Functional Medicine Practitioner Referrals

Finding a doctor or practitioner who can work with you as a partner is often not a simple or easy task, but there are more and more practitioners who apply the principles of Functional and Integrative Medicine in their practices. I have provided a list of organizations that can help you find a practitioner to help guide you. However, the background, training, and scope of practice differ considerably from person to person. Therefore you still must thoroughly investigate each practitioner's level of knowledge, training, skill, and scope of practice. This information is presented to start you on your inquiry. It is still your responsibility to fully investigate the qualifications and training of the practitioner you choose.

The Institute for Functional Medicine

(800) 228-0622
www.functionalmedicine.org

The Institute for Functional Medicine is a nonprofit educational institution dedicated to training health professionals in the principles and practice of Functional Medicine. Functional Medicine is a science-based health-care approach that assesses and treats underlying causes of illness through individually tailored therapies to restore health and improve function. It is the medicine of the future.

The Consortium of Academic Health Centers for Integrative Medicine

www.imconsortium.org

The Consortium of Academic Health Centers for Integrative Medicine includes forty-one highly esteemed academic medical centers dedicated to research, education, and clinical care in Integrative Medicine.

The Center for Mind-Body Medicine

www.cmbm.org

The Center for Mind–Body Medicine is a nonprofit educational organization dedicated to reviving the spirit and transforming the practice of medicine. The center works to create a more effective, comprehensive, and compassionate model of health care and health education. The center model combines the precision of modern science with the wisdom of the world's healing traditions, to help health professionals heal themselves, their patients and clients, and their communities.

American College for Advancement in Medicine

(800) 532-3688
www.acam.org

Autism Research Institute

www.autism.com

American Holistic Medical Association (AHMA)

www.holisticmedicine.org

International Society for Orthomolecular Medicine

www.orthomed.org

Orthomolecular.org

Website resource for practitioners
www.orthomolecular.org

The American Association of Naturopathic Physicians

www.naturopathic.org

American Dietetic Association

www.eatright.org

Nutrition in Complementary Care (NCC)

www.complementarynutrition.org

National Association of Nutrition Professionals

www.nanp.org

Brain Exercise Tools
Brain Age

www.brainage.com

Brain Age is a Nintendo DS brain exercise tool that exercises your mind with word puzzles, memory games, math problems, and more to keep your brain active and healthy.

The Healthy Brain Kit

By Andrew Weil and Gary Small

Clinically proven tools to boost your memory, sharpen your mind, and keep your brain young.

Heavy Metal Toxicity
American Board of Clinical Metal Toxicology

www.abcmt.org

Amalgam Removal
International Academy of Oral Medicine & Toxicology

www.iaomt.org

American Academy of Biological Dentistry

www.biologicaldentistry.org

Relaxation Sources
Jon Kabat-Zinn, Ph.D., a pioneer in mind-body medicine and bringing mindfulness tools to medical centers, has a wonderful guided mindfulness audio program. I recommend his program called Series 3.

www.mindfulnesstapes.com

Healing Rhythms

www.wilddivine.com

Healing Rhythms is a personal training tool that uses your body's own biometrics to teach you stress management and relaxation techniques for a more balanced lifestyle.

Belleruth Naparastek's Guided Imagery Center

www.healthjourneys.com

Academy for Guided Imagery

www.academyforguidedimagery.com

Benson-Henry Institute for Mind Body Medicine

www.mbmi.org

Tools for Relaxation and Healing
emWave Personal Stress Reliever

www.emwave.com

A scientifically validated stress relief technology to help you balance your emotions, mind, and body using the science of heart-rate variability.

Resperate

www.resperate.com

A small personal biofeedback device to train yourself to relax.

Northern Light Technologies

www.northernlighttechnologies.com

Light therapy is a simple, medically recognized, efficient treatment to fight Seasonal Affective Disorder (SAD), the milder winter blues, and some sleep disorders.

Sunlight Saunas (source of far-infrared saunas)

www.sunlightsaunas.com

Restorative and Educational Retreats
Kripalu Center for Yoga & Health

www.kripalu.org

Omega Institute

www.eomega.org

Shambhala Mountain Center

www.shambhalamountain.org

I believe that clear, complete instructions in the plan are necessary for achieving an UltraMind. I also believe that much more detail and guidance are necessary than can be provided in a book. That is why I have created a FREE online companion workbook to help you succeed. It is *The UltraMind Solution Companion Guide*. It contains additional resources and tools you need to succeed, including:

- **Recipes**—A delicious collection of nourishing recipes that will allow you to follow the exact healthy eating plan outlined in *The UltraMind Solution*.
- **Shopping Lists**—A handy list of everything you need to shop for based on the recipes provided, including the foods you should enjoy and the foods you should stay away from.
- **Helpful Trackers**—A handy set of charts so you can track how much your mind, body, and spirit improve as you progress through this program. It's important for you not only to feel better but to see how much progress you've made.
- **Handy Checklists**—A series of checklists that will allow you to easily keep track of all the steps you should take during the preparation phase, the actual six-week program itself, what to do afterward, shopping lists, and more, so you can track the progress that you've made.
- **Testing Guide**—For those of you who seek medical care, this important section will outline a series of advanced tests that your doctor can order to help better pinpoint the underlying cause of your health problems.
- **Supplement Guide**—One of the most useful tools in here, this will help you organize what supplements you are supposed to take and when to take them to minimize any confusion.

**To download the guide, simply go to
www.ultramind.com/guide.**

In addition to the downloadable guide, I've put together a special website that includes many of the time-saving, program-enhancing tools that the guide has but also allows you to connect with others on the UltraMind Solution.

One of the wonderful things about the Internet is it allows me to stay in touch with many more people than I otherwise could. At the same time it allows all of you—people who are going through the same struggles and successes while fixing your broken brain and regaining your health—to stay in touch with one another.

When you join the UltraMind community, you'll get access to:

- **Recipe Exchange**—A recipe exchange so you can share your best recipes with others and search for delicious recipes that others have contributed.
- **Message Boards**—Message boards that allow you to connect with others to share advice and tips for getting the most out of the program.
- **Trackers**—An integrated module that allows you to track your mind, health, weight, and other vital statistics all online, securely and privately.
- **Private Journal**—A private online journal where you can record your daily thoughts as well as a public blog that you can use to share thoughts with others.
- **Food Log**—A detailed food log so you can track reactions to foods you might be allergic to that might be making you toxic and inflamed.
- **Share Your Success**—A place where you can post your own success story and see and be motivated by the hundreds of success stories posted by others.

To join the UltraMind community, please go to www.ultramind.com/join.

Here's a list of other books and resources that you'll find helpful on your path toward achieving UltraWellness—lifelong health and vitality.

- ❖ *UltraMetabolism*—This is Dr. Hyman's full eight-week plan to boost your metabolism. In this groundbreaking book, Dr. Hyman reveals the same plan that he uses with his patients to help them reprogram their genes for weight loss and health. You can download a free sneak preview at www.ultramind.com/um.

- ❖ *The UltraMetabolism Cookbook*—This is the cookbook that follows the main UltraMetabolism book and provides more than two hundred nourishing recipes to help you turn on your fat-burning DNA. These easy-to-prepare, delicious recipes will help ease you on to your path toward an UltraMetabolism. You can download a free preview by going to www.ultramind.com/cookbook.

- ❖ *The UltraSimple Diet*—This is an accelerated one-week version of Dr. Hyman's weight loss plan, focused on helping you lose up to ten pounds in seven days. Dr. Hyman reveals the two most powerful underlying factors that may be causing you to be sick and overweight and lays out a detailed, step-by-step, one-week plan to overcome them. You can download a free preview at www.ultramind.com/usd.

- ❖ **Other Solutions**—Please visit www.ultrawellness.com/store to see a complete list of other health solutions offered by Dr. Hyman, including *The UltraThyroid Solution, The Detox Box, The 5 Forces of Wellness,* and *Nutrigenomics*.

Chapter 1: Broken Brains

1. Demyttenaere, K., et al. WHO World Mental Health Survey Consortium. 2004. Prevalence, severity, and unmet need for treatment of mental disorders in the World Health Organization, World Mental Health Surveys. *JAMA* 21:2581–90.

2. World Health Initiative on Depression in Public Health. www.who.int/mental_health/management/depression/depressioninph/en/

3. Mental Health: A Report of the Surgeon General. Rockville, MD. U.S. Department of Health and Human Services, Substance Abuse and Mental Health Services Administration, Center for Mental Health Services, National Institutes of Health, National Institute of Mental Health, 1999.

4. Belfer, M. L. 2008. Child and adolescent mental disorders: the magnitude of the problem across the globe. *J Child Psychol Psychiatry* 49 (3):226–36.

5. An Unhealthy America, Economic Burden of Chronic Disease (October 2007). http://www.milkeninstitute.org/publications/publications.taf?function=detail&ID=38801020&cat=ResRep

6. Serafetinides, E. A. 1971. Cost of psychiatric illness versus cost of psychiatric research. *Am J Psychiatry* 148:951.

7. Froehlich, T. E., et al. 2007. Prevalence, recognition, and treatment of Attention-Deficit/Hyperactivity Disorder in a national sample of U.S. children. *Arch Pediatr Adolesc Med* 161 (9):857–64.

8. Zuvekas, S. H., B. Vitiello, G. S. Norquist. 2006. Recent trends in stimulant medication use among U.S. children. *Am J Psychiatry* 63 (4):579–85.

9. Wazana, A., M. Bresnahan, and J. Kline. 2007. The autism epidemic: Fact or artifact? *J Am Acad Child Adolesc Psychiatry* 46 (6):721–30.

10. Grizzle, K. L. 2007. Developmental dyslexia. *Pediatr Clin North Am* 54 (3):507–523, vi.

11. Hibbeln, J. R. 2007. From homicide to happiness—a commentary on omega-3 fatty acids in human society. Cleave Award Lecture. *Nutr Health* 19 (1–2):9–19.

12. Tiemeir, H., et al. 2002. Vitamin B_{12} folate, and homocysteine in depression: the Rotterdam Study. *Am J Psychiatry* 159 (12):2099–101.

13. Davis, J. D., and G. Tremont. 2007. Neuropsychiatric aspects of hypothyroidism and treatment reversibility. *Minerva Endocrinol* 32 (1):49–65. Review.

14. Zachi, E. C., et al. 2007. Neuropsychological dysfunction related to earlier occupational exposure to mercury vapor. *Braz J Med Biol Res* 40 (3):425–33.

15. Paulose-Ram, R., et al. 2007. Trends in psychotropic medication use among U.S. adults. *Pharmacoepidemiol Drug Saf* 16 (5):560–70.

16. Papakostas, G. I. 2007. Limitations of contemporary antidepressants: tolerability. *J Clin Psychiatry* 68 Suppl 10:11–7.

17. Turner, E. H., et al. 2008. Selective publication of antidepressant trials and its influence on apparent efficacy. *N Engl J Med* 358 (3):252–60.

Chapter 2: The Accidental Psychiatrist

1. Adi-Japha, E., et al. 2007. ADHD and dysgraphia: underlying mechanisms. *Cortex* 43 (6):700–9.
2. McCann, D., A. Barrett, and A. Cooper. 2007. Food additives and hyperactive behaviour in 3-year-old and 8/9-year-old children in the community: a randomised, double-blinded, placebo-controlled trial. *Lancet*.
3. Stevenson, J. 2006. Dietary influences on cognitive development and behaviour in children. *Proc Nutr Soc* 65 (4):361–65.
4. Sinn, N. 2007. Physical fatty acid deficiency signs in children with ADHD symptoms. *Prostaglandins Leukot Essent Fatty Acids*.
5. Mousain-Bosc, M., et al. 2006. Improvement of neurobehavioral disorders in children supplemented with magnesium-vitamin B_6. I. Attention deficit hyperactivity disorders. *Magnes Res* 19 (1):46–52.
6. Randle, H.W., and R. K. Winkelmann. 1980. Pityriasis rubra pilaris and celiac sprue with malabsorption. *Cutis* 25 (6):626–27.
7. Holick, M. F. 2007. Vitamin D deficiency. *N Engl J Med* 357 (3):266–81. Review.
8. Wintergerst, E. S., S. Maggini, and D. H. Hornig. Contribution of selected vitamins and trace elements to immune function. *Ann Nutr Metab* (2007) 51 (4):301–23.
9. Altura, B. M., and B. T. Altura. 2001. Tension headaches and muscle tension: Is there a role for magnesium? *Med Hypotheses* 57 (6):705–13.
10. Vargas, D. L., et al. 2005. Neuroglial activation and neuroinflammation in the brain of patients with autism. *Ann Neurol* 57 (1):67–81.
11. Lenoir, M., et al. 2007. Intense sweetness surpasses cocaine reward. *PLoS ONE* 2 (1):e698.
12. Drisko, J., et al. 2006. Treating irritable bowel syndrome with a food elimination diet followed by food challenge and probiotics. *J Am Coll Nutr* 25 (6):514–22.
13. Sedghizadeh, P. P., et al. 2002. Celiac disease and recurrent aphthous stomatitis: A report and review of the literature. *Oral Surg Oral Med Oral Pathol Oral Radiol Endod* 94 (4):474–78.
14. Macdonald, T. T., and G. Monteleone. 2005. Immunity, inflammation, and allergy in the gut. *Science* 307 (5717):1920–1925.
15. Cheuk, D. K., and V. Wong. 2006. Attention-deficit hyperactivity disorder and blood mercury level: A case-control study in Chinese children. *Neuropediatrics* 37 (4):234–40.
16. Banerjee, T. D., F. Middleton, and S. V. Faraone. 2007. Environmental risk factors for attention-deficit hyperactivity disorder. *Acta Paediatr* 96 (9):1269–1274.
17. Braun, J. M., et al. 2006. Exposures to environmental toxicants and attention deficit hyperactivity disorder in U.S. children. *Environ Health Perspect* 114 (12):1904–1909.
18. Institute for Functional Medicine. *Textbook of Functional Medicine*. Gig Harbor, Wa.: Institute for Functional Medicine, 2005.

Chapter 3: The Myths of Psychiatry and Neurology

1. Laing, R. D. *The Voice of Experience* (New York: Pantheon, 1982).
2. Rosenhan, D. L. 1973. On being sane in insane places. *Science* 179 (70): 250–58.
3. Laplace, Pierre-Simon. *1749–1827: A Life in Exact Science, Charles Coulston Gillispie* (Princeton: Princeton University Press, 2000).
4. Green, P. H., and B. Jabri. 2003. Coeliac disease. *Lancet* 362 (9381):383–91. Review.
5. Farrell, R. J., and C. P. Kelly. 2002. Celiac sprue. *N Engl J Med* 346 (3):180–88. Review.

6. Bushara, K. O. 2005. Neurologic presentation of celiac disease. *Gastroenterology* 128 (4 Suppl 1):S92–97. Review.

7. Millward, C., et al. 2004. Gluten- and casein-free diets for autistic spectrum disorder. *Cochrane Database Syst Rev* 2:CD003498. Review.

8. Grosjean, B., and G. E. Tsia. 2007. NMDA neurotransmission as a critical mediator of borderline personality disorder. *J Psychiatry Neurosci* 32 (2):103–15. Review.

9. Niederhofer, H., and K. Pittschieler. 2006. A preliminary investigation of ADHD symptoms in persons with celiac disease. *J Atten Disord* 10 (2):200–4.

10. Martin, A., and D. Leslie. 2003. Trends in Psychotropic Medication Costs for Children and Adolescents, 1997–2000. *Arch Pediatr Adolesc Med* 157: 997–1004.

11. Scheffler, R. M., et al. 2007. The global market for ADHD medications. *Health Aff* 26 (2):450–57.

12. Bhatara, V., et al. 2004. National trends in concomitant psychotropic medication with stimulants in pediatric visits: Practice versus knowledge. *Atten Disord* 7 (4):217–26.

13. Kaufman, D. W., et al. 2002. Recent patterns of medication use in the ambulatory adult population of the United States. The Slone Survey. *JAMA* 287:337–44.

14. Herbert, M. R. 2005. Autism, a brain disorder, or a disorder that affects the brain? *Clin Neuropsychiatry* 2 (6):354–79.

15. U.C. Davis work, MIND institute work, Pardo C., Johns Hopkins.

16. Selkoe, D. J., American College of Physicians; American Physiological Society. 2004. Alzheimer's disease: mechanistic understanding predicts novel therapies. *Ann Intern Med* 140 (8):627–38. Review.

17. Yaffe, K., et al. 2004. The metabolic syndrome, inflammation, and risk of cognitive decline. *JAMA* 292 (18):2237–2242.

18. Ehninger, D., and G. Kempermann. 2007. Neurogenesis in the adult hippocampus. *Cell Tissue Res*.

Chapter 4: Why You Are Suffering from Brain Damage

1. Johnson, R. J., et al. 2007. Potential role of sugar (fructose) in the epidemic of hypertension, obesity and the metabolic syndrome, diabetes, kidney disease, and cardiovascular disease. *Am J Clin Nutr* 86 (4):899–906.

2. George A. Bray, S. J. Nielsen, and B. M. Popkin. 2004. Consumption of high-fructose corn syrup in beverages may play a role in the epidemic of obesity. *Am. J. Clinical Nutrition* 79:537–43.

3. Lenoir, M., et al. 2007. Intense sweetness surpasses cocaine reward. *PLoS ONE* 2 (1):e698.

4. Holford, P. *Optimum Nutrition for the Mind* (Laguna Beach: Basic Health Publications, 2004).

5. Morris, M. C., et al. 2003. Dietary fats and the risk of incident Alzheimer disease. *Arch Neurol* 60 (2):194–202.

6. Ibid., 194–200.

7. Trejo, J. L., et al. 2002. Sedentary life impairs self-reparative processes in the brain: The role of serum insulin-like growth factor-I. *Rev Neurosci* 13 (4):365–74. Review.

8. Vaynman, S., and F. Gomez-Pinilla. 2006. Revenge of the "sit": How lifestyle impacts neuronal and cognitive health through molecular systems that interface energy metabolism with neuronal plasticity. *J Neurosci Res* 84 (4):699–715. Review.

9. Cotman, C. W., N. C. Berchtold, and L. A. Christie. 2007. Exercise builds brain health: Key roles of growth factor cascades and inflammation. *Trends Neurosci* 30 (9):464–72. Epub August 31, 2007.

10. Blumenthal, J. A., et al. 2007. Exercise and pharmacotherapy in the treatment of major depressive disorder. *Psychosom Med* 69 (7):587–96.

11. Swaab, D. F., A. M. Bao, and P. J. Lucassen. 2005. The stress system in the human brain in depression and neurodegeneration. *Ageing Res Rev* 4(2):141–94. Review.

12. Doraiswamy, P. M., and G. L. Xiong. 2007. Does meditation enhance cognition and brain longevity? *Ann NY Acad Sci.*

13. Gilliland, K., and D. Andress. 1981. Ad lib caffeine consumption, symptoms of caffeinism, and academic performance. *Am J Psychiatry* 138 (4):512–14.

14. O'Keefe, J. H., K. A. Bybee, and C. J. Lavie. 2007. Alcohol and cardiovascular health: the razor-sharp double-edged sword. *J Am Coll Cardiol* 50 (11):1009–1014. Review.

15. Anttila, T., et al. 2004. Alcohol drinking in middle age and subsequent risk of mild cognitive impairment and dementia in old age: A prospective population based study. *BMJ* 329 (7465):539.

16. Mukamal, K. J., et al. 2003. Prospective study of alcohol consumption and risk of dementia in older adults. *JAMA* 289 (11):1405–1413.

17. Volkow, N. D., et al. 1992. Decreased brain metabolism in neurologically intact healthy alcoholics. *Am J Psychiatry* 149 (8):1016–1022.

18. Brunnemann, K., and D. Hoffmann. 1991. Analytical studies on tobacco-specific N-nitrosamines in tobacco and tobacco smoke. *Crit Rev Toxicol* 21:235–40.

19. Pergadia, M., et al. 2004. Double-blind trial of the effects of tryptophan depletion on depression and cerebral blood flow in smokers. *Addict Behav* 29 (4):665–71.

20. De Mendelssohn, A. S. Kasper, and J. Tauscher. 2004. [Neuroimaging in substance abuse disorders] *Nervenarzt* 75 (7):651–62. Review.

21. Littarru, G. P., and P. Langsjoen. 2007. Coenzyme Q10 and statins: Biochemical and clinical implications. *Mitochondrion* 7 Suppl:S168–74. Epub March 27, 2007. Review.

22. Valuck, R. J., and J. M. Ruscin. 2004. A case-control study on adverse effects: H2 blocker or proton pump inhibitor use and risk of vitamin B_{12} deficiency in older adults. *J Clin Epidemiol* 57 (4):422–28.

23. Dial, S., et al. 2005. Use of gastric acid-suppressive agents and the risk of community acquired *Clostrium difficile*–associated disease. *JAMA* (23):2989–2995.

24. Yang, Y. X., et al. 2006. Long-term proton pump inhibitor therapy and risk of hip fracture. *JAMA* 296 (24):2947–2953.

25. Ruscin, J. M., R. L. Page, and R. J. Valuck. 2002. Vitamin B(12) deficiency associated with histamine(2)-receptor antagonists and a proton-pump inhibitor. *Ann Pharmacother* 36 (5):812–16.

26. Laine, L., et al. 2000. Review article: potential gastrointestinal effects of long-term acid suppression with proton pump inhibitors. *Aliment Pharmacol Ther* 14 (6):651–68. Review.

27. Atkuri, K. R., J. J. Mantovani, and L. A. Herzenberg. 2007. N—Acetylcysteine—a safe antidote for cysteine/glutathione deficiency. *Curr Opin Pharmacol* 7 (4):355–59. Epub June 29, 2007.

28. Ross, E. A., N. J. Szabo, and I. R. Tebbett. 2000. Lead content of calcium supplements. *JAMA* 284 (11):1425–1429.

29. Thompson, W. W., et al. 2007. Vaccine Safety Datalink Team. Early thimerosal exposure and neuropsychological outcomes at 7 to 10 years. *N Engl J Med* 357 (13):1281–1292.

30. Deppisch, L. M., et al. 1999. Andrew Jackson's exposure to mercury and lead: Poisoned president? *JAMA* 282 (6):569–71.

31. Guzzi, G., et al. 2006. Dental amalgam and mercury levels in autopsy tissues: Food for thought. *Am J Forensic Med Pathol* 27 (1):42–45.

32. Harris, H. H., et al. 2008. Migration of mercury from dental amalgam through human teeth. *J Synchrotron Radiat* 15 (Pt 2):123–28.

33. Schober, S. E., et al. 2003. Blood mercury levels in US children and women of childbearing age, 1999–2000. *JAMA* 289 (13):1667–1674.

34. www.cfsan.fda.gov/~acrobat/hgstak56.pdf

35. Cory-Slechta, D. A. 2005. Studying toxicants as single chemicals: Does this strategy adequately identify neurotoxic risk? *Neurotoxicology* 26 (4):491–510. Review.

36. www.archive.ewg.org/reports/bodyburden2/execsumm.php

37. www.vm.cfsan.fda.gov/~dms/eafus.html.

38. Alavanja, M. C., J. A. Hoppin, and F. Kamel. 2004. Health effects of chronic pesticide exposure: Cancer and neurotoxicity. *Annu Rev Public Health* 25:155–97. Review.

39. Curl, C. L., R. A. Fenske, and K. Elgethun. 2003. Organophosphorus pesticide exposure of urban and suburban preschool children with organic and conventional diets. *Environ Health Perspect* 111 (3):377–82.

40. Roberts, E. M., et al. 2007. Maternal residence near agricultural pesticide applications and autism spectrum disorders among children in the California Central Valley. *Environ Health Perspect* 115 (10):1482–1489.

41. Grandjean, P., et al. 2006. Pesticide exposure and stunting as independent predictors of neurobehavioral deficits in Ecuadorian school children. *Pediatrics* 117 (3):e546–56.

42. McCann, D., et al. 2007. Food additives and hyperactive behaviour in 3-year-old and 8/9-year-old children in the community: A randomised, double-blinded, placebo-controlled trial. *Lancet* 370 (9598):1560–1567.

43. Wang, B. L., et al. 2007. Unmetabolized VOCs in urine as biomarkers of low level exposure in indoor environments. *J Occup Health* 49 (2):104–10.

44. Uzun, N., and Y. Kendirli. 2005. Clinical, socio-demographic, neurophysiological and neuropsychiatric evaluation of children with volatile substance addiction. *Child Care Health Dev* 31 (4):425–32.

45. Shoemaker, R. C., and D. E. House. 2006. Sick building syndrome (SBS) and exposure to water-damaged buildings: Time series study, clinical trial and mechanisms. *Neurotoxicol Teratol* 28 (5): 573–88. Epub August 7, 2006.

46. Campbell, A. W., et al. 2003. Neural autoantibodies and neurophysiologic abnormalities in patients exposed to molds in water-damaged buildings. *Arch Environ Health* 58 (8):464–74.

47. Rea, W. J., et al. 2003. Effects of toxic exposure to molds and mycotoxins in building-related illnesses. *Arch Environ Health* 58 (7):399–405.

48. Bellinger, D. C. 2007. Children's cognitive health: The influence of environmental chemical exposures. *Altern Ther Health Med* 13 (2):S140–44. Review.

49. Needleman, H. L., and C. A. Gatsonis. 1990. Low-level lead exposure and the IQ of children. A meta-analysis of modern studies. *JAMA* 263 (5):673–78.

50. Needleman, H. L., et al. 1990. The long-term effects of exposure to low doses of lead in childhood. An 11-year follow-up report. *N Engl J Med* 322 (2):83–88.

51. Canfield, R. L., et al. 2003. Intellectual impairment in children with blood lead concentrations below 10 microg per deciliter. *N Engl J Med* 348 (16):1517–1526.

52. Stewart, W. F., and B. S. Schwartz. 2007. Effects of lead on the adult brain: A 15-year exploration. *Am J Ind Med* 50 (10):729–39.

53. Menke, A., et al. 2006. Blood lead below 0.48 micromol/L (10 microg/dL) and mortality among US adults. *Circulation* 114 (13):1388–1394.

54. Romano, C., and M. L. Grossi-Bianchi. 1968. Aphasia and dementia in childhood chronic lead encephalopathy: A curable form of acquired mental impairment. *Panminerva Med* 10 (11):448–50.

55. Choi, B. H. 1989. The effects of methylmercury on the developing brain. *Prog Neurobiol* 32 (6):447–70. Review.

56. Krewski, D., et al. 2007. Recent advances in research on radiofrequency fields and health: 2001–2003. *J Toxicol Environ Health B Crit Rev* 10 (4):287–318. Review.

57. Feychting, M. F., et al. 2003. Occupational magnetic field exposure and neurodegenerative disease. *Epidemiology* 14 (4):413–19; Discussion, 427–28.

58. Ahlbom, A. 2001. Neurodegenerative diseases, suicide and depressive symptoms in relation to EMF. *Bioelectromagnetics* Suppl 5:S132–43.

Chapter 6: Key #1: Optimize Nutrition

1. Freeman, M. P., et al. 2006. Omega-3 fatty acids: evidence basis for treatment and future research in psychiatry. *J Clin Psychiatry* 67 (12):1954–1967. Review.

2. Hibbeln, J. R., L. R. Nieminen and W. E. Lands. 2004. Increasing homicide rates and linoleic acid consumption among five Western countries, 1961–2000. *Lipids* 39 (12):1207–1213.

3. Gesch, C. B., et al. 2002. Influence of supplementary vitamins, minerals and essential fatty acids on the antisocial behaviour of young adult prisoners: Randomised, placebo-controlled trial. *Br J Psychiatry* 181:22–28.

4. Freeman, M. P. 2006. Omega-3 fatty acids and perinatal depression: a review of the literature and recommendations for future research. *Prostaglandins Leukot Essent Fatty Acids* 75 (4–5):291–97.

5. Richardson, A. I. 2004. Long-chain polyunsaturated fatty acids in childhood developmental and psychiatric disorders. *Lipids* 39 (12):1215–1222. Review.

6. Megson, M. N. 2000. Is autism a G-alpha protein defect reversible with natural vitamin A? *Med Hypotheses* 54 (6):979–83.

7. Parker, G., et al. 2006. Omega-3 fatty acids and mood disorders. *Am J Psychiatry* (2006) 163 (6):969–78. Review. Erratum in *Am J Psychiatry* 163 (10):1842.

8. Crook, T. H., et al. 1997. Effects of phosphatidylserine in age-associated memory impairment. *Neurology* 41 (5):644–49.

9. Hellhammer, J., et al. 2004. Effects of soy lecithin phosphatidic acid and phosphatidylserine complex (PAS) on the endocrine and psychological responses to mental stress. *Stress* 7 (2):119–26.

10. Kidd, P. M. 1999. A review of nutrients and botanicals in the integrative management of cognitive dysfunction. *Altern Med Rev* 4 (3):144–61. Review.

11. Shaw, P., et al. 2007. Polymorphisms of the dopamine D4 receptor, clinical outcome, and cortical structure in attention-deficit/hyperactivity disorder. *Arch Gen Psychiatry* 64 (8):921–31.

12. Nyman, E. S., et al. 2007. ADHD candidate gene study in a population-based birth cohort: Association with DBH and DRD2. *J Am Acad Child Adolesc Psychiatry* 46 (12):1614–1621.

13. Sharma, A., et al. 1999. D4 dopamine receptor-mediated phospholipid methylation and its implications for mental illnesses such as schizophrenia. *Mol Psychiatry* 4 (3):235–46.

14. Das, U. N. 2008. Folic acid and polyunsaturated fatty acids improve cognitive function and prevent depression, dementia, and Alzheimer's disease. But how and why. *Prostaglandins Leukot Essent Fatty Acids* 78 (1):11–19.

15. Deijen, J. B. et al. 1999. Tyrosine improves cognitive performance and reduces blood pressure in cadets after one week of a combat training course. *Brain Res Bull* 48 (2):203–9.

16. Delgado, P. L., et al. 1990. Serotonin function and the mechanism of antidepressant action. Reversal of antidepressant-induced remission by rapid depletion of plasma tryptophan. *Arch Gen Psychiatry* 47 (5):411–18.

17. Coppen, A., and C. Bolander-Gouaille. 2005. Treatment of depression: time to consider folic acid and vitamin B_{12}. *J Psychopharmacol* 19 (1):59–65. Review.

18. Roberts, S. H., et al. 2007. IT. Folate Augmentation of Treatment—Evaluation for Depression (FolATED); Protocol of a randomised controlled trial. *BMC Psychiatry* 7 (1):65.

19. Tiihonen, J., et al. 2006. Antidepressants and the risk of suicide, attempted suicide, and overall mortality in a nationwide cohort. *Arch Gen Psychiatry* 63 (12):1358–1367.

20. Abdou, A. M., et al. 2006. Relaxation and immunity enhancement effects of gamma-aminobutyric acid (GABA) administration in humans. *Biofactors* 26 (3):201–8.

21. El Idrissi, A., et al. 2003. Prevention of epileptic seizures by taurine. *Adv Exp Med Biol* 526:515–25.

22. Courtney, C., et al. 2004. AD2000 Collaborative Group. Long-term donepezil treatment in 565 patients with Alzheimer's disease (AD2000): randomised double-blind trial. *Lancet* 363 (9427):2105–2115.

23. Hampl, J. S., C. A. Taylor, and C. S. Johnston. 2004. Vitamin C deficiency and depletion in the United States: the Third National Health and Nutrition Examination Survey, 1988 to 1994. *Am J Public Health* 94 (5):870–75.

24. Noble, J. M., A. Mandel, and M. C. Patterson. 2007. Scurvy and rickets masked by chronic neurologic illness: revisiting "psychologic malnutrition." *Pediatrics* 119 (3):e783–90.

25. Ames, B. N. 2004. A role for supplements in optimizing health: the metabolic tune-up. *Arch Biochem Biophys* 423 (1):227–34. Review.

26. Kaplan, B. J. et al. 2007. Vitamins, minerals, and mood. *Psychol Bull* 133 (5):747–60.

27. Seshadri, S., et al. 2002. Plasma homocysteine as a risk factor for dementia and Alzheimer's disease. *N Engl J Med* 346 (7):476–83.

28. Ames, B. 2002. High-dose vitamin therapy stimulates variant enzymes with decreased coenzyme binding affinity (increased km): relevance to genetic disease and polymorphisms. *Am J Clin Nutr* 75:616–58.

29. Fairfield, K. 2002. Vitamins for chronic disease prevention in adults, scientific review. *JAMA* 287:3116–3126.

30. Vasquez, A. 2004. The clinical importance of vitamin D (cholecalciferol): A paradigm shift with implications for all health care providers, alternative therapies.

31. Holick, M. 2004. Vitamin D: importance in the prevention of cancers, type 1 diabetes, heart disease and osteoporosis. *Am J Clin Nutr* 79:362–71.

32. Heaney, R. 2003. Long-latency deficiency disease: insights from calcium and vitamin D. *Am J Clin Nutr* 78:912–19.

33. Mischoulon, D., and M. F. Raab. 2007. The role of folate in depression and dementia. *J Clin Psychiatry* 68 Suppl 10:28–33. Review.

34. James, S. J., et al. 2004. Metabolic biomarkers of increased oxidative stress and

impaired methylation capacity in children with autism. *Am J Clin Nutr* 80 (6):1611–17.

35. Triantafyllou, N. I., et al. 2007. Folate and vitamin B$_{12}$ levels in levodopa-treated Parkinson's disease patients: Their relationship to clinical manifestations, mood and cognition. *Parkinsonism Relat Disord.*

36. Reif, A., B. Pfuhlmann, and K. P. Lesch. 2005. Homocysteinemia as well as methyl-enetetrahydrofolate reductase polymorphism are associated with affective psychoses. *Prog Neuropsychopharmacol Biol Psychiatry* (7):1162–1168.

37. Herbert, V. 1962. Experimental nutritional folate deficiency in man. *Trans Assoc Am Physicians* 75:307–20.

38. Tolmunen, T., et al. 2007. Dietary folate and depressive symptoms are associated in middle-aged Finnish men. *J Nutr* 133 (10):3233–3236.

39. Penninx, B. W., et al. 2000. Vitamin B(12) deficiency and depression in physically disabled older women: Epidemiologic evidence from the Women's Health and Aging Study. *Am J Psychiatry* 157 (5):715–21.

40. Papakostas, G. I., et al. 2004. Serum folate, vitamin B$_{12}$, and homocysteine in major depressive disorder, Part 1: predictors of clinical response in fluoxetine-resistant depression. *J Clin Psychiatry* 65 (8):1090–1095.

41. Alpert, J. E., et al. 2002. Folinic acid (Leucovorin) as an adjunctive treatment for SSRI-refractory depression. *Ann Clin Psychiatry* 14 (1):33–38.

42. Corrada, M. M., C. H. Kawas, and J. Hallfrisch. 2005. Reduced risk of Alzheimer's disease with high folate intake: the Baltimore Longitudinal Study of Aging. *Alzheimer's and Dementia* 1:11–18.

43. Clarke, R., et al. 2007. Low vitamin B-12 status and risk of cognitive decline in older adults. *Am J Clin Nutr.* 86 (5):1384–1391.

44. Waly, M., et al. 2004. Activation of methionine synthase by insulin-like growth factor-1 and dopamine: a target for neurodevelopmental toxins and thimerosal. *Mol Psychiatry* 9 (4):358–70.

45. Gerrior, S., and L. Bente. 2007. "Nutrient Content of the U.S. Food Supply, 1909–94." U.S. Department of Agriculture, Center for Nutrition Policy and Promotion. Home Economics Report No. 53.

46. Alpaslan, M., and H. Gunduz. 2000. The effects of growing conditions on oil content, fatty acid composition and tocopherol content of some sunflower varieties produced in Turkey. *Die Nahrung* (Germany): 44 (6):434–37.

47. Composition of Foods: Raw, Processed, Prepared. USDA National Nutrient Database for Standard Reference, Release 15. U.S. Department of Agriculture, Agricultural Research Service, Beltsville Human Nutrition Research Center, Nutrient Data Laboratory (2002), www.ars.usda.gov.

48. Wilkins, C. H., et al. 2006. Vitamin D deficiency is associated with low mood and worse cognitive performance in older adults. *Am J Geriatr Psychiatry* 14 (12):1032–40.

49. Gloth, F. M. III, W. Alam, and B. Hollis. 1999. Vitamin D vs. broad spectrum phototherapy in the treatment of seasonal affective disorder. *J Nutr Health Aging* 3 (1):5–7.

50. Cannell, J. J. 2008. Autsim and vitamin D. *Med Hypotheses* 70 (4):750–59.

51. Autier, P., and S. Gandini. 2007. Vitamin D supplementation and total mortality: a metaanalysis of randomized controlled trials. *Arch Intern Med* 167 (16):1730–1737. Review.

52. Holick, M. F. 2006. Vitamin D deficiency. *N Engl J Med* 357 (3):266–81. Review.

53. Holick, M. 2004. Sunlight and vitamin D for bone health and prevention of au-

toimmune diseases, cancers and cardiovascular disease. *Am J Clin Nutr* (80) suppl: 1678S–1688S.

54. Tong, G. M., and R. K. Rude. 2005. Magnesium deficiency in critical illness. *J Intensive Care Med* 20 (1):3–17. Review.

55. www.who.int/publications/cra/chapters/volume1/0257–0280.pdf

56. Nowak, G., B. Szewczyk, and A. Pilc. 2005. Zinc and depression. An update. *Pharmacol Rep* 57 (6):713–18. Review.

57. Heleniak, E. P., and S. W. Lamola 1986. A new prostaglandin disturbance syndrome in schizophrenia: delta-6-pyroluria. *Med Hypotheses* 19 (4):333–38. Review.

58. Hoffer, A., and M. Mahon. 1961. The presence of unidentified substances in the urine of psychiatric patients. *J Neuropsychiatr* 2:331–62.

59. McGinnis, W. R., et al. 2008. Discerning the Mauve Factor, pending publication Alter Thera Health Med.

60. Benton, D., and R. Cook. 1990. Selenium supplementation improves mood in a double-blind crossover trial. *Psychopharmacology* (Berl). 102 (4):549–50.

Chapter 7: Key #2: Balance Your Hormones

1. Cordain, L., et al. 2005. Origins and evolution of the Western diet: Health implications for the 21st century. *Am J Clin Nutr* 8 (2):341–54. Review.

2. http://www.cspinet.org/new/sugar_limit.html.

3. Kinoshita, J.; Alzheimer Research Forum. 2006. Alzheimer Research Forum live discussion: Insulin resistance: a common axis linking Alzheimer's, depression, and metabolism? *J Alzheimers Dis* 9 (1): 89–93.

4. Yaffe, K., et al. 2004. The metabolic syndrome, inflammation, and risk of cognitive decline. *JAMA* 292 (18):2237–2242.

5. *NY Times,* January 14, 2003.

6. Silverman, D. H., et al. 2001. Positron emission tomography in evaluation of dementia: Regional brain metabolism and long-term outcome. *JAMA* 286 (17):2120–127.

7. Timonen, M. et al. 2007. Insulin resistance and depressive symptoms in young adult males: Findings from Finnish military conscripts. *Psychosom Med* 69 (8):723–28.

8. Hyman, M. A. 2006. Systems biology: The gut-brain-fat cell connection and obesity. *Altern Ther Health Med* 12 (1):10–16. Review.

9. Abbott, R. D., et al. 2004. Walking and dementia in physically capable elderly men. *JAMA* 292 (12):1447–453.

10. Camaris, G., et al. 2000. The Colorado Thyroid Disease Prevalence Study. *Arch Intern Med* 160:526–34.

11. Chueire, V. B., J. H., Romaldini and L. S. Ward. 2007. Subclinical hypothyroidism increases the risk for depression in the elderly. *Arch Gerontol Geriatr* 44 (1):21–28. Epub 2006 May 5.

12. Montero-Pedrazuela, A. et al. 2006. Modulation of adult hippocampal neurogenesis by thyroid hormones: implications in depressive-like behavior. *Mol Psychiatry* 11 (4):361–71.

13. Thomsen, A. F., et al. 2005. Increased risk of developing affective disorder in patients with hypothyroidism: a register-based study. *Thyroid* 15 (7):700–7.

14. Bauer, M., A. Heinz, and P. C. Whybrow. 2002. Thyroid hormones, serotonin and mood: of synergy and significance in the adult brain. *Mol Psychiatry* 7 (2):140–56. Review.

15. Van Boxtel, M. P., et al. 2004. Thyroid function, depressed mood, and cognitive per-

formance in older individuals: the Maastricht Aging Study. *Psychoneuroendocrinology* 29 (7):891–98.

16. Miller, K. J., et al. 2006. Memory improvement with treatment of hypothyroidism. *Int J Neurosci* 116 (8):895–906.

17. Rack, S. K., and E. H. Makela. 2000. Hypothyroidism and depression: a therapeutic challenge. *Ann Pharmacother* 34 (10):1142–1145.

18. Bunevicius, R., et al. 1999. Effects of thyroxine as compared with thyroxine plus tri-iodothyronine in patients with hypothyroidism. *N Engl J Med* 340 (6):424–29.

19. Abraham, G., R. Miley, and J. Lawson. 2006. T3 augmentation of SSRI resistant depression. *J Affect Disord* 91 (2–3):211–15. Epub 2006 February 17.

20. Cooper-Kazaz, R., et al. 2007. Combined treatment with sertraline and liothyronine in major depression: A randomized, double-blind, placebo-controlled trial. *Arch Gen Psychiatry* 64 (6):679–88.

21. Porterfield, S. P. 1994. Vulnerability of the developing brain to thyroid abnormalities: environmental insults to the thyroid system. *Environ Health Perspect* 102 Suppl 2:125–30. Review.

22. Otake, T., et al. 2007. Thyroid hormone status of newborns in relation to utero exposure to PCBs and hydroxylated PCB metabolites. *Environ Res* 105 (2):240–46. Epub 2007 May 8.

23. Galletti, P. M., and G. Joyet. 1958. Effect of fluorine on thyroidal iodine metabolism in hyperthyroidism. *J Clin Endocrinol Metab* 18 (10): 1102–1110.

24. Rasheed, P., and L. S. Al-Sowielem. 2003. Prevalence and predictors of premenstrual syndrome among college-aged women in Saudi Arabia. *Ann Saudi Med* 23 (6):381–87.

25. Tan, R. S., and S. J. Pu. 2001. The andropause and memory loss: is there a link between androgen decline and dementia in the aging male? *Asian J Androl* 3 (3): 169–74. Review.

26. Rich-Edwards, J. W., et al. 2007. Milk consumption and the prepubertal somatotropic axis. *Nutr J* 6:28.

27. Milk, hormones and human health, 10/23–25/2006, Boston. *J Mammary Gland Biol Neoplasia* (2007) 12 (4):315.

28. Pape-Zambito, D. A., A. L. Magliaro, and R. S. Kensinger, 2007. Concentrations of 17beta-estradiol in Holstein whole milk. *J Diary Sci.* 90 (7):3308–3313.

29. Osterlund, M. K., M. R. Witt, and J. A. Gustafsson. 2005. Estrogen action in mood and neurodegenerative disorders: estrogenic compounds with selective properties—the next generation of therapeutics. *Endocrine* 28 (3):235–42. Review.

30. Pluchino, N., et al. 2001. Progesterone and progestins: effects on brain, allopregnanolone and beta-endorphin. *J Steroid Biochem Mol Biol* 102 (1–5):205–13. Epub 2006 October 18. Review.

31. Schulman, M. M., et al. 2007. The burden of testosterone deficiency syndrome in adult men: economic and quality-of-life impact. *J Sex Med* 4 (4 Pt 1):1056–1069. Links.

32. Bernhardt, P. C., et al. 1998. Testosterone changes during vicarious experiences of winning and losing among fans at sporting events. *Physiol Behav* 65 (1):59–62.

33. Sternbach, H. 1998. Age-associated testosterone decline in men: clinical issues for psychiatry. *Am J Psychiatry* 155 (10):1310–1318. Review.

34. Beauchet, O. 2001. Testosterone and cognitive function: current clinical evidence of a relationship. *Eur J Endocrinol* 155 (6):773–81. Review.

35. Wu, C. Y., T. J. Yu, and M. J. Chen. 2000. Age-related testosterone level changes and male andropause syndrome. *Chang Gung Med J* 23 (6):348–53.

36. Goldstat, R., et al. 2003. Transdermal testosterone therapy improves well-being, mood, and sexual function in premenopausal women. *Menopause* 10 (5):390–98.

37. Srinivasan, V., et al. 2006. Melatonin in mood disorders. *World J Biol Psychiatry* 7 (3):138–51. Review.

38. Blackman, M. R., et al. 2007. Growth hormone and sex steroid administration in healthy aged women and men: a randomized-controlled trial. *JAMA* 288 (18):2282–2292.

39. Van Cauter, E., R. Leproult, and L. Plat. 2000. Age-related changes in slow wave sleep and REM sleep and relationship with growth hormone and cortisol levels in healthy men. *JAMA* 284 (7):861–68.

40. Harrington, J. M. 1994. Shift work and health—a critical review of the literature on working hours. *Ann Acad Med* 23 (5):699–705. Review.

41. Scott, J. P., L. R. McNaughton, and R. C. Polman. 2006. Effects of sleep deprivation and exercise on cognitive, motor performance and mood. *Physiol Behav* 87 (2):396–408. Epub 2006 January 3.

42. Young, T., J. Skatrud, and P. E. Peppard. 2004. Risk factors for obstructive sleep apnea in adults. *JAMA* 291 (16):2013–2016. Review.

Chapter 8: Key #3: Cool Off Inflammation

1. Elenkov, I. J., et al. 2005. Cytokine dysregulation, inflammation and well-being. *Neuroimmunomodulation* 12 (5):255–69.

2. Herbert, M. 2006. Autism: A brain disorder, or a disorder that affects the brain? *Clinical Neuropsychiatry* 2 6:354–79.

3. Ibid. 2005. Large brains in autism: The challenge of pervasive abnormality. *Neuroscientist* 11 (5):417–40. Review.

4. Vargas, D. L., et al. 2005. Neuroglial activation and neuroinflammation in the brain of patients with autism. *Ann Neurol* (2005) 57 (1):67–81. Erratum in *Ann Neurol* 57 (2):304.

5. Ashwood, P., J. Wills, J. Van de Water. 2006. The immune response in autism: a new frontier for autism research. *J Leukoc Biol* 80 (1):1–15. Review.

6. Das, U. N. 2007. Is depression a low-grade systemic inflammatory condition? *Am J Clin Nutr* 85 (6):1665–666.

7. Anisman, H., and Z. Merali. 2003. Cytokines, stress and depressive illness: brain-immune interactions. *Ann Med* 35 (1):2–11. Review.

8. Müller, N., and M. J. Schwarz. 2007. Immunological aspects of depressive disorders. *Nervenarzt* 78 (11):1261–273.

9. Bode, L., and H. Ludwig. 2003. Borna disease virus infection, a human mental-health risk. *Clin Microbiol Rev* 16 (3):534–45. Review.

10. Groves, D. A., and V. J. Brown. 2005. Vagal nerve stimulation: a review of its applications and potential mechanisms that mediate its clinical effects. *Neurosci Biobehav Rev* 29 (3):493–500. Review.

11. Parker, G., et al. 2006. Omega-3 fatty acids and mood disorders. *Am J Psychiatry* 163 (6):969–78. Review.

12. Blumenthal, J. A., et al. 2007. Exercise and pharmacotherapy in the treatment of major depressive disorder. *Psychosom Med* 69 (7):587–96. Epub 2007 September 10.

13. Papakostas, G. I., et al. 2005. Brain MRI white matter hyperintensities and one-carbon cycle metabolism in nongeriatric outpatients with major depressive disorder (Part II). *Psychiatry Res* 140 (3):301–7. Epub 2005 November 16.

14. Hoekstra, P. J., and R. B. Minderaa. 2005. Tic disorders and obsessive-compulsive disorder: Is autoimmunity involved? *Int Rev Psychiatry* 17 (6):497–502. Review.

15. Griffin, W. S. 2006. Inflammation and neurodegenerative diseases. *Am J Clin Nutr* 83 (2):470S–74S. Review.

16. McIntyre, R. S., et al. 2007. Should depressive syndromes be reclassified as "metabolic syndrome type II"? *Ann Clin Psychiatry* 19 (4):257–64.

17. Ibid. 2006. Managing psychiatric disorders with antidiabetic agents: Translational research and treatment opportunities. *Expert Opin Pharmacother* 7 (10):1305–1321.

18. Hunter, J. O. 1991. Food allergy—or enterometabolic disorder? *Lancet* 338 (8765):495–96.

19. King, D. S. 1981. Can allergic exposure provoke psychological symptoms? A double-blind test. *Biol Psychiatry* 16 (1):3–19.

20. Ludvigsson, J. F., et al. 2007. Coeliac disease and risk of mood disorders—a general population-based cohort study. *J Affect Disord* 99 (1–3):117–26. Epub 2006 October 6.

21. Ludvigsson, J. F., et al. 2007. Coeliac disease and risk of schizophrenia and other psychosis: A general population cohort study. *Scand J Gastroenterol* 42 (2):179–85.

22. Margutti, P., F. Delunardo, and E. Ortona. 2006. Autoantibodies associated with psychiatric disorders. *Curr Neurovasc Res* 3 (2):149–57. Review.

23. Hu, W. T., et al. 2006. Cognitive impairment and celiac disease. *Arch Neurol* 63 (10):1440–1446.

24. Wilders-Truschnig, M., et al. 2007. IgG antibodies against food antigens are correlated with inflammation and intima media thickness in obese juveniles. *Exp Clin Endocrinol Diabetes* 116 (4):241–45.

25. Liu, Y., T. Heiberg, and K. L. Reichelt. 2007. Towards a possible aetiology for depressions? *Behav Brain Funct* 14 (3):47.

26. MacDonald, T. T., and G. Monteleone. 2005. Immunity, inflammation, and allergy in the gut. *Science* 307:1920–1925.

27. Atkinson, W., et al. 2007. Food elimination based on IgG antibodies in irritable bowel syndrome: A randomised controlled trial. *Gut* 53 (10):1459–1464.

Chapter 9: Key #4: Fix Your Digestion

1. www.digestive.niddk.nih.gov/statistics/statistics.htm

2. Benarroch, E. E. 2007. Enteric nervous system: Functional organization and neurologic implications. *Neurology* 13 69(20):1953–957. Review.

3. Sandler, R. H., et al. 2000. Relief of psychiatric symptoms in a patient with Crohn's disease after metronidazole therapy. *Clin Infect Dis* 30 (1):213–14.

4. Lin, H. 2004. Small intestinal bacterial overgrowth: A framework for understanding irritable bowel syndrome *JAMA* 292:852–58.

5. Orr, W. C., S. Elsenbruch and M. J. Harnish. 2000. Autonomic regulation of cardiac function during sleep in patients with irritable bowel syndrome. *Am J Gastroenterol* 95:2865–2871.

6. Anisman, H., and Z. Merali. 2003. Cytokines, stress and depressive illness: Brain-immune interactions. *Ann Med* 35:2–11.

7. Banks, W. A., S. A. Farr, and J. E. Morley. 2002–2003. Entry of blood-borne cytokines into the central nervous system: Effects on cognitive processes. *Neuroimmunomodulation* 10:319–27.

8. Rivier, C. 1993. Effect of peripheral and central cytokines on the hypothalamic-pituitary-adrenal axis in the rat. *Ann NY Acad Sci* 697:97–105.

9. Carlson, S. L., et al. 1987. Alternations of monoamines in specific central autonomic nuclei following immunization in mice. *Brain Behav Immun* 1:52–63.

10. Shattock, P., and P. Whiteley. 2002. Biochemical aspects in autism spectrum disorders: Updating the opioid-excess theory and presenting new opportunities for biomedical intervention. *Expert Opin Ther Targets* 6 (2):175–83. Review.

11. Pimentel, M., et al. 2006. The effect of a nonabsorbed oral antibiotic (rifaximin) on the symptoms of the irritable bowel syndrome: A randomized trial. *Ann Intern Med* 145 (8):557–63.

12. Av, S. P. 2007. Hepatic encephalopathy: Pathophysiology and advances in therapy. *Trop Gastroenterol* 28 (1):4–10. Review.

13. Jansson-Nettelbladt, E., et al. 2006. Endogenous ethanol fermentation in a child with short bowel syndrome. *Acta Paediatr* 95 (4):502–4.

14. Kidd, P. M. 2002. Autism, an extreme challenge to integrative medicine. Part 2: Medical management. *Altern Med Rev* 7 (6):472–99. Review.

15. Sandler, R. H., et al. 2000. Short-term benefit from oral vancomycin treatment of regressive-onset autism. *J Child Neurol* 15 (7):429–35.

16. Parracho, H. M., et al. 2005. Differences between the gut microflora of children with autistic spectrum disorders and that of healthy children. *J Med Microbiol.* 54 (Pt. 10):987–91.

17. Walsh, W. J., L. B. Glab, and M. L. Haakenson. 2004. Reduced violent behavior following biochemical therapy. *Physiol Behav* 82 (5):835–39.

18. Ibid.

19. Benton, D. 2001. The impact of diet on antisocial, violent and criminal behaviour. *Neurosci Biobehav Rev* 31 (5):752–74. Epub 2007 March 4. Review.

20. Wakefield, A. J., et al. 2002. Review article: The concept of entero-colonic encephalopathy, autism and opioid receptor ligands. *Aliment Pharmacol Ther* 16 (4):663–74.

21. Aytac, U., and N. H. Dang. 2004. CD26/dipeptidyl peptidase IV: A regulator of immune function and a potential molecular target for therapy. *Curr Drug Targets Immune Endocr Metabol Disord* 4 (1):11–8. Review.

22. Mentlein, R. 1999. Dipeptidyl-peptidase IV (CD26)—role in the inactivation of regulatory peptides. *Regul Pept* 85 (1):9–24. Review.

23. Shattock, P., and P. Whiteley. 2002. Biochemical aspects in autism spectrum disorders: Updating the opioid-excess theory and presenting new opportunities for biomedical intervention. *Expert Opin Ther Targets* 6 (2):175–83.

24. Ek, J., M. Stensrud, and K. L. Reichelt. 1999. Gluten-free diet decreases urinary peptide levels in children with celiac disease. *J Pediatr Gastroenterol Nutr* 29 (3):282–85.

25. Liu, Y., T. Heiberg, and K. L. Reichelt. 2007. Towards a possible aetiology for depressions? *Behav Brain Funct* 14 3:47.

26. Wakefield, A. I., et al. 2005. The significance of ileo-colonic lymphoid nodular hyperplasia in children with autistic spectrum disorder. *Eur J Gastroenterol Hepatol* 17 (8):827–36.

27. Uhlmann, V., et al. 2002. Potential viral pathogenic mechanism for new variant inflammatory bowel disease. *Mol Pathol* 55 (2):84–90.

28. Kawashima, H., et al. 2002. Detection and sequencing of measles virus from peripheral mononuclear cells from patients with inflammatory bowel disease and autism. *Dig Dis Sci* 45 (4):723–29.

29. Bradstreet, J. J., et al. 2004. Detection of measles virus genomic RNA in cerebrospinal fluid of children with regressive autism: A report of three cases. *J. Am Phys Surgeons* 38–45.

30. Taylor, B., et al. 1999. Autism and measles, mumps, and rubella vaccine: no epidemiological evidence for a causal association. *Lancet* 353 (9169):2026–2029.

31. Millward, C., et al. 2004. Gluten- and casein-free diets for autistic spectrum disorder. *Cochrane Database Syst Rev* (2):CD003498. Review.

32. Hu, W. T., et al. 2006. Cognitive impairment and celiac disease. *Arch Neurol* 63 (10):1440–446.

33. Kalaydijian, A. E., et al. 2006. The gluten connection: The association between schizophrenia and celiac disease. *Acta Psychiatr Scand* 113 (2):82–90. Review.

34. www.gut.bmjjournals.com/cgi/content/abstract/53/10/1459 (Food elimination based on IgG antibodies in irritable bowel syndrome: a randomised controlled trial).

35. Shaheen, N., and F. Ransohoff. 2002. Gastroesophageal reflux, barrett esophagus, and esophageal cancer: Scientific Review. *JAMA* 287: 1972–1981.

36. www.en.wikipedia.org/wiki/List_of_top_selling_drugs

37. Ruscin, J. M., R. L. Page, and R. J. Valuck. 2002. Vitamin B_{12} deficiency associated with histamine(2)-receptor antagonists and a proton-pump inhibitor. *Ann Pharmacother* 36 (5):812–16.

38. Dial, S., et al. 2005. Use of gastric acid-suppressive agents and the risk of community acquired *Clostrium difficile*-Associated Disease. *JAMA* 294 (23):2989–2995.

Chapter 10: Key #5: Enhance Detoxification

1. www.cdc.gov/nchs/fastats/lcod.htm.

2. Plassman, H. I., et al. 2008. Prevalence of cognitive impairment without dementia in the United States. *Ann Intern Med* 148 (6):427–34.

3. Tsai, M. S., et al. 1994. Apolipoprotein E: risk factor for Alzheimer disease. *Am J Hum Genet.* 54 (4):643–49.

4. Godfrey, M. E., D. P. Wojcik, and C. A. Krone. 2003. Apolipoprotein E genotyping as a potential biomarker for mercury neurotoxicity. *J Alzheimer's Dis* 5 (3):189–95.

5. Clarkson, T. W., L. Magos, and G. Myers. 2003. The toxicology of mercury—current exposures and clinical manifestations. *N Engl J Med* 349 (18):1731–1737. Review.

6. Wojcik, D. P., et al. 2006. Mercury toxicity presenting as chronic fatigue, memory impairment and depression: diagnosis, treatment, susceptibility, and outcomes in a New Zealand general practice setting (1994–2006). *Neuro Endocrinol Lett* 27 (4):415–23.

7. Stroombergen, M. C., and R. H. Waring. 1999. Determination of glutathione S-transferase mu and theta polymorphisms in neurological disease. *Hum Exp Toxicol* 18 (3):141–45.

8. Bernardini, S., et al. 2005. Glutathione S transferase P1 *C allelic variant increases susceptibility for late-onset Alzheimer disease: Association study and relationship with apolipoprotein E epsilon4 allele. *Clin Chem* 51 (6):944–51. Epub 2005 April 1.

9. Spalletta, G., et al. 2007. Glutathione S-transferase P1 and T1 gene polymorphisms predict longitudinal course and age at onset of Alzheimer disease. *Am J Geriatr Psychiatry* 15 (10):879–87.

10. Gundacker, C., et al. 2007. Glutathione-S-transferase polymorphism, metallothionein expression, and mercury levels among students in Austria. *Sci Total Environ* 385 (1–3):37–47. Epub 2007 Aug 22.

11. Dorszewska, J., et al. 2007. Oxidative DNA damage and level of thiols as related to polymorphisms of MTHFR, MTR, MTHFD1 in Alzheimer's and Parkinson's diseases. *Acta Neurobiol Exp* (Wars) 67 (2):113–29.

12. Rodríguez, E., et al. 2006. Cholesteryl ester transfer protein (CETP) polymorphism

modifies the Alzheimer's disease risk associated with APOE epsilon4 allele. *J Neurol* 253 (2):181–85. Epub 2005 Aug 17.

13. Mutter, J., et al. 2007. Mercury and Alzheimer's disease. *Fortschr Neurol Psychiatr* 75 (9):528–38.

14. Torres-Alanis, O., et al., 2000. Urinary excretion of trace elements in humans after sodium 2,3-dimercaptopropane-1-sulfonate challenge test. *J Toxicol Clin Toxicol* 38 (7):697–700.

15. www.iaomt.org/articles/category_view.asp?intReleaseID=271&catid=30

16. Huse, D. M., et al. 2005. Burden of illness in Parkinson's disease. *Mov Disord* 20 (11):1449–1454.

17. Tanner, C. M., et al. 1999. Parkinson disease in twins: An etiologic study. *JAMA* 281 (4):341.

18. Cummings, J. L. 2007. Understanding Parkinson Disease. *JAMA* (1999) 281:376–78.

19. Ayala, A., et al. Mitochondrial toxins and neurodegenerative diseases. *Front Biosci* (12):986–1007. Review.

20. Kobal Grum, D., et al. 2006. Personality traits in miners with past occupational elemental mercury exposure. *Environ Health Perspect* 114 (2):290–96.

21. Elbaz, A., C. Dufouil and A. Alpérovitch. 2007. Interaction between genes and environment in neurodegenerative diseases. *C. R. Biol* 330 (4):318–28. Epub 2007 Apr 9. Review.

22. Skaper, S. D. 2007. The brain as a target for inflammatory processes and neuroprotective strategies. *Ann NY Acad Sci* 1122:23–34.

23. Cummings, J. L. 1999. Understanding Parkinson's disease. *JAMA* 281 (4):376–78.

24. Schapira, A. H., and C. W. Olanow. 2004. Neuroprotection in Parkinson disease: mysteries, myths, and misconceptions. *JAMA* 291 (3):358–64. Review.

25. Berg, D. 2006. Marker for a preclinical diagnosis of Parkinson's disease as a basis for neuroprotection. *J Neural Transm Suppl* (71):123–32.

26. Menke, A., et al. 2006. Blood level below 0.48 micromal/L (10 microg/dL) and mortality among U.S. adults. *Circulation* 114 (13):1388–1394.

27. Lindh, U., et al. 2002. Removal of dental amalgam and other metal alloys supported by antioxidant therapy alleviates symptoms and improves quality of life in patients with amalgam-associated ill health. *Neuro Endocrinol Lett* 23 (5–6):459–82.

28. Zachi, E. C., M. A. Faria and A. Taub. 2007. Neuropsychological dysfunction related to earlier occupational exposure to mercury vapor. *Braz J Med Biol Res* Mar 40 (3):425–33.

29. Kokayi, K., et al. 2006. Findings of and treatment for high levels of mercury and lead toxicity in ground zero rescue and recovery workers and lower Manhattan residents. *Explore* (NY) 2 (5):400–7.

30. Ritvo, E. R., et al. 1986. Retinal pathology in autistic children—a possible biological marker for a subtype? *J Am Acad Child Psychiatry* 25 (1):137.

31. Megson, M. N. 2000. Is autism a G-alpha protein defect reversible with natural vitamin A? *Med Hypotheses* 54 (6):979–83.

32. Peixoto, N. C., et al. 2007. Metallothionein, zinc, and mercury levels in tissues of young rats exposed to zinc and subsequently to mercury. *Life Sci* 81 (16):1264–1271. Epub 2007 September 16.

33. http://www.autism.com/triggers/vaccine/heavymetals.pdf

34. Holmes, A. S., M. F. Blaxill and B. E. Haley. 2003. Reduced levels of mercury in first baby haircuts of autistic children. *Int J Toxicol* 22 (4):277–85.

35. Adams, J. B., et al. 2007. Mercury, lead, and zinc in baby teeth of children with autism versus controls. *J Toxicol Environ Health A* 70 (12):1046–1051.

36. Geier, D. A, and M. R. Geier. 2007. A prospective study of mercury toxicity bio-markers in autistic spectrum disorders. *J Toxicol Environ Health A* 70 (20):1723–1730.

37. Echeverria, D., et al. 2006. The association between a genetic polymorphism of co-proporphyrinogen oxidase, dental mercury exposure and neurobehavioral response in humans. *Neurotoxicol Teratol* 28 (1):39–48.

38. Heyer, N. J., et al. 2004. Chronic low-level mercury exposure, BDNF polymor-phism, and associations with self-reported symptoms and mood. *Toxicol Sci* 81 (2):354–63. Epub 2004 July 14.

39. Echeverria, D., et al. 2005. Chronic low-level mercury exposure, BDNF polymor-phism, and associations with cognitive and motor function. *Neurotoxicol Teratol* 27 (6):781–96.

40. Dringen, R., and J. Hirrlinger. 2003. Glutathione pathways in the brain. *Biol Chem* 384 (4):505–16. Review.

41. Bolt, H. M., and R. Thier. 2006. Relevance of the deletion polymorphisms of the glutathione S-transferases GSTT1 and GSTM1 in pharmacology and toxicology. *Curr Drug Metab* 7 (6):613–28. Review.

42. Dröge, W., and R. Breitkreutz. 2000. Glutathione and immune function. *Proc Nutr Soc* 59 (4):595–600. Review.

43. Atkuri, K. R., et al. 2007. N-acetylcysteine—a safe antidote for cysteine/glutathione deficiency. *Curr Opin Pharmacol* 7 (4):355–59. Epub 2007 June 29. Review.

44. Nuttall, S., et al. 1998. Glutathione: in sickness and in health. *Lancet* 351 (9103): 645–46.

Chapter 11: Key #6: Boost Energy Metabolism

1. Shao, I., et al. 2008. Mitochondrial involvement in psychiatric disorders. *Ann Med* 40 (4):281–95.

2. Lin, M. T., and M. F. Beal. 2006. Mitochondrial dysfunction and oxidative stress in neurodegenerative diseases. *Nature* 443 (7113):787–95. Review.

3. Chauhan, A., and V. Chauhan. 2006. Oxidative stress in autism. *Pathophysiology* 13 (3):171–81.

4. Bourre, J. M. 2006. Effects of nutrients (in food) on the structure and function of the nervous system: Update on dietary requirements for brain. Part 2: macronutri-ents. *J Nutr Health Aging* 10 (5):386–99. Review.

5. Razmara, A., et al. 2007. Estrogen suppresses brain mitochondrial oxidative stress in female and male rats. *Brain Res* 1176:71–81. Epub 2007 Aug 24.

6. Psarra, A. M., S. Solakidi, and C. E. Sekeris. 2006. The mitochondrion as a primary site of action of steroid and thyroid hormones: Presence and action of steroid and thyroid hormone receptors in mitochondria of animal cells. *Mol Cell Endocrinol* 246 (1–2):21–33. Epub 2006 Jan 4. Review.

7. Psarra, A. M., S. Solakidi, and C. E. Sekeris. 2006. The mitochondria as a primary site of action of regulatory agents involved in neuroimmunomodulation. *Ann NY Acad Sci* 1088:12–22. Review.

8. Corda, S., et al. 2001. Rapid reactive oxygen species production by mitochondria in endothelial cells exposed to tumor necrosis factor-alpha is mediated by ceramide. *Am J Respir Cell Mol Biol* 24 (6):762–68.

9. Yin, Z., et al. 2007. Methylmercury induces oxidative injury, alterations in perme-ability and glutamine transport in cultured astrocytes. *Brain Res* 1131(1):1–10. Epub 2006 December 19.

10. Lombard, J. 1998. Autism: A mitochondrial disorder? *Med Hypotheses* 50 (6):497–500. Review.

11. Clark-Taylor, T., and B. E. Clark-Taylor. 2004. Is autism a disorder of fatty acid metabolism? Possible dysfunction of mitochondrial beta-oxidation by long chain acyl-CoA dehydrogenase. *Med Hypotheses* 62 (6):970–75.

12. Leuner, K., et al. 2007. Mitochondrial dysfunction: the first domino in brain aging and Alzheimer's disease? *Antioxid Redox Signal* 9 (10):1659–1675. Review.

13. Yamashita, H., and M. Matsumoto. 2007. Molecular pathogenesis, experimental models and new therapeutic strategies for Parkinson's disease. *Regen Med* 2 (4):447–55.

14. Muqit, M. M., S. Gandhi, and N. W. Wood. 2006. Mitochondria in Parkinson disease: back in fashion with a little help from genetics. *Arch Neurol* 63 (5):649–54.

15. Moretti, A., A. Gorini, and R. F. Villa. 2003. Affective disorders, antidepressant drugs and brain metabolism. *Mol Psychiatry* 8 (9):773–85. Review.

16. Kato, T. 2007. Mitochondrial dysfunction as the molecular basis of bipolar disorder: Therapeutic implications. *CNS Drugs* 21 (1):1–11. Review.

17. Trushina, E., and C. T. McMurray. 2007. Oxidative stress and mitochondrial dysfunction in neurodegenerative diseases. *Neuroscience* 145 (4):1233–1248. Epub 2007 February 14. Review.

18. Villmann, C., and C. M. Becker. 2007. On the hypes and falls in neuroprotection: Targeting the NMDA receptor. *Neuroscientist* 13 (6):594–615. Epub 2007 October 2.

19. Mattson, M. P. 2007. Calcium and neurodegeneration. *Aging Cell* 6 (3):337–50. Epub 2007 February 28. Review.

20. Baur, J. A., et al. 2006. Resveratrol improves health and survival of mice on a high-calorie diet. *Nature* 444 (7117):337–42. Epub 2006 November 1.

21. Petersen, K. F., and G. I. Shulman. 2006. Etiology of insulin resistance. *Am J Med* 119 (5) Suppl 1:S10–16. Review.

22. Petersen, K. F., et al. 2004. Impaired mitochondrial activity in the insulin-resistant offspring of patients with type 2 diabetes. *N Engl J Med* 350 (7):664–71.

23. Lagouge, M., et al. 2006. Resveratrol improves mitochondrial function and protects against metabolic disease by activating SIRT1 and PGC-1alpha. *Cell* (Epub ahead of print).

24. Hipkiss, A. R. 2008. Energy metabolism, altered proteins, sirtuins and ageing: converging mechanisms? *Biogerontology* 9 (1):49–55.

25. Whitmer, R. A. 2007. Type 2 diabetes and risk of cognitive impairment and dementia. *Curr Neurol Neurosci Rep* 7 (5):373–80. Review.

26. McIntyre, R. S., et al. 2007. Should depressive syndromes be reclassified as "metabolic syndrome Type II"? *Ann Clin Psychiatry* 19 (4):257–64. Review.

27. Binienda, Z., et al. 2005. L-carnitine and neuroprotection in the animal model of mitochondrial dysfunction. *Ann NY Acad Sci* (1053):174–82.

28. Ames, B. N. 2003. The metabolic tune-up: Metabolic harmony and disease prevention. *J Nutr* 133 (5 Suppl 1):1554S–1548S.

29. Liu, J., et al. 2002. Memory loss in old rats is associated with brain mitochondrial decay and RNA/DNA oxidation: Partial reversal by feeding acetyl-L-carnitine and/or R-alpha-lipoic acid. *Proc Natl Acad Sci USA* 99 (4):2356–2361.

30. Liu, J., and B. N. Ames. 2005. Reducing mitochondrial decay with mitochondrial nutrients to delay and treat cognitive dysfunction, Alzheimer's disease, and Parkinson's disease. *Nutr Neurosci* 8 (2):67–89.

31. Shea, T. B. 2007. Effects of dietary supplementation with N-acetylcysteine, acetyl-L-carnitine and S-adenosyl methionine on cognitive performance and aggression in normal mice and mice expressing human ApoE4. *Neuromolecular Med* 9 (3):264–69.

32. Engelhart, M. J., et al. 2002. Dietary intake of antioxidants and risk of Alzheimer disease. *JAMA* 287 (24):3223–3229.

33. Dai, Q., et al. 2006. Fruit and vegetable juices and Alzheimer's disease: The Kame Project. *Am J Med* 119 (9):751–59.

34. Mythri, R. B., et al. 2007. Mitochondrial complex I inhibition in Parkinson's disease: How can curcumin protect mitochondria? *Antioxid Redox Signal* 9 (3):399–408.

35. Beal, M. F. 2004. Mitochondrial dysfunction and oxidative damage in Alzheimer's and Parkinson's diseases and coenzyme Q10 as a potential treatment. *J Bioenerg Biomembr* 36 (4):381–86. Review.

36. Shults, C. W., et al. 2002. Parkinson Study Group. Effects of coenzyme Q10 in early Parkinson disease: Evidence of slowing of the functional decline. *Arch Neurol* 59 (10):1541–1550.

37. Young, A. J., et al. 2007. Coenzyme Q10: A review of its promise as a neuroprotectant. *CNS Spectr* 12 (1):62–68. Review.

38. Rosenberg, R. N. 2002. Mitochondrial therapy for Parkinson disease. *Arch Neurol* 59 (10):1523.

39. Littarru, G. P., and P. Langsjoen. 2007. Coenzyme Q10 and statins: Biochemical and clinical implications. *Mitochondrion* 7 Suppl:S168–74. Epub 2007 March 27. Review.

40. Sewright, K. A., P. M. Clarkson, and P. D. Thompson. 2007. Statin myopathy: Incidence, risk factors, and pathophysiology. *Curr Atheroscler Rep* 9 (5):389–96.

41. Draeger, A., et al. 2006. Statin therapy induces ultrastructural damage in skeletal muscle in patients without myalgia. *J Pathol* 210 (1):94–102.

42. Phillips, P. S., et al. 2002. Scripps Mercy Clinical Research Center. Statin-associated myopathy with normal creatine kinase levels. *Ann Intern Med* 137 (7):581–85.

43. www.news.bbc.co.uk/2/hi/health/3931157.stm

44. Beal, M. F. 2003. Bioenergetic approaches for neuroprotection in Parkinson's disease. *Ann Neurol* Suppl 3:S39–47; discussion S47–48.

45. Moreira, P. I., et al. 2007. Lipoic acid and N-acetyl cysteine decrease mitochondrial-related oxidative stress in Alzheimer disease patient fibroblasts. *J Alzheimers Dis* 12 (2):195–206.

46. McGinnis, W. R. 2005. Oxidative stress in autism. *Altern Ther Health Med* 11 (1):19.

Chapter 12: Key #7: Calm Your Mind

1. Lantz, P. M., et al. 1998. Socioeconomic Factors, Health Behaviors, and Mortality: Results From a Nationally Representative Prospective Study of US Adult, *JAMA* 279:1703–1708.

2. Karasek, R. 2006. The stress-disequilibrium theory: chronic disease development, low social control, and physiological de-regulation. *Med Lav* 97 (2):258–71. Review.

3. Sapolsky, Robert M. *Why Zebras Don't Get Ulcers: An Updated Guide to Stress, Stress-Related Diseases, and Coping* (New York: Holt/Owl, 1994; 2004).

4. McEwen, B. S. 1998. Protective and damaging effects of stress mediators. *N Engl J Med* 338 (3):171–79. Review.

5. Uno, H., et al. 1994. Neurotoxicity of glucocorticoids in the primate brain. *Horm Behav* 28 (4):336–48.

6. Gillespie, C. F., and C. B. Nemeroff. 2005. Hypercortisolemia and depression. *Psychosom Med* 67 Suppl 1:S26–28. Review.

7. Pruessner, J. C., et al. 2005. Self-esteem, locus of control, hippocampal volume, and cortisol regulation in young and old adulthood. *Neuroimage* 28 (4):815–26. Epub 2005 July 14.

8. Lupien, S. I., et al. 2007. The effects of stress and stress hormones on human cognition: Implications for the field of brain and cognition. *Brain Cogn* 65 (3):209–37. Epub 2007 April 26.

9. Yehuda, R. 2002. Post-traumatic stress disorder. *N Engl J Med* 346 (2):108–14. Review.

10. McEwen, B. S. 2006. Protective and damaging effects of stress mediators: central role of the brain. *Dialogues Clin Neurosci* 8 (4):367–81. Review.

11. Brown, D. P. 2007. The energy body and its functions: Immunosurveillance, longevity, and regeneration. *Ann NY Acad Sci*. Epub 2007 September 28.

12. Starkman, M. N., et al. 1992. Hippocampal formation volume, memory dysfunction, and cortisol levels in patients with Cushing's syndrome. *Biol Psychiatry* 32 (9):756–65.

13. Starkman, M. N., et al. 1999. Decrease in cortisol reverses human hippocampal atrophy following treatment of Cushing's disease. *Biol Psychiatry* 46 (12):1595–1602.

14. Ibid., et al. 2003. Improvement in learning associated with increase in hippocampal formation volume. *Biol Psychiatry* 53 (3):233–38.

15. Cameron, H. A., and R. D. McKay. 1999. Restoring production of hippocampal neurons in old age. *Nat Neurosci* 2 (10):894–97.

16. Hansen, A. L., B. H. Johnsen, and J. F. Thayer. 2003. Vagal influence on working memory and attention. *Int J Psychophysiol* 48 (3):263–74.

17. Chahine, T., et al. 2007. Particulate air pollution, oxidative stress genes, and heart rate variability in an elderly cohort. *Environ Health Perspect* 115 (11):1617–1622.

18. Sloan, R. P., et al. 2007. RR interval variability is inversely related to inflammatory markers: The CARDIA study. *Mol Med* 13 (3–4):178–84.

19. Pavlov, V. A., and K. J. Tracey. 2005. The cholinergic anti-inflammatory pathway. *Brain Behav Immun* 19 (6):493–99. Review.

20. Theise, N. D., and R. Harris. 2006. Postmodern biology: (adult) (stem) cells are plastic, stochastic, complex, and uncertain. *Handb Exp Pharmacol* (174):389–408. Review.

21. Lamming, D. W., J. G. Wood, and D. A. Sinclair. 2004. Small molecules that regulate lifespan: Evidence for xenohormesis. *Mol Microbiol* 53 (4):1003–1009. Review.

22. Yun, A. I., and J. D. Doux. 2007. Unhappy meal: How our need to detect stress may have shaped our preferences for taste. *Med Hypotheses* 69 (4):746–51.

23. Bazar, K. A., et al. 2006. Obesity and ADHD may represent different manifestations of a common environmental oversampling syndrome: A model for revealing mechanistic overlap among cognitive, metabolic, and inflammatory disorders. *Med Hypotheses* 66 (2):263–69. Review.

24. Kallio, P., et al. 2007. Dietary carbohydrate modification induces alterations in gene expression in abdominal subcutaneous adipose tissue in persons with the metabolic syndrome: The FUNGENUT Study. *Am J Clin Nutr* 85 (5):1417–1427.

25. WHO Initiative on Depression in Public Health, http://www.who.int/mental_health/management/depression/depressioninph/en/. Accessed March 10, 2008.

26. Palpant, R. G., R. Steimnitz, T. H. Bornemann, and K. Hawkins. 2006. The Carter Center Mental Health Program: Addressing the public health crisis in the field of mental health through policy change and stigma reduction. *Preventing Chronic Disease* 3:1–6.

Chapter 14: Eating Right for Your Brain

1. Philpot, W. *Brain Allergies: The Psychonutrient and Magnetic Connections* (New York: McGraw-Hill, 2000).
2. Campbell, T. C. 1990. A study on diet, nutrition and disease in the People's Republic of China. Part I. *Bol Asoc Med* P R 82 (3):132–34.
3. Campbell, T. C. 1990. A study on diet, nutrition and disease in the People's Republic of China. Part II. *Bol Asoc Med* P R 82 (7):316–18. Review.

Chapter 15: Tuning Up Your Brain Chemistry with Supplements

1. Kaplan, B. J., et al. 2007. Vitamins, minerals, and mood. *Psychol Bull* 33 (5):747–60.
2. Bourre, J. M. 2006. Effects of nutrients (in food) on the structure and function of the nervous system: Update on dietary requirements for the brain. Part 1: Micronutrients. *J Nutr Health Aging* 10 (5):377–85. Review.
3. Ibid., 2006. Part 2: Macronutrients. *J Nutr Health Aging* 10 (5):386–99. Review.

Chapter 16: The UltraMind Lifestyle

1. Galvin, J. A., et al. 2006. The relaxation response: reducing stress and improving cognition in healthy aging adults. *Complement Ther Clin Pract* 12 (3):186–91.
2. Hankey, A. 2006. Studies of advanced stages of meditation in the Tibetan buddhist and vedic traditions. I: A comparison of general changes. *Evid Based Complement Alternat Med* 3 (4):513–21.
3. Davidson, R. J., et al. 2003. Alterations in brain and immune function produced by mindfulness meditation. *Psychosom Med* 65 (4):564–70.
4. Gordon, J. S. 2006. Healing the wounds of war: Gaza diary. *Altern Ther Health Med* 12 (1):18–21.
5. Verghese, J., et al. 2003. Leisure activities and the risk of dementia in the elderly. *N Eng J Med* 348 (25):2508–2516.

Chapter 17: Living Clean and Green

1. Galletti, P. M., and G. Joyet. 1958. Effect of fluorine on thyroidal iodine metabolism in hyperthyroidism. *J Clin Endocrinol Metab* 18 (10):1102–1110.
2. Xanthis, A., et al. 2007. Advanced glycosylation end products and nutrition—a possible relation with diabetic atherosclerosis and how to prevent it. *J Food Sci* 72 (8):R125–29.

Chapter 23: Key #2: Balance Your Hormones

1. Persky, V. W., et al. 2002. Effect of soy protein on endogenous hormones in post-menopausal women. *Am J Clin Nutr* 75 (1):145–53. Erratum in *Am J Clin Nutr* 76 (3):695.
2. Galletti, P. M., and G. Joyet. 1958. Effect of fluorine on thyroidal iodine metabolism in hyperthyroidism. *J Clin Endocrinol Metab* 18 (10):1102–1110.
3. Gaby, A. R. 2004. Sublaboratory hypothyroidism and the empirical use of *Armour thyroid Altern Med Rev* 9 (2):157–79.
4. Goglia, F. 2005. Biological effects of 3,5-diiodothyronine (T[2]). *Biochemistry (Mosc)* 70 (2):164–72.

Chapter 24: Key #3: Cool Off Inflammation

1. Smith, J. K. 1999. Long-term exercise and atherogenic activity of blood mononuclear cells in persons at risk of developing ischemic heart disease. *JAMA* 281 (18):1722–1727.
2. Church, T. S. 2003. Reduction of C-reactive protein levels through use of a multivitamin *Am J Med* 115 (9):702–7.

Chapter 28: Key #7: Calm Your Mind

1. Gortner, E. M., S. S. Rude, and J. W. Pennebaker. 2006. Benefits of expressive writing in lowering rumination and depressive symptoms. *Behav Ther* 37 (3):292–303.

Conclusion: The Future of Medicine

1. Ernst, E., et al. 2001. Mind-body therapies: are the trial data getting stronger? *Altern Ther Health Med* 13 (5):62–64.
2. Cohen, S., D. Janicki-Deverts, and G. E. Miller. 2001. Psychological stress and disease. *JAMA* 298 (14):1685–1687.

INDEX

Page numbers in *italics* refer to illustrations.

MARK HYMAN, M.D.

Dr. Hyman is editor in chief of *Alternative Therapies in Health and Medicine*, the most prestigious journal in the field of Integrative Medicine, and the medical editor of *Natural Solutions*. He is the coauthor of the *New York Times* bestselling book published by Scribner *Ultraprevention: The Six-Week Plan That Will Make You Healthy for Life* and *The Detox Box: A Program for Greater Health and Vitality* (Sounds True, 2004), *The 5 Forces of Wellness: The Ultraprevention System for Living an Active, Age-Defying, Disease-Free Life* (Nightingale-Conant, 2005), and *NutriGenomics: The New Science of Health* (2006). His book *UltraMetabolism: The Simple Plan for Automatic Weight Loss* (Scribner, March 2006), a *New York Times* bestseller, focuses on a cutting-edge personalized—or "nutrigenomic"—approach to weight loss and metabolism. A companion PBS pledge special produced by WLIW features this approach. His book *The UltraSimple Diet,* a *New York Times* bestseller, is a one-week anti-inflammatory detoxification program (Pocket Books, March 2007). *The UltraMetabolism Cookbook* was released in November 2007.

A guest on the *Today* show, *Good Morning America, The Early Show*, and *The View* with Barbara Walters, Dr. Hyman has also appeared on CNN, FOX, PBS, and NPR, as well as many other television and radio stations. He has written for and is quoted regularly in leading consumer magazines, including *Parade, Elle, Fitness, Glamour, Family Circle, US Weekly, Women's World, First for Women, Health, Natural Health, Self, Shape*, and *Town & Country*.

For nearly ten years, Dr. Hyman was the co-medical director at Canyon Ranch in Lenox, Massachusetts, an internationally acclaimed health resort. He is the founder and medical director of the UltraWellness Center in Lenox (www.ultrawellnesscenter.com). His website www.ultrawellness .com empowers health-care consumers, allowing them to take advantage of the medicine of the future today. He is on the board of advisers and faculty of Food As Medicine, Center for Mind-Body Medicine. He is also vice chair of the board of directors and on the faculty of the Institute for Functional Medicine and collaborates with the Harvard Medical School's Division for Research and Education in Complementary and Integrative Medicine.

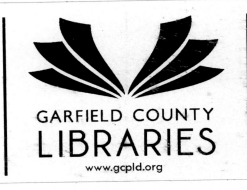